Endoscopic Approach to the Patient with Biliary Tract Disease

Editor

JACQUES VAN DAM

GASTROINTESTINAL ENDOSCOPY CLINICS OF NORTH AMERICA

www.giendo.theclinics.com

Consulting Editor
CHARLES J. LIGHTDALE

April 2013 • Volume 23 • Number 2

ELSEVIER

1600 John F. Kennedy Boulevard • Suite 1800 • Philadelphia, Pennsylvania, 19103-2899

http://www.theclinics.com

GASTROINTESTINAL ENDOSCOPY CLINICS OF NORTH AMERICA Volume 23, Number 2
April 2013 ISSN 1052-5157, ISBN-13: 978-1-4557-7093-9

Editor: Kerry Holland
Developmental Editor: Donald Mumford

Gastrointestinal Endoscopy Clinics of North America (ISSN 1052-5157) is published quarterly by Elsevier Inc., 360 Park Avenue South, New York, NY 10010-1710. Months of issue are January, April, July, and October. Business and Editorial Offices: 1600 John F. Kennedy Blvd., Suite 1800, Philadelphia, PA, 19103-2899. Periodicals postage paid at New York, NY and additional mailing offices. Subscription prices are $319.00 per year for US individuals, $441.00 per year for US institutions, $169.00 per year for US students and residents, $351.00 per year for Canadian individuals, $538.00 per year for Canadian institutions, $445.00 per year for international individuals, $538.00 per year for international institutions, and $235.00 per year for Canadian and foreign students/residents. To receive student/resident rate, orders must be accompanied by name of affiliated institution, date of term, and the *signature* of program/residency coordinator on institution letterhead. Orders will be billed at individual rate until proof of status is received. Foreign air speed delivery is included in all *Clinics* subscription prices. All prices are subject to change without notice. **POSTMASTER:** Send address change to *Gastrointestinal Endoscopy Clinics of North America*, Elsevier Health Sciences Division, Subscription Customer Service, 3251 Riverport Lane, Maryland Heights, MO 63043. **Customer Service: 1-800-654-2452 (US). From outside the United States, call 1-314-447-8871. Fax: 1-314-447-8029. E-mail: JournalsCustomerService-usa@elsevier.com (for print support) or JournalsOnlineSupport-usa@elsevier.com (for online support).**

Reprints. For copies of 100 or more, of articles in this publication, please contact the Commercial Reprints Department, Elsevier Inc., 360 Park Avenue South, New York, NY 10010-1710. Tel. (212) 633-3812; Fax: (212) 482-1935; E-mail: reprints@elsevier.com.

Gastrointestinal Endoscopy Clinics of North America is covered in *Excerpta Medica, MEDLINE/PubMed (Index Medicus), and MEDLINE/MEDLARS.*

Printed in the United States of America.

Contributors

CONSULTING EDITOR

CHARLES J. LIGHTDALE, MD
Professor, Department of Medicine, Columbia University Medical Center, New York, New York

EDITOR

JACQUES VAN DAM, MD, PhD
Professor of Medicine (Clinical Scholar), Keck School of Medicine, University of Southern California, Los Angeles, California

AUTHORS

ZAREE BABAKHANIAN, MD
Fellow, Division of Gastrointestinal and Liver Diseases, Keck School of Medicine of USC, Los Angeles, California

JOHN BAILLIE, MB, ChB, FRCP, FASGE
Director of Medical Gastroenterology, Carteret General Hospital, Morehead City, North Carolina

YAN G. BAKMAN, MD
Instructor, Advanced Therapeutic Endoscopy Fellow, Division of Gastroenterology, Hepatology and Nutrition, University of Minnesota, Minneapolis, Minnesota

SUBHAS BANERJEE, MD
Director of Endoscopy and Associate Professor of Medicine, Division of Gastroenterology and Hepatology, Stanford University School of Medicine, Stanford, California

TODD H. BARON Sr, MD, FASGE
Professor of Medicine, Division of Gastroenterology and Hepatology, Mayo Clinic, South West Rochester, Minnesota

WILLIAM R. BRUGGE, MD
Professor of Medicine, Gastrointestinal Unit, Massachusetts General Hospital, Harvard Medical School, Boston, Massachusetts

BRYAN BALMADRID, MD
Digestive Disease Institute, Virginia Mason Medical Center, Seattle, Washington

JAMES BUXBAUM, MD
Division of Gastrointestinal and Liver Diseases, Keck School of Medicine; Director of Endoscopy, Los Angeles County Hospital, University of Southern California, Los Angeles, California

TOMAS DAVEE, MD
Resident Physician, Department of Internal Medicine, Stanford University Medical Center, Stanford, California

JOHN A. DONOVAN, MD
Assistant Professor of Clinical Medicine, Division of Gastrointestinal and Liver Diseases, Keck School of Medicine, University of Southern California, Los Angeles, California

MARTIN L. FREEMAN, MD, FACG, FASGE
Professor of Medicine, Interim Director, Division of Gastroenterology, Hepatology and Nutrition, University of Minnesota, Minneapolis, Minnesota

MUHAMMAD K. HASAN, MD
Center for Interventional Endoscopy, Florida Hospital, Orlando, Florida

LINDA ANN HOU, MD
Gastroenterology/Liver Fellow, Division of Gastrointestinal and Liver Diseases, Department of Medicine, LAC+USC Medical Center, Keck School of Medicine, University of Southern California, Los Angeles, California

TAKAO ITOI, MD
Department of Gastroenterology and Hepatology, Tokyo Medical University, Tokyo, Japan

MICHEL KAHALEH, MD, AGAF, FACG, FASGE
Professor of Clinical Medicine, Chief Endoscopy, Medical Director, Pancreas Program, Division of Gastroenterology and Hepatology, Weill Cornell Medical College, New York, New York

HYUNG-KEUN KIM, MD
Division of Gastroenterology, Department of Internal Medicine, Uijeongbu St. Mary's Hospital, College of Medicine, The Catholic University of Korea, Guemo-dong, Uijeongbu, Republic of Korea; Cedars-Sinai Medical Center, Los Angeles, California

RAJAN KOCHAR, MD, MPH
Clinical Instructor, Advanced Endoscopy, Division of Gastroenterology and Hepatology, Stanford University School of Medicine, Stanford, California

RICHARD KOZAREK, MD
Digestive Disease Institute, Virginia Mason Medical Center, Seattle, Washington

ALEXANDER LEE, MD
Fellow in Gastroenterology, Division of Gastroenterology, University of California, San Francisco, San Francisco, California

WESLEY D. LEUNG, MD
ERCP Fellow, Division of Gastroenterology/Hepatology, Indiana University Medical Center, Indianapolis, Indiana

QUIN Y. LIU, MD
Assistant Professor of Clinical Pediatrics, Keck School of Medicine, University of Southern California; Director of Interventional Endoscopy, Division of Gastroenterology and Nutrition, Children's Hospital Los Angeles, Los Angeles, California

SIMON K. LO, MD
Cedars-Sinai Medical Center; David Geffen School of Medicine at UCLA, Los Angeles, California

JOHN Y. NASR, MD
Clinical Assistant Professor of Medicine, Division of Gastroenterology, Hepatology, and Nutrition, University of Pittsburgh Medical Center, Pittsburgh, Pennsylvania

VIVIEN NGUYEN, MD
Fellow in Pediatric Gastroenterology, Division of Gastroenterology and Nutrition, Children's Hospital Los Angeles, Los Angeles, California

ISAAC RAIJMAN, MD, AGAF, FASGE, FACP
President, Digestive Associates of Houston; Clinical Associate Professor of Medicine, Baylor College of Medicine; Clinical Associate Professor of Medicine, University of Texas Health Science Center, Houston, Texas

SAVREET SARKARIA, MD
Assistant Professor of Clinical Medicine, Division of Gastroenterology and Hepatology, Weill Cornell Medical College, New York, New York

MICHAEL SAUNDERS, MD
Clinical Professor of Medicine, Director, Digestive Disease Center, Division of Gastroenterology, University of Washington Medical Center, Seattle, Washington

JANAK N. SHAH, MD
Paul May and Frank Stein Interventional Endoscopy Center, Director of Pancreatic and Biliary Endoscopy, California Pacific Medical Center, Associate Clinical Professor of Medicine, University of California, San Francisco, San Francisco, California

STUART SHERMAN, MD
Professor of Medicine and Radiology, Division of Gastroenterology/Hepatology, Indiana University Medical Center, Indianapolis, Indiana

ADAM SLIVKA, MD, PhD
Professor of Medicine, Associate Chief of Division of Gastroenterology, Hepatology, and Nutrition, University of Pittsburgh Medical Center, Pittsburgh, Pennsylvania

SUBHA SUNDARARAJAN, MD
Fellow in Gastroenterology, Division of Gastroenterology and Hepatology, Weill Cornell Medical College, New York, New York

JACQUES VAN DAM, MD, PhD
Professor of Medicine (Clinical Scholar), Keck School of Medicine, University of Southern California, Los Angeles, California

SHYAM VARADARAJULU, MD
Medical Director, Center for Interventional Endoscopy, Florida Hospital, Orlando, Florida

KEVIN WEBB, MD
Division of Gastroenterology, University of Washington Medical Center, Seattle, Washington

WON JAE YOON, MD
Research Fellow, Gastrointestinal Unit, Massachusetts General Hospital, Boston, Massachusetts

Contents

Advances in biliary imaging have improved making accurate diagnoses of the presence and causes of biliary obstruction. Abdominal ultrasound is a useful screening tool because it is highly specific for choledocholithiasis. New developments in CT and MRI have also been useful in the diagnosis of biliary disease. Although diagnosis of biliary disease can be achieved in a noninvasive manner, there are limitations to modern MRI and CT cholangiographic techniques; their use may not be necessary or cost effective. MRI and CT imaging of the biliary tract provides opportunities for less-invasive diagnostic techniques but should be used judiciously before interventional endoscopy.

Infection of the biliary tract, or cholangitis, is a potentially life-threatening condition. Bile duct stones are the most common cause of biliary obstruction predisposing to cholangitis. The key components in the pathogenesis of cholangitis are biliary obstruction and biliary infection. Several underlying mechanisms of bactibilia have been proposed. Characteristic clinical features of cholangitis include abdominal pain, fever, and jaundice. A combination of clinical features with laboratory tests and imaging studies are frequently used to diagnose cholangitis. Endoscopic retrograde cholangiopancreatography is the best diagnostic test. Less invasive imaging tests may be performed initially in clinically stable patients with uncertain diagnoses.

Endoscopic retrograde cholangiopancreatography allows intervention for a variety of diseases of the biliary tract. Cannulation of the bile duct is the prerequisite step for biliary intervention. Although obtaining biliary access is straightforward in many cases, it can occasionally be challenging. Multiple devices, all with additional wire-guided techniques, have been developed to aid cannulation. More advanced techniques have also been developed to aid biliary access if it is unsuccessful with standard devices. Multimodality techniques can be used if other approaches fail.

This article provides an evidence-based discussion of these approaches, and provides insight into their appropriate application.

Miniature endoscopes that can be introduced into the bile duct through the duodenoscope during endoscopic retrograde cholangiopancreatography were developed to allow nonsurgical management of difficult biliary stones. The direct visualization enabled by these cholangioscopes of the biliary epithelium provides additional data in the assessment of biliary strictures. Cholangioscopy allows assessment of the biliary lumen, biliary epithelium, targeted tissue acquisition, targeted therapy, and wire guidance.

It is imperative for gastroenterologists to understand the different formations of bile duct stones and the various medical treatments available. To minimize the complications of endoscopic retrograde cholangiopancreatography (ERCP), it is critical to appropriately assess the risk of bile duct stones before intervention. Biliary endoscopists should be comfortable with the basic techniques of stone removal, including sphincterotomy, mechanical lithotripsy, and stent placement. It is important to be aware of advanced options, including laser and electrohydraulic stone fragmentation, and papillary dilatation for problematic cases. The timing and need for ERCP in those who require a cholecystectomy is also a consideration.

Differentiating between malignant and benign bile duct strictures is often challenging. Endoscopic retrograde cholangiopancreatography with brush cytology and/or endobiliary forceps biopsy is routinely performed. Advanced cytologic methods such as fluorescence in situ hybridization or digital image analysis increases the sensitivity of cytology. Endoscopic ultrasonography enables detailed examination of tissues surrounding the bile duct stricture and offers the advantage of fine-needle aspiration. Intraductal ultrasonography enables detailed evaluation of bile duct wall layers, and cholangioscopy offers direct visualization of the bile duct lesions. Novel techniques of probe-based confocal laser endomicroscopy and optical coherence tomography have introduced the era of in vivo histology.

The use of endoscopic retrograde cholangiopancreatography for treating benign biliary strictures has become the standard of practice, with surgery and percutaneous therapy reserved for selected patients. The gold-standard endoscopic therapy is dilation of the stricture followed by placing and exchanging progressively larger and more numerable plastic stents over a 1-year period. Newer modalities, including the use of fully covered

Since its original description by Oddi in 1887, the sphincter of Oddi has been the subject of much study. Furthermore, the clinical syndrome of sphincter of Oddi dysfunction (SOD) and its therapy are controversial areas. Nevertheless, SOD is commonly diagnosed and treated by physicians. This article reviews the epidemiology, clinical manifestations, and current diagnostic and therapeutic modalities of SOD.

Endoscopic retrograde cholangiopancreatography (ERCP) is currently the standard of care for biliary drainage. In the hands of experienced endoscopists, conventional ERCP has a failed cannulation rate of 3% to 5%. Failures have traditionally been referred for either percutaneous transhepatic biliary drainage (PTBD) or surgery. Both PTBD and surgery have higher than desirable complication rates. Endoscopic ultrasound-guided biliary drainage (EUS-BD) is a novel and attractive alternative after failed ERCP. Many groups have reported on the feasibility, efficacy, and safety of this technique. This article reviews the indications and technique currently practiced in EUS-BD, including EUS-guided rendezvous, EUS-guided choledocho-duodenostomy, and EUS-guided hepaticogastrostomy.

Acute cholecystitis is a commonly encountered medical emergency that is managed surgically with excellent results. Recent experiences with endoscopic cystic duct stent placement and cholecystectomy using the NOTES (Natural Orifice Transluminal Endoscopic Surgery) approach have inspired endoscopists to identify other less invasive means for treating cholecystitis. The ability to access and drain obstructive bile ducts in real time using endoscopic ultrasound guidance has led to recent reports of successful gallbladder drainage using similar techniques. This article discusses the current state of the endoscopic management of acute and acalculous cholecystitis, and outlines a consensus approach to the management of these patients.

Laparoscopic cholecystectomy (LC) is complicated by bile duct injury in 0.3% to 0.6% of cases. These injuries range from simple leaks from the cystic duct stump that can almost always be managed by endoscopic stenting to complex strictures, transections, and even resections of the bile duct, often with concomitant vascular damage leading to ischemia. The management of LC-related biliary injuries requires a multidisciplinary approach involving an endoscopist experienced in the use of ERCP, a skilled interventional radiologist, and a surgeon with specific training in the management of hepatobiliary injuries.

Biliary complications occur after liver transplantation. These complications can be effectively and safely managed using endoscopic approaches and can prevent unnecessary and potentially morbid surgery.

Endoscopic retrograde cholangiopancreatography (ERCP) in surgically altered anatomy can be technically challenging, because of three main problems that must be overcome: (1) endoscopically traversing the altered luminal anatomy, (2) cannulating the biliary orifice from an altered position, and (3) performing biliary interventions with available ERCP instruments. This article addresses the most common and most challenging variations in anatomy encountered by a gastroenterologist performing ERCP. It also highlights the innovations and progress that have been made in coping with these anatomic variations, with special attention paid to altered anatomy from bariatric surgery.

Congenital biliary tract anomalies typically present with neonatal cholestasia. In children and adults, endoscopic retrograde cholangiopancreatography (ERCP) and endoscopic ultrasound are used to evaluate and treat choledochal cysts. Contrarily, endoscopy has traditionally played a minor role in the diagnosis of the cholestatic infant. Recent studies support the incorporation of ERCP into the diagnostic algorithm for biliary atresia and neonatal cholestasis. But at present, most pediatric liver centers do not consider its use essential. This article reviews the congenital biliary tract anomalies in which endoscopy has been shown to contribute to the evaluation of the cholestatic infant.

GASTROINTESTINAL ENDOSCOPY CLINICS OF NORTH AMERICA

FORTHCOMING ISSUES

July 2013
Advanced Imaging in Endoscopy
Sharmila Anandasabapathy, MD,
Editor

October 2013
Pancreatic Diseases
Martin Freeman, MD, *Editor*

January 2014
EUS-guided Tissue Acquisition
Shyam Varadarajulu, MD
and Robert Hawes, MD, *Editors*

RECENT ISSUES

January 2013
Endolumenal Therapy
Steven A. Edmundowicz, MD, *Editor*

October 2012
Celiac Disease
Peter H.R. Green, MD and
Benjamin Lebwohl, MD, *Editors*

July 2012
Therapeutic ERCP
Michel Kahaleh, MD, *Editor*

RELATED INTEREST

Clinics in Liver Disease, August 2012 (Vol. 16, No. 3)
Nonalcoholic Fatty Liver Disease
Arun J. Sanyal, MBBS, MD, *Editor*

Foreword

The Best Endoscopic Methods in Biliary Disease

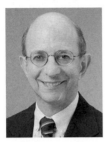

Charles J. Lightdale, MD
Consulting Editor

The biliary tract is subject to a multiplicity of ills spanning an incidence of common to rare. Imaging of the biliary system with ultrasound, computed tomography, and magnetic resonance imaging has brought tremendous diagnostic power to biliary diseases, and laparoscopic cholecystectomy led a revolution in abdominal surgery. For gastrointestinal endoscopists, the biliary system has become a prime area for diagnosis and even more so for therapy. The endoscopic procedures of greatest value involve combining endoscopy with fluoroscopy in endoscopic retrograde cholangiopancreatography (ERCP) and combining endoscopy with high-frequency ultrasonography in endoscopic ultrasonography (EUS).

In the United States, ERCP and EUS are performed mostly by interventional gastroenterologists, whereas in other areas of the world larger numbers of radiologists and surgeons also practice these procedures. Recently, direct endoscopic examination of the bile ducts with peroral cholangioscopy has become widely available, and advanced imaging technology has allowed visualization at the cellular level. A dazzling array of therapeutic devices have been developed to perform endoscopic papillotomy and ampullectomy, remove stones, dilate strictures, ablate malignant tissue, and implant temporary and permanent stents. Once limited to academic medical centers, endoscopic treatment of biliary disease is now widely practiced in a community setting. The field is still young and attracts an increasing number of trainees, many willing to devote additional time in advanced training programs to master the techniques involved. Certainly, endoscopic methods have resulted in tremendous benefit to those suffering from bile duct disorders.

Dr Jacques Van Dam is the Guest Editor for this issue of the *Gastrointestinal Endoscopy Clinics of North America*. He has focused brilliantly on this subject and selected

Gastrointest Endoscopy Clin N Am 23 (2013) xiii–xiv
http://dx.doi.org/10.1016/j.giec.2013.01.006
1052-5157/13/$ – see front matter © 2013 Published by Elsevier Inc.

giendo.theclinics.com

an outstanding group of experts in biliary disease to author articles that fully cover the field. Here is the latest information coupled with wise advice regarding when and how to best apply endoscopic methods. Gastroenterologists, surgeons, radiologists, at all levels of experience, if you deal with biliary disease, this volume is for you.

Charles J. Lightdale, MD
Department of Medicine
Division of Digestive and Liver Diseases
Columbia University Medical Center
161 Fort Washington Avenue, Room 812
New York, NY 10032, USA

E-mail address:
CJL18@columbia.edu

Preface

Endoscopic Advances in Biliary Disease

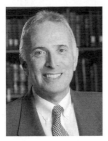

Jacques Van Dam, MD, PhD
Editor

This time, something a little bit different. More often than not, *Gastrointestinal Endoscopy Clinics of North America* focuses on a particular instrument or procedure. And most of the time, this makes sense. Alternatively, some issues have focused on a particular disorder and how endoscopists may best intervene diagnostically or therapeutically. This approach also has merit.

In this issue, however, we have targeted a familiar organ system and assembled the world's leading experts in reviewing its various pathologies, benign and malignant, mechanical and physiological, infectious, iatrogenic, and congenital. We review not a single endoscopic procedure, but rather go to our endoscope cabinet to determine which of our exceptional tools is best suited to a specific task. And in doing so, we evaluate each instrument's strengths and flaws, limitations, and complications.

Patients with biliary tract disease are responsible for more hospitalizations in the United States than any other gastrointestinal disorder. Cholecystitis is treated in more than one half million Americans each year, which is just a fraction of the 20-25 million estimated to have gallstones. And although there has been a historical demarcation between surgical and endoscopic treatment of biliary tract disease, the introduction of endoscopic ultrasound (EUS) and the vision of a few innovative endoscopists have opened the possibility of less invasive approaches to diseases previously thought managed only by surgical intervention.

I am grateful to the internationally renowned experts who have graciously given their time and expertise to this monograph. The reader will not only benefit from their years of experience but also learn the newest technologies available now and those that may become the new standard in the future. EUS-guided biliary drainage, photodynamic therapy and radiofrequency ablation of bile duct cancers, and deep enteroscopic techniques to reach the postoperative biliary tree are but a few examples.

The world is becoming a smaller place. Information now travels over distances and at speeds not contemplated by earlier generations of physicians. Access to this

Gastrointest Endoscopy Clin N Am 23 (2013) xv–xvi
http://dx.doi.org/10.1016/j.giec.2013.01.005
1052-5157/13/$ – see front matter © 2013 Published by Elsevier Inc.

giendo.theclinics.com

monograph and others like it is available to physicians who may not yet have in their endoscopy facilities the tools and approaches detailed in this issue. However, it is essential that all those who seek to treat patients with biliary tract disease understand the mechanisms of its various diseases and learn how rapidly advancing technology is changing how we diagnose and treat our patients.

I wish to thank my mentor Dr Michael V. Sivak Jr, who not only taught me the advanced interventional skills I use every day in my endoscopic practice but also demonstrated by his example the importance of advancing the field and the imperative of passing along those advances to the next generations of endoscopists. I am also grateful to Charles Lightdale and Kerry Holland for the opportunity to contribute yet another monograph in this series. I appreciate their confidence in the outcome of this issue. And I thank Lesley Simon for her invaluable editorial skills and tireless effort in reviewing the authors' contributions.

Jacques Van Dam, MD, PhD
Professor of Medicine (Clinical Scholar)
Keck School of Medicine
University of Southern California
1510 San Pablo Street
HCC1:Suite 322R, M/C 9198
Los Angeles, CA 90033, USA

Pre-ERCP Imaging of the Bile Duct and Gallbladder

Linda Ann Hou, MD[a], Jacques Van Dam, MD, PhD[b],*

KEYWORDS

- Biliary imaging • Abdominal ultrasound • Computerized tomography • MRI • MRCP

KEY POINTS

- Initial evaluation of suspected biliary obstruction should include liver biochemical tests and a transabdominal ultrasound (US).
- Patients with suspicion of choledocholithiasis should be risk stratified; those who are high risk should undergo endoscopic retrograde cholangiopancreatography (ERCP) without further radiologic imaging. Patients with intermediate risk of choledocholithiasis should undergo endoscopic ultrasonography (EUS), magnetic resonance cholangiopancreatography (MRCP), or intraoperative cholangiography, depending on the availability.
- Patients with suspected malignancy should undergo a CT scan or an MRI/MRCP to evaluate extent of disease, followed by further endoscopic diagnosis and/or therapy, if technically feasible.

INTRODUCTION

Biliary diseases and conditions associated with biliary obstruction affect a significant portion of the worldwide population, and accurate diagnosis of the presence and cause of biliary obstruction is central to providing cost-effective work-up and treatment. Since its advent in 1968, ERCP has become the gold standard in the setting of biliary obstruction. It is one of many invasive direct cholangiography techniques, with a reported complication rate of 1% to 9% and a mortality rate from 0.2% to 0.5%.[1]

Advances in biliary radiology with US, CT, and MRI technology in recent years, however, have allowed accurate, noninvasive imaging of the biliary tree and pancreas. In the setting of obstructive jaundice, imaging helps assess the severity and cause of

[a] Division of Gastrointestinal and Liver Diseases, Department of Medicine, LAC+USC Medical Center, Keck School of Medicine, University of Southern California, 1983 Marengo Avenue, D & T Building, Room B4H100, Los Angeles, CA 90033, USA; [b] Keck School of Medicine, University of Southern California, 1510 San Pablo Street, HCC1: Suite 322R, M/C 9198, Los Angeles, CA 90033, USA
* Corresponding author. Keck School of Medicine, University of Southern California, 1510 San Pablo Street, HCC1: Suite 322R, M/C 9198, Los Angeles, CA 90033.

Gastrointest Endoscopy Clin N Am 23 (2013) 185–197
http://dx.doi.org/10.1016/j.giec.2012.12.011
1052-5157/13/$ – see front matter © 2013 Elsevier Inc. All rights reserved.

giendo.theclinics.com

the obstruction. In some cases, a multimodality imaging approach may be necessary. This article focuses on the general approach to patients with suspected biliary obstruction and discusses the applications of various imaging modalities that may be useful before performing ERCP.

ABDOMINAL ULTRASOUND

Abdominal US is widely recommended as the initial imaging test in evaluating patients presenting with jaundice because it is noninvasive, safe, inexpensive, and widely available. In addition, US is portable and allows for bedside imaging.

US for Gallstones

Gallstones appear as echogenic foci that cast acoustic shadows and seek gravitational dependence (**Fig. 1**).[2] The accuracy of US in the diagnosis of cholelithiasis has been well established,[3] with sensitivities reported at approximately 96%,[4] although the size and number of gallstones cannot be accurately determined on US. The sensitivity of US in diagnosing gallbladder stones is comparable to that of MRCP (97.7%), although it is less sensitive (27% compared with 50% for MRCP) for detecting microlithiasis or biliary sludge.[5] US has also been shown accurate in diagnosing complications of gallstones, in particular cholecystitis, and provided a definitive diagnosis in nearly 80% of patients with suspected cholecystitis in one study.[6]

Even though US has a high specificity (100% in multiple studies[7]) for choledocholithiasis, it is insensitive: sensitivity of US ranges from 22% to 33%[8,9] for detecting common bile duct stones. US, however, is able to detect dilatation of the common bile duct (sensitivity, 77%[10]), a finding often seen with choledocholithiasis. Biliary dilatation greater than 6 mm often indicates biliary obstruction in patients with an intact gallbladder.[11] With a normal-caliber duct (<6 mm), gallstones were found in only 6% of cases at time of surgery, although 37.5% of patients with duct diameters greater than 5 mm had stones at time of surgery.[12] In patients who are postcholecystectomy, the predictive value of duct dilatation for duct stones was 71% and the predictive value of nondilated ducts in excluding stones was 83%. Therefore, US should not be considered an adequate screening test for choledocholithiasis.

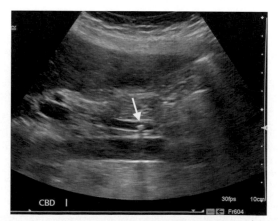

Fig. 1. Abdominal US image of common bile duct stone (*white arrow*).

US is limited in its ability to detect common bile duct stones for many reasons. Intestinal gas often obscures the distal common duct, preventing detection of ampullary stones. Also, calculi require surrounding bile for sonographic contrast, so it can be difficult to visualize stones in normal-caliber bile ducts.[13] Operator experience also plays a major role in sensitivity: when the examination is performed by an expert operator, sensitivity is nearly double (77%–90%) that of an operator with little experience (37%–47%).[14]

Although US has limitations, it can be useful in establishing the best ERCP strategy for endoscopists to use on patients undergoing laparoscopic cholecystectomy. Unnecessary diagnostic ERCPs can be avoided with rigid criteria. The recent algorithm proposed by the American Society for Gastrointestinal Endoscopy states that a normal abdominal US, with normal levels of serum alkaline phosphatase and bilirubin on initial patient presentation, has a negative predictive value of 95% to 96% for common bile duct stones.[15]

US for Malignancy

Evaluating patients who have suspected malignant biliary obstruction is more complex, because the cause, level of obstruction, and extent of the malignancy all need to be addressed. The presence of metastases is particularly important, because it dictates clinical management. In this scenario, the drawbacks of US remain, including the dependency on the operator's interpretive skill and suboptimal imaging because of obesity or intestinal gas.

Abdominal US has a sensitivity of 71% at defining the etiology of biliary obstruction and is particularly sensitive for detecting the level of biliary obstruction in jaundice (sensitivity 88%–90%).[9] The sensitivity of US has increased to 90% for the diagnosis of primary gallbladder cancer, with the infiltrating type still the most difficult to find.[16]

US, however, is less sensitive for diagnosing other tumors, including pancreatic carcinoma, ampullary carcinoma, and cholangiocarcinoma, with a rate less than 50%[9] in defining cause. The most common finding is dilatation of the common bile duct, often as an indirect sign of tumor, and small carcinomas of the distal duct are often not well visualized. Malignancy is reported as the most common cause of obstruction at the suprapancreatic level or proximal to the level of porta hepatis. Although the sensitivity of US for detecting bile duct cancer has been reported as high (over 90% in one study[17]), further imaging is needed if a malignancy is suspected, particularly for staging purposes.

Using US to assess the spread of bile duct cancers has only been reported with Klatskin tumors. Although US with Doppler has been fairly reliable in detecting the invasion of Klatskin tumors into the liver, portal vein, and bile ducts, it has not been helpful in detecting lymph node and peritoneal metastases,[18] and further endoscopic or radiologic imaging is required. The sensitivity of US for diagnosing pancreatic tumors is also variable, reported between 48% and 89%, with low specificity and accuracy, particularly if the tumor is less than 2 cm in diameter.[14]

CT

CT, although usually not the first imaging modality used to evaluate patients with biliary obstruction, can be helpful in diagnosing biliary disease. CT allows for detailed evaluation of the biliary tract, particularly with the advent of modern CT cholangiographic techniques that include the use of biliary excreted contrast material.

CT for Gallstones

Again, CT is usually not the first modality of choice for detecting cholelithiasis, although it can be depicted on CT scan. The appearance of gallstones on CT imaging varies with the chemical composition of the stone, because those stones that are heavily calcified show up radiopaque, but soft tissue attenuation stones can be difficult to visualize. Approximately 10% to 20% of gallstones are composed of pure cholesterol, which are low in density, and, because they are isoattenuating with bile, are hard to see on CT images.[19] This can account for many false-negative CT scans.

Compared with US, CT imaging is better able to accurately demonstrate the location (97%) and cause (94%) of biliary obstruction; however, US is still more sensitive, specific, and accurate for diagnosis of cholelithiasis and has been shown to have a much higher positive predictive value (75% vs 50% for CT) and negative predictive value (97% vs 89% for CT) for diagnosing acute biliary disease.[20] US, therefore, may be more useful than CT for initial screening of acute biliary disease.

Optimization of CT technique, including using thin sections[21] and unenhanced helical CT, can improve the detection of filling defects and has been shown to have greater sensitivity, specificity, and accuracy for the diagnosis of choledocholithiasis.[22] Overall, the sensitivity of CT for choledocholithiasis is reported as between 65% and 88%,[23] with conventional CT imaging having a specificity reported as high as 73% to 97%.[15]

CT cholangiography combines the use of helical CT imaging with the use of intravenous biliary contrast material to generate cholangiographic images of opacified bile ducts. These intravenous contrast materials, such as iopanoic acid, are excreted into bile, but often require the preimaging administration of antihistaminic drugs. In the United States, intravenous contrast-enhanced CT cholangiography has been used mostly to define second-order or third-order bile duct anatomy before living liver transplant donation.[24]

CT cholangiography is helpful for patients with suspected choledocholithiasis (sensitivity 86%–93%, specificity 100%).[25] It has also been shown to have sensitivity in diagnosing bile duct stones comparable with magnetic resonance cholangiography (>90%) and higher than unenhanced helical CT.[26]

CT cholangiography has its limitations, however. In one study comparing CT cholangiography with fiberoptic cholangioscopy, common bile duct stones less than 5 mm in diameter were missed by CT cholangiography in several cases and subsequently detected by invasive cholangioscopy.[27] Furthermore, the excretion of these noninvasive contrast materials, such as iopodic acid, can have variable effects. In particular, patients with liver insufficiency and high serum bilirubin levels (levels >3 mg/dL) often have CT cholangiographic images with insufficient opacification of bile ducts.[28] Concerns regarding the higher doses of radiation, compared with conventional helical CT, and the potential toxicity of the contrast agents have limited the use of CT cholangiography.

CT for Malignancy

Although CT is not the best imaging technique for choledocholithiasis, it is frequently performed during the work-up of jaundice. The sensitivity of CT in detecting gallbladder carcinoma has been reported as greater than 90%.[29] The finding of a mass with variable enhancement is associated with an ill-defined contour of the gallbladder wall or possibly even a fungate mass within the gallbladder itself. Helical CT has been accurate in diagnosing and staging of T2 tumors,[30] but the accuracy of CT for local staging is higher for tumors presenting as a mass lesion as opposed to tumors that present, on imaging, as thickened wall. Overall, dual-phase helical CT has been useful for determining the resectability of gallbladder carcinoma.[31]

Cholangiocarcinoma is often depicted on CT scan as an abrupt termination of bile duct dilatation. The multidetector technique that enables reformations with quality images has been helpful in showing the site and cause of obstruction (97% accuracy for determining the level; 94% accuracy for cause of obstruction[32]), but sensitivity can still be low (40%).[33] CT is more sensitive in detecting hilar carcinoma, but it may not detect small masses. Tumors can have nonspecific appearances, with variable enhancement patterns, although they usually present as patchy peripheral enhancement that is most prominent during the portal venous phase. Usually, cholangiocarinomas are of lesser attenuation than liver parenchyma on unenhanced CT, but appearances can still be nonspecific. Thin sections on imaging with newer helical multidetector CT are more sensitive for detecting subtle, small cholangiocarcinomas as the cause of biliary obstruction.[32]

MAGNETIC RESONANCE CHOLANGIOPANCREATOGRAPHY

MRI offers inherent advantages over CT imaging: there is no risk of radiation or additional contrast, and the appearance of gallstone does not seem affected by their internal composition. MRCP, which uses heavy T2 weighting and rapid image acquisition, provides accurate imaging of the biliary tree and pancreatic duct and has been available as a noninvasive alternative to diagnostic ERCP for 20 years. The T2 weighting allows for bile and pancreatic juice to appear bright, with a high-signal intensity that contrasts with nearby hepatic and pancreatic tissue that appears dark with a low-signal intensity. Because MRCP is noninvasive and does not carry any of the morbidity and mortality associated with ERCP, it has been widely adopted for use in the work-up of biliary obstruction. It also does not require sedation, as endoscopic US and ERCP do, so MRCP avoids risks associated with sedation. Some patients undergoing MRCP, however, may ultimately require diagnostic (tissue/cytology sampling) or therapeutic (sphincterotomy, removal of gallstones, or stent placement) ERCP. Decision-analysis models on the value of MRCP have not demonstrated a reduction in the number of ERCPs in patients with choledocholithiasis or other biliary diseases.[34,35]

MRCP for Gallstones

Gallstones are well depicted on MRCP, regardless of their location and appear, on T2 images, as foci of low-signal intensity surrounded by bright bile (**Fig. 2**). Several studies have demonstrated that the sensitivity and specificity for MRCP in diagnosing choledocholithiasis is high (85%–92% and 93%–97%).[36,37] In one study, however, sensitivity decreased to 64% with stones less than 5 mm in diameter,[38] even though MRCP can demonstrate calculi as small as 2 mm.[39] Multiple studies show that, even with thin-section 3-D imaging techniques, the sensitivity for stones that are 3 mm or smaller may be less than 50%.[40,41] Additional limitations have also been reported, such as mistaking multiple impacted stones (with minimal surrounding bile) for a stricture[42] or cholangitis[41] or misidentifying pneumobilia for stones because pneumobilia also manifests as a signal void.

MRI is still useful, however, because it offers information about adjacent anatomy and allows for biliary imaging in patients with surgically altered anatomy, such as those with biliary enteric anastomoses, Roux-en-Y anastomoses, and hepaticojejunostomies, which make ERCP difficult or impossible to perform. The most recent recommendations from the American Society for Gastrointestinal Endoscopy,[15]

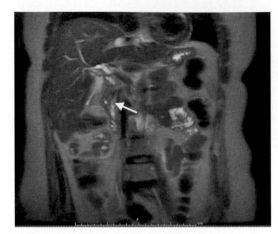

Fig. 2. MRCP image of common bile duct stone (*white arrow*).

adopted from the algorithm proposed by Tse and colleagues,[43] acknowledge the role of MRCP in the preoperative evaluation of patients with an intermediate risk for choledocholithiasis.

MRCP for Malignancy

Many types of tumors cause malignant biliary obstruction. Pancreatic cancer, the most common cause of malignant biliary obstruction, is frequently associated with dilatation of both the common bile duct and pancreatic duct (double-duct sign), which can be seen on multiple modalities of imaging, including MRCP. MRI and MRCP may also define an extrahepatic mass or thickening of the bile duct wall and are, therefore, helpful in diagnosing cholangiocarcinoma and gallbladder carcinoma. MRI and MRCP are also useful in staging. Gastrointestinal tumors metastases, hepatocellular carcinoma, lymphoma, and other malignancies may also cause biliary obstruction through liver metastases, lymph node metastases, or infiltration by continuity.[44] For patients with pancreatic cancer, MRI combined with MRCP protocols have been established for differential diagnosis and staging and assisting surgeons in determining resectability.[45] In a prospective study comparing MRCP with ERCP for detecting pancreatic cancer, MRCP was considered superior to ERCP (sensitivity, 84% vs 70%).[46]

The MRCP depiction of bile duct carcinoma is usually an irregular biliary stricture or obstruction with dilatation above it. MRI may demonstrate the morphology and length of stricture or even a polypoid change; benign strictures tend to have smooth, symmetric luminal narrowing and involve shorter bile duct segments compared with malignant strictures, although there may be a tendency to overestimate the degree and length of stenosis on MRCP.[47]

In cases of gallbladder carcinoma, MRCP may be a better choice than ERCP, because MRCP can demonstrate the filling defect within the gallbladder. On ERCP, the gallbladder is usually not visualized because of the obliteration of the cystic duct in these patients. Patients with gallbladder carcinoma often present with biliary obstruction (50%) caused by lymphadenopathy or invasion or compression of the bile duct by the tumor. The sensitivity of MRCP for bile duct invasion is only approximately 70%,[48] because MRCP imaging is unlikely to pick up microinvasion. MRCP was found, however, more useful than ERCP in diagnosing Klatskin tumors, because

MRCP offers more information about the biliary tree proximal to the area of obstruction. Furthermore, MRCP was superior in identifying the anatomic extent of Klatskin tumors.[49]

Although MRCP may be helpful in identifying the presence of biliary obstruction, it is less reliable in differentiating malignancy from benign causes of biliary obstruction. In a recent meta-analysis, MRCP's accuracy in identifying malignancy is 88%, lower than the rates for choledocholithiasis (92%) and biliary obstruction in general (97%).[36] This is possibly due to the lower spatial resolution for depicting biliary strictures (smooth vs irregular, tapering vs abrupt) compared with direct cholangiography.[50] And although MRCP is highly accurate for imaging the biliary system, ampullary lesions are problematic: interference from intraluminal gas, duodenal contractions, or even juxta-ampullary diverticula can lead to an incorrect diagnosis.[51] ERCP is more sensitive because it offers a direct view of the papilla and the ability to take biopsies.

Especially for patients with pancreatic or biliary cancer, the advantage of ERCP is its ability to serve both diagnostic and therapeutic functions at the same time. Patients who are surgical candidates can undergo tissue sampling with needle aspiration, brush cytology, or forceps biopsy; for patients who are not surgical candidates, stenting can be performed for palliation.

ENDOSCOPIC ULTRASONOGRAPHY

EUS allows for endoscopic visualization and US imaging of the extrahepatic bile duct. EUS is able to yield high-resolution images (0.1 mm) because of the endoscope probe's proximity to the internal structures—an advantage compared with transadominal US, especially in obese patients.

EUS for Gallstones

Both linear and radial echoendoscopes have been used for detecting choledocholithiasis.[52] EUS is more sensitive, specific, and accurate than abdominal US and CT in diagnosing choledocholithiasis, especially those bile ducts containing with small stones (sensitivity: EUS, 91%; US, 27%; CT, 27%).[7] A meta-analysis pooling 27 studies assessed the performance of EUS in detecting choledocholithiasis compared with ERCP, intraoperative cholangiograms, or surgical common bile duct exploration (as gold standard), and EUS was reported to have 89% to 94% sensitivity and 94% to 95% specificity.[53] A separate meta-analysis pooled data from 5 randomized, prospective, blinded trials that compared EUS with MRCP for detecting choledocholithiasis and found that the aggregate sensitivities of EUS and MRCP were 93% and 85%, respectively, and there was no significant difference between the specificities of the modalities (EUS, 96%; MRCP, 93%).[37] In particular, EUS has also shown highly accurate in evaluating the bile duct and choledocholithiasis in patients with acute pancreatitis, with an accuracy reported as 97% and 100%.[54] Complications with EUS performed for diagnostic purposes are low, reported as 0.3% in a large study of 42,000 patients.[55]

Because EUS is able to produce high-resolution images, it is more sensitive than MRCP in detecting small stones. If EUS demonstrates gallstones, therapeutic ERCP can, theoretically, be performed immediately after the EUS, allowing for a single session of sedation. MRCP, alternatively, is performed by a radiologist in a different location and usually on a different day, so if MRCP detects a gallstone, treatment may be delayed. Because of the technical skill required by the endosonographer and the specialized equipment, however, EUS is limited in its availability, whereas MRCP is widely available. Another potential disadvantage of EUS is that, in certain clinical situations, the US transducer cannot be positioned into the duodenum (ie, altered anatomy in postsurgical patients), and this precludes the effective use of EUS for detecting choledocholithiasis.

Many studies have evaluated the role of EUS in reducing the number of unnecessary invasive and potentially risky ERCPs for patients suspected of having choledocholithiasis. Performing EUS first, before ERCP, can eliminate the need for ERCP in 60% to 73% of patients,[15] according to the results of several recent trials. An EUS-first strategy has also been shown cost-effective: a prospective study of 455 patients found EUS cost-effective for patients with an estimated likelihood of choledocholithiasis less than 61%, whereas the ERCP-first method was more cost-effective for patients at higher risk.[56] A comparison of intraoperative cholangiography, ERCP, and EUS in patients scheduled to undergo laparoscopic cholecystectomy also found the EUS-first strategy cost-effective when patients were at a medium risk (11%–55%) for common bile duct stones.[57] In patients with suspected gallstone pancreatitis, EUS also had a sensitivity of 91% and accuracy of 97% for detecting choledocholithiasis, similar to ERCP,[54] and has also been associated with a trend toward less morbidity.[58] An EUS-first strategy has been associated with reduced costs in patients with severe acute biliary pancreatitis.[59]

EUS for Malignancy

The high-resolution EUS images of the bile duct and pancreas are helpful in evaluating suspected malignancy. In a recent meta-analyses summarizing the performance of EUS in assessing biliary obstruction, EUS had a high overall sensitivity (88%; 95% CI, 85%–91%) and specificity (90%; 87%–93%) for biliary obstruction (area under curve 0.97), but the sensitivity and specificity were higher for choledocholithiasis than for malignancy (sensitivity, 89% vs 78%; specificity, 94% vs 84%).[60] Even so, EUS performs better than MRCP in cases of suspected malignant biliary obstruction, because MRCP had low specificity (76%), positive predictive value (25%), and accuracy (61%; CI, 0.41–0.78) for the diagnosis of biliary stricture compared with EUS (100%; 100%; 89% CI, 0.72–0.98).[61] In another prospective study comparing the diagnostic accuracy of malignant strictures in CT, MRCP, and EUS to ERCP, the sensitivity and specificity were higher in MRCP (85%, 71%) than EUS (79%, 62%), but EUS was able to correctly diagnose benign strictures (on absence of visible mass) in the majority of the cases in which MRCP provided a false-positive diagnosis.[62]

SUMMARY AND RECOMMENDATIONS

Recent advances in biliary imaging with US, CT, and MRI technology have expanded the role of noninvasive imaging of the biliary and pancreatic trees in causes of biliary obstruction (**Table 1**). US remains an inexpensive and sensitive initial screening test for causes of biliary obstruction, and CT and MRI play important roles in evaluating suspected malignancy before ERCP. Although MRCP has been widely adopted because of its availability, high sensitivity, and specificity, it still has some limitations, particularly in the setting of imaging for small gallstones and, so far, has not shown to significantly decrease the number of ERCPs performed in choledocholithiasis. An EUS-first strategy for choledocholithiasis has, alternatively, been shown cost-effective and to decrease the number of ERCPs performed.

Recommendations
- Initial evaluation of suspected biliary obstruction should include liver biochemical tests and a transabdominal US.

Table 1
The sensitivities for different imaging modalities for common bile duct stones and malignancy

	US		CT		MRCP		EUS	
	Sens	Spec	Sens	Spec	Sens	Spec	Sens	Spec
Common bile duct stones	22%–33%[8,9]	100%[7]	65%–88%[23]	73%–97%[15]	85%–92%[36,37] <50% for Stones <3 mm[40,41]	93%–97%[36,37]	81%–94%[7]	94%–95%[53]
Malignancy	71%[16]	Unknown	40%–94%[33]	97%[32]	84%[46]	76%–88%[36]	78%[60]	84%[60]

Abbreviations: Sens, sensitivity; Spec, Specificity.

- Patients with suspected choledocholithiasis should be risk stratified; those who are high risk should undergo ERCP without further imaging. Patients who are at intermediate risk should undergo EUS, MRCP, or fluoroscopic cholangiography, depending on the availability.
- Patients with suspected malignancy should undergo a CT scan or an MRI/MRCP to evaluate extent of disease, followed by further endoscopic diagnosis/therapy if technically feasible.

REFERENCES

1. Mallery JS, Baron TH, Dominitz JA, et al. Complications of ERCP. Gastrointest Endosc 2003;57(6):633–8.
2. Gore RM, Yaghmai V, Newark GM, et al. Imaging benign and malignant disease of the gallbladder. Radiol Clin North Am 2002;40(6):1307–23.
3. Bartrum RJ, Crow JC, Foote SR. Ultrasonic and radiographic cholecystography. N Engl J Med 1977;296(10):538–41.
4. Everhart JE, Khare M, Hill M, et al. Prevalence and ethnic differences in gallbladder disease in the United States. Gastroenterology 1999;117(3):632–9.
5. Calvo MM, Bujanda L, Heras I, et al. Magnetic resonance cholangiography versus ultrasound in the evaluation of the gallbladder. J Clin Gastroenterol 2002;34:233–6.
6. Teefy SA, Baron RL, Bigler SA. Sonography of the gallbladder: significance of striated (layered) thickening of the gallbladder wall. AJR Am J Roentgenol 1991;156:945–7.
7. Sugiyama M, Atomi Y. Endoscopic ultrasonography for diagnosing choledocholithiasis: a prospective comparative study with ultrasonography and computed tomography. Gastrointest Endosc 1997;45(2):143–8, 143–6.
8. Einstein DM, Lapin SA, Ralls PW, et al. The insensitivity of sonography in the detection of choledocholithiasis. AJR Am J Roentgenol 1984;142:725–8.
9. Blackbourne LH, Earnhardt RC, Sistrom CL, et al. The sensitivity and role of ultrasound in the evaluation of biliary obstruction. Am Surg 1994;60(9):683–90.
10. Pedersen OM, Nordgard K, Kvinnsland S. Value of sonography in obstructive jaundice. Limitations of bile duct caliber as an indext of obstruction. Scand J Gastroenterol 1987;22:975–81.
11. Parulekar S. Ultrasound evaluation of comon bile duct size. Radiology 1979;133:703–7.
12. Majeed AW, Ross B, Johnson AG, et al. Common duct diameter as an independent predictor of choledocholithiasis; is it useful? Clin Radiol 1999;54:170–2.
13. Callen PW, Filly RA. Ultrasound in the evaluation of patients with right upper quadrant pain. Clin Diagn Ultrasound 1981;7:21–32.
14. Gandolfi G, Torresan F, Solmi L, et al. The role of ultrasound in biliary and pancreatic diseases. Eur J Ultrasound 2003;16(3):141–59.
15. American Society for Gastrointestinal Endoscopy. The role of endoscopy in the evaluation of suspected choledocholithiasis. Gastrointest Endosc 2010;71:1–9.
16. Oikarinen H. Diagnostic imaging of carcinomas of the gallbladder and the bile ducts. Acta Radiol 2006;47(4):345–58.
17. Bloom CM, Langer B, Wilson SR. Role of US in the detection, characterization, and staging of cholangiocarcinoma. Radiographics 1999;19:1199–218.
18. Hann LE, Greatrex KV, Bach AM, et al. Cholangiocarcinoma at the hepatic hilus: sonographic findings. Am J Roentgenol 1997;168:985–9.

19. Gore RM, Nemcek AA, Vogelzang RL. Choledocholithiasis. In: Gore RM, Levine MS, Laufer I, editors. Textbook of gastrointestinal radiology, vol. 2. Philadelphia: Saunders; 1994. p. 1660–74.

20. Harvey RT, Miller WT. Acute biliary disease: initial CT and follow-up US versus Initial US and follow-up CT. Radiology 1999;213:831–6.

21. Yeh BM, Liu PS, Soto JA, et al. MR Imaging and CT of the biliary tract. Radiographics 2009;29:1669–88.

22. Neitlich JD, Topazian M, Smith RC, et al. Detection of choledocholithiasis: comparison of unenhanced helical CT and endoscopic retrograde cholangiopancreatography. Radiology 1997;203:753–7.

23. Anderson SW, Rho E, Soto JA. Detection of biliary duct narrowing and choledocholithiasis: accuracy of portal venous phase multidetector CT. Radiology 2008; 247:418–27.

24. Wang ZJ, Yeh BM, Roberts JP, et al. Living donor candidates for right hepatic lobe transplantation: evaluation at CT cholangiography—initial experience. Radiology 2005;235:899–904.

25. Soto JA, Velez SM, Guzman J. Choledocholithiasis: diagnosis with oral-contrast enhanced CT cholangiography. AJR Am J Roentgenol 1999;172:943–8.

26. Soto JA, Alvarez O, Munera F, et al. Diagnosing bile duct stones: comparison of unenhanced helical CT, oral contrast-enhanced CT cholangiography, and MR cholangiography. AJR Am J Roentgenol 2000;175:1127–34.

27. Koito K, Namieno T, Hirokawa N, et al. Virtual CT cholangioscopy: comparison with fiberoptic cholangioscopy. Endoscopy 2001;33:676–81.

28. Stockberger SM, Sherman S, Kopecky KK. Helical CT cholangiography. Abdom Imaging 1996;21:98–104.

29. Ohtani T, Shirai Y, Tsukada K, et al. Spread of gallbladder carcinoma, CT evaluation with pathologic correlation. Abdom Imaging 1996;21:195–201.

30. Yoshimitsu K, Honda H, Shinozaki K, et al. Helical CT of the local spread of carcinoma of the gallbladder: evaluation according to the TMN system in patients who underwent surgical resection. AJR Am J Roentgenol 2002;179:423–8.

31. Kumaran V, Gulati S, Paul B, et al. The role of dual-phase helical CT in assessing resectability of carcinoma of the gallbladder. Eur Radiol 2002;12:1993–9.

32. Baron RL. Computed tomography of the bile ducts. Semin Roentgenol 1997;32: 172–87.

33. Yamashita Y, Takahashi M, Kanazawa S, et al. Hilar cholangiocarinoma: an evaluation of subtypes with CT and angiography. Acta Radiol 1992;33:351–5.

34. Arguedas MR, Dupont AW, Wilcox CM. Where do ERCP, endoscopic ultrasound, magnetic resonance cholangiopancreatography, and intraoperative cholangiography fit in the management of acute biliary pancreatitis? A decision analysis model. Am J Gastroenterol 2001;96:2892–9.

35. Sahai AV, Devonshire D, Yeoh KG, et al. The decision-making value of magnetic resonance cholangiopancreatography in patients see in a referral center for suspected biliary and pancreatic disease. Am J Gastroenterol 2001;96:2074–80.

36. Romagnuolo J, Bardou M, Rahme E, et al. Magnetic resonance cholangiopancreatography: a meta-analysis of test performance in suspected biliary disease. Ann Intern Med 2003;139:547–57.

37. Verma D, Kapadia A, Eisen GM, et al. EUS vs MRCP for detection of choledocholithiasis. Gastrointest Endosc 2006;64:248–54.

38. Boraschi P, Neri E, Barccini G, et al. Choledocholithiasis: diagnostic accuracy of MR cholangiopancreatography. Three year experience. Magn Reson Imaging 1999;17:1245–53.

39. Fulcher AS, Turner MA, Capps GW, et al. Half-Fourier RARE MR cholangiopancreatography: experience in 300 subjects. Radiology 1998;207:21–32.
40. Nandalur KR, Hussain HK, Weadock WJ, et al. Possible biliary disease: diagnostic performance of high spatial-resolution isotropic 3D T2-weighted MRCP. Radiology 2008;249:883–90.
41. Laokpessi A, Bouillet P, Sautereau D, et al. Value of magnetic resonance cholangiography in the preoperative diagnosis of common bile duct stones. Am J Gastroenterol 2001;26:2354–9.
42. Irie H, Honda H, Kuroiwa T, et al. Pitfalls inMR cholangiopancreatographic interpretation. Radiographics 2001;21:23–7.
43. Tse F, Barkun JS, Barkun AN. The elective evaluation of patients with suspected choledocholithiasis undergoing laparoscopic cholecystectomy. Gastrointest Endosc 2004;60:437–48.
44. Yeh TS, Jan YY, Tseng HH, et al. Malignant perihilar biliary obstruction: magnetic perihilar biliary obstruction: magnetic resonance cholangiopancreatographic findings. Am J Gastroenterol 2000;95:432–40.
45. Catalano C, Pavone P, Laghi A, et al. Pancreatic adenocarcinoma: combination of MR imaging, MR angiography and MR cholangiopanreatography for the diagnosis and assessment of resectability. Eur Radiol 1998;98:428–34.
46. Adamek HE, Albert J, Breer H, et al. Pancreatic cancer detection with magnetic resonance cholaniopancreatography and endoscopic retrograde cholangiopancreatography: a prospective controlled study. Lancet 2000;356:190–3.
47. Hoeffel C, Azizi L, Lewin M, et al. Normal and pathologic features of the postoperative biliary tract at 3D MR cholangiopancreatopgraphy and MR imaging. Radiographics 2006;26:1603–20.
48. Yoshimitsu K, Honda H, Jimi M, et al. MR diagnosis of adenomyomatosis of the gallbladder and differentiation from gallbladder carcinoma: importance of showing Rokitansky-Aschoff sinuses. AJR Am J Roentgenol 1999;172:1535–40.
49. Yeh TS, Jan YY, Tseng JK, et al. Malignant perihilar biliary obstruction: magnetic resonance cholangiopanceratographic findings. Am J Gastroenterol 2000;95: 432–40.
50. Mehta SN, Reinhold C, Barkun AN. Magnetic resonance cholangiopancreatogarphy. Gastrointest Endosc Clin N Am 1997;7:247–70.
51. David V, Reinhold C, Hochman M, et al. Pitfalls in the interpretation of MR cholangiopancreatography. AJR Am J Roentgenol 1998;170:1055–9.
52. Kohut M, Nowakowska Dulawa E, Marek T, et al. Accuracy of linear endoscopic ultrasonography in the evaluation of patients with suspected common bile duct stones. Endoscopy 2002;34:299–303.
53. Tse F, Liu L, Barkun AN, et al. EUS: a meta-analysis of test performance in suspected choledocholithiasis. Gastrointest Endosc 2008;67:235–44.
54. Chak A, Hawes RH, Cooper GS, et al. Prospective assessment of the utility of EUS in the evaluation of gallstone pancreatitis. Gastrointest Endosc 1999;49: 599–604.
55. Rosch T, Dittler HJ, Fockens P, et al. Major complications of endoscopic ultrasonography: results of a survey of 42,105 cases. Gastrointest Endosc 1993;39:341.
56. Buscarini E, Tansini P, Vallisa D, et al. EUS for suspected choledocholithiasis: do benefits outweigh costs? A prospective controlled study. Gastrointest Endosc 2003;57:510–8.
57. Sahai AV, Mauldin PD, Marsi V, et al. Bile duct stones and laparaoscopic cholecystectomy: a decision analysis to assess the roles of intraoperative cholangiography, EUS, and ERCP. Gastrointest Endosc 1999;49:334–43.

58. Liu CL, Fan ST, Lo CM, et al. Comparison of earl endoscopic ultrasonography cholangiography for patients with intermediate probability of bile duct stones: a prospective randomized trial. Gastrointest Endosc 2009;69:244–52.

59. Romagnuolo J, Currie G, Calgary Advanced Therapeutic Endoscopy Center Study Group. Noninvastive vs. selective invasive biliary imaging for acute biliary pancreatitis: an economic evaluation by using decision tree analysis. Gastrointest Endosc 2005;61:86–97.

60. Garrow D, Miller S, Sinha D, et al. Endoscopic ultrasound: a meta-analysis of test performance in suspected biliary obstruction. Clin Gastroenterol Hepatol 2007; 5(5):616–23.

61. Sheiman JM, Carlos RC, Barnett JL, et al. Can endoscopic ultrasound or magnetic resonance cholangiopancreatography replace ERCP in patients with suspected biliary disease? A prospective trial and cost analysis. Am J Gastroenterol 2001;96(10):2900–4.

62. Rosch T, Meining A, Fruhmorgen S, et al. A prospective comparison of the diagnostic accuracy of ERCP, MRCP, CT and EUS in biliary strictures. Gastrointest Endosc 2002;55:870–6.

Infections of the Biliary Tract

Rajan Kochar, MD, MPH, Subhas Banerjee, MD*

KEYWORDS

- Cholangitis • Biliary drainage • Choledocholithiasis • Oriental cholangiohepatitis
- Ascariasis • Fascioliasis • *Clonorchis* • AIDS cholangiopathy
- Management of cholangitis

KEY POINTS

- Infection of the biliary tract or cholangitis is a potentially life-threatening systemic disease that results from a combination of bile duct obstruction and infection. Choledocholithiasis is the most common cause of acute cholangitis.
- Other important causes include benign and malignant bile duct strictures, instrumentation or surgery involving the biliary tree, and rare causes including infection with hepatobiliary parasites, acquired immune deficiency syndrome cholangiopathy, and recurrent pyogenic cholangitis.
- Several mechanisms have been proposed to contribute to the pathogenesis of cholangitis, including bacterial ascension from the small bowel (ascending cholangitis), bacterial translocation through the bowel wall followed by hematogenous seeding, and bacterial contamination of portal blood.
- The most common organisms responsible for cholangitis are enteric gram-negative bacteria including *Escherichia coli* and *Klebsiella*, and gram-positive bacteria such as enterococci. Infection with multiple bacteria and anaerobic organisms is common in elderly patients and those with abnormal postsurgical biliary anatomy.
- In the absence of established diagnostic criteria, a combination of clinical features, laboratory tests, and imaging studies are used to accurately diagnose acute cholangitis.

INTRODUCTION

Infection of the biliary tract, also known as cholangitis, is a systemic process characterized by inflammation and infection in the bile ducts. Other terms used for this condition include ascending cholangitis and suppurative cholangitis. Acute cholangitis is potentially a life-threatening emergency, characterized by obstruction and infection of the biliary tree. Charcot[1] first described cholangitis in 1877 and coined the term

Financial disclosure: None.
Division of Gastroenterology and Hepatology, Stanford University School of Medicine, 300 Pasteur Drive, MC 5244, Stanford, CA 94305, USA
* Corresponding author.
E-mail address: subhas.banerjee@stanford.edu

Gastrointest Endoscopy Clin N Am 23 (2013) 199–218
http://dx.doi.org/10.1016/j.giec.2012.12.008
1052-5157/13/$ – see front matter © 2013 Elsevier Inc. All rights reserved.

hepatic fever to describe the malady. The cardinal clinical features of cholangitis, namely right upper quadrant abdominal pain, fever with chills, and jaundice, are therefore known as the Charcot triad.

Cholangitis typically results from a combination of biliary obstruction and infection. Bile duct stones, or choledocholithiasis, constitute the single most common obstructive cause predisposing to cholangitis, accounting for ~80% of cases.[2,3] Several other causes of biliary obstruction may result in cholangitis, including benign and malignant biliary strictures, pancreatitis, and biliary parasites. The clinical presentation may range from mild forms responsive to medical treatment alone, to severe life-threatening forms requiring intensive care and emergent biliary drainage. In the past few decades, the prognosis of patients with acute cholangitis has improved with advances in intensive care, antibiotic therapy, and biliary drainage procedures. The mortality has reduced from more than 50% in the 1970s[4,5] to less than 10% since the 1980s.[6,7] However, untreated patients with severe cholangitis continue to have a significant mortality.

Early diagnosis is crucial to determining the type and timing of treatment. Consensus guidelines (Tokyo Guidelines) have been created for the diagnosis, severity assessment, and treatment of cholangitis.[8,9] However, cholangitis remains largely a clinical diagnosis relying on clinical features, laboratory tests, and radiologic studies. Early biliary decompression is the focus of therapy for acute cholangitis, and prompt medical treatment that includes intravenous fluids, appropriate antibiotics, and correction of electrolyte abnormalities and coagulopathy is required.

This article presents a comprehensive overview of the pathogenesis, diagnosis, and management of cholangitis, with a focus on endoscopic therapy. In addition, a brief review of rare causes of cholangitis, including acquired immune deficiency syndrome (AIDS) cholangiopathy, parasitic infections of the biliary tract, and recurrent pyogenic cholangitis, is also presented.

ACUTE ASCENDING CHOLANGITIS
Pathogenesis/Mechanism

Cholangitis implies infection in the setting of partial or complete obstruction of the biliary tree. This closed-space infection results in multiplication of organisms, increased intraluminal pressure in the biliary tree,[10–12] and, often, hematogenous seeding causing bacteremia.[13]

The biliary tree is normally sterile as a consequence of several anatomic and physiologic mechanisms.[14,15] A competent sphincter of Oddi prevents intestinal contents from refluxing into the bile duct, and anterograde flow of bile periodically flushes the biliary system, keeping it free of organisms. Further, components of bile, including bile salts and immunoglobulin A (IgA), have antibacterial properties. Bile salts are bacteriostatic, promoting sterility of the biliary tree directly and also by limiting the growth of bacteria within the duodenum.[16,17] Tight junctions between hepatocytes separate the bile canaliculi from hepatic sinusoids, thereby protecting the biliary tree from bacteremia. In addition, Kupffer cells within the hepatic sinusoids maintain the sterility of the biliary system by phagocytosing organisms.[14]

The term ascending cholangitis comes from the presumed duodenal origin of the bacteria that ascend to infect the biliary tree.[12,18] Several current theories suggest additional routes of infection in cholangitis. These theories include bacterial seeding of the biliary tree through the portal venous system,[19] via the periductal lymphatics,[20] by secretion from the liver,[21] and from an infected gall bladder.[22]

Organisms might reach the biliary tree by ascent from the duodenum. This theory is supported by the low incidence of bactibilia in patients with complete neoplastic obstruction of the biliary system compared with the higher incidence in patients with intermittent obstruction caused by choledocholithiasis.[18,21,23] In addition, clinically significant infection may follow instrumentation in these patients, especially when adequate biliary drainage is not achieved.[24] In contrast, it has been argued that, if this theory is correct, patients with neoplastic obstruction should harbor bacteria that ascended before developing complete biliary obstruction.[21] Evidence in favor of a portal source includes animal studies on mice with ligated bile ducts that developed cholangitis on introduction of bacteria into the portal or systemic venous blood.[19,25] Further support in favor of a portal source is evidence for increase in bacterial translocation across the intestinal wall in patients with obstructive jaundice. However, patients with complete neoplastic obstruction have low rates of bactibilia, which suggests additional alternate routes of seeding the biliary tree.

Complete biliary obstruction creates a state of immune dysfunction.[26] Studies indicate that absence of bile salts and IgA in the intestine leads to a change in the bacterial flora that colonizes the small intestine. Under normal circumstances, colonization of the duodenum and jejunum with coliforms is limited,[27,28] but this has been shown to change in studies of bile duct–ligated rats, indicating a shift in the small bowel flora with *Escherichia coli* predominating.[29] In addition to the change in the bacterial flora of the duodenum, intestinal bacteria are more likely to translocate in rodents with ligated bile ducts.[30] The increased translocation may be in part caused by the absence of bile salts. Bile salts have a detergent effect on bacterial endotoxins, and therefore their absence may be responsible for increased translocation of endotoxins.[31] Several changes in neutrophil function have also been noted in patients with obstructive jaundice with reduced phagocytosis, impaired adhesion, and abnormal response to cytokines. All these changes may diminish the neutrophil response to infection.[3,26] In addition, some studies have shown impaired phagocytic function of Kupffer cells in animal models of biliary obstruction, with recovery when the obstruction is relieved.[32]

Bile duct obstruction leads to increased pressure in the biliary tree, which is thought to play a role in the pathogenesis of cholangitis.[10,11] Patients with high biliary pressures as measured during surgery have higher rates of bacteremia, morbidity, and mortality compared with those with lower ductal pressures.[11] Animal studies suggest that high biliary pressure enables bacteria to enter the lymphatics and the bloodstream by distorting the tight junctions between hepatocytes and blunting of the microvillus border of the hepatocytes.[13,33]

Cause

"Every gallstone is a tomb-stone erected to the evil memory of the germs that lie dead within it."

—Lord Moynihan.

Choledocholithiasis is the most common underlying cause of cholangitis in the Western world.[2,3,34] Bile duct stones typically cause intermittent obstruction, allowing bacterial entry into the bile duct, and also act as a nidus for bacterial adhesion and growth. Most bile duct stones migrate from the gall bladder. Up to 15% of patients with symptomatic cholelithiasis may have additional choledocholithiasis.[34,35] Primary de novo bile duct stones are usually pigmented bilirubin stones thought to result from bile stasis and low-level infection. These de novo bile duct stones are more common in Asian populations and in the elderly with dilated bile ducts as a consequence of postsurgical changes or periampullary duodenal diverticula.[34–37]

Other causes of biliary obstruction, such as benign and malignant stenoses, extrinsic compression from pancreatitis, biliary stent obstruction, and parasitic infection, may also put the patient at risk for developing cholangitis. **Table 1** summarizes the most common causes of biliary obstruction leading to cholangitis.

Microbiology

Cholangitis is usually caused by enteric bacteria. Bile cultures are positive in more than 80% of patients with cholangitis; however, the rates of bacteremia vary and positive blood cultures may be detected in 20% to 80% of patients with cholangitis. Polymicrobial isolates are found in 30% to 90% of patients and are more likely in those with an abnormal biliary tree caused by earlier surgery and in patients who have undergone earlier instrumentation of the biliary tree.[3,4,38–40] The most common organisms are *E coli* (25%–50%), *Klebsiella* (15%–20%), and *Enterobacter* species (5%–10%).[3] *Enterococcus* is the most common gram-positive bacterium causing cholangitis and is found in 10% to 20% of patients. Anaerobes may be present in 5% to 10% of patients and are usually found in mixed infections. The most common anaerobic bacteria isolated include *Bacteroides* species followed by *Clostridia* organisms.[8] Elderly patients and patients with surgically altered anatomy, including bilioenteric anastomosis, are more likely to have anaerobic mixed infections.[3,40,41] Hepatobiliary parasites including *Ascaris*, *Opisthorchis*, *Clonorchis*, and *Fasciola* are important causes of biliary obstruction, especially in Asia, and cause cholangitis by superimposed bacterial infection.[42] Viral infection of the biliary tract has been reported in

Table 1 Causes of acute cholangitis		
Gallstones	Secondary choledocholithiasis (origin in gallbladder) Primary bile duct stones (pigmented) Complicated stones (eg, Mirizzi syndrome)	
Bile duct strictures	**Benign** Postoperative: orthotopic liver transplant (anastomotic/ nonanastomotic), complicated cholecystectomy, sump syndrome Pancreatitis: acute (edema), chronic (scarring, fibrosis) Primary sclerosing cholangitis Autoimmune cholangitis Congenital anomalies: choledochal cysts, biliary atresia	**Malignant** Pancreatic cancer Cholangiocarcinoma Ampullary/duodenal neoplasm Gallbladder carcinoma Metastatic lymph nodes
Biliary instrumentation	ERCP with incomplete drainage Hemobilia Bile duct stent obstruction	
Infection	**Parasitic infection** Ascariasis Hepatobiliary flukes: *Opisthorchis*, *Clonorchis*, *Fasciola*)	**Others** Viral infection (AIDS cholangiopathy) Recurrent pyogenic cholangitis (Oriental cholangiohepatitis) Fungal infection (candida cholangitis)

Abbreviation: ERCP, endoscopic retrograde cholangiopancreatography.

patients with hepatitis C and human immunodeficiency virus (HIV).[43] AIDS cholangiopathy in patients with HIV caused by *Cryptosporidium*, microsporidia, *Cyclospora*, or cytomegalovirus infection is less common now with the advent of effective retroviral therapy.[44] Isolation of *Candida* from the biliary tract is rare, and has been reported in immunosuppressed patients at risk for candidemia.[45]

Clinical Features and Diagnosis

The Charcot triad of fever, abdominal pain, and jaundice is typically present in 50% to 70% of patients with cholangitis, and in as few as 20% in some series.[34] The Reynold pentad (Charcot triad with the addition of hypotension and altered mental status) is encountered even less frequently, in only 4% to 8% of patients with cholangitis. Fever and abdominal pain together are seen in up to 80% of the patients and jaundice in 60% to 70%.[46] Thus, many patients with acute cholangitis do not present with the classic signs and symptoms, and further diagnostic testing may be required to establish the diagnosis. A high clinical suspicion must be held for elderly patients, who often have an atypical presentation, and for patients with known anatomic abnormalities or history of hepatobiliary disease including previous biliary surgery or instrumentation. It may be difficult to distinguish between cholangitis and acute cholecystitis and a combination of clinical presentation, laboratory testing and imaging studies is required to guide management.

Laboratory data

Laboratory data in acute cholangitis typically reflect inflammation and cholestasis. Markers of inflammation and infection, including leukocytosis with a left shift and increased C-reactive protein (CRP), may be present. Blood cultures are positive in some patients and usually grow enteric bacteria. Liver function test abnormalities reflect a cholestatic pattern with hyperbilirubinemia and increased alkaline phosphatase (ALP) and gamma glutamyl transferase (GGT).[46,47] The degree of hyperbilirubinemia varies with the cause and duration of obstruction and is usually greater in malignant obstruction.[48] Serum transaminases are increased to a variable degree and often a transient spike of AST/ALT levels greater than 1000 IU/mL may be observed caused by choledocholithiasis.[46,49]

Diagnostic criteria and severity assessment

The severity of acute cholangitis varies significantly from a mild, self-limiting form to life-threatening forms with hemodynamic instability and septic shock. Accurate diagnosis and early severity assessment are imperative to guide the type and timing of therapy. Patients with mild cholangitis may be treated medically and observed, but patients with severe cholangitis require urgent biliary drainage.

Standard diagnostic criteria for acute cholangitis are lacking and some physicians base their diagnosis on clinical features, whereas others rely more on imaging studies or endoscopic confirmation of biliary obstruction and pus in the biliary tree. Diagnostic criteria called the Tokyo Guidelines have been proposed in the past and were recently updated. These criteria combine clinical features, laboratory data, and imaging studies in an attempt to establish the diagnosis (**Box 1**) and severity of acute cholangitis with greater accuracy.[8,9] **Table 2** compares the sensitivity and specificity of these criteria with the Charcot triad.[9]

Imaging studies

There are several imaging modalities that may be considered in patients with acute cholangitis to determine the cause of biliary obstruction. These modalities include abdominal ultrasound (US), computed tomography (CT) scan of the abdomen,

---

Box 1
Updated Tokyo Guidelines: diagnostic criteria for acute cholangitis

A. Systemic inflammation

    A-1. Fever (>38°C) and/or shaking chills

    A-2. Laboratory data: evidence of inflammation (white blood cells <4 or >10 thousand per microliter, CRP>1 mg/L2)

B. Cholestasis

    B-1. Jaundice (total bilirubin >2 mg/dL)

    B-2. Laboratory data: ALP, GGT, AST, ALT > 1.5 × upper limit of normal

C. Imaging

    C-1. Biliary dilation

    C-2. Evidence of cause on imaging (stricture, stone, stent, and so forth.)

Definite diagnosis: 1 item each in A, B, and C

Suspected diagnosis: 1 item in A plus 1 item in either B or C

---

magnetic resonance cholangiopancreatography (MRCP), endoscopic US (EUS), endoscopic retrograde cholangiopancreatography (ERCP), and percutaneous transhepatic cholangiography (PTC). Although ERCP is the most sensitive diagnostic test for cholangitis and also offers the ability to treat the condition, the procedure and associated need for sedation/anesthesia carry significant risks in these already ill patients; therefore, noninvasive imaging studies or lower-risk endoscopic tests, such as EUS, are often performed first.

The choice of imaging modality and the order in which they are performed depends primarily on the clinical stability of the patient and the suspected cause of obstruction. A transabdominal US is typically the initial imaging study of choice. It is highly sensitive and specific for evaluating the gallbladder and for detecting biliary ductal dilatation; however, its ability to detect bile duct stones is low, with a sensitivity ranging from 20% to 50%.[50–52] A CT scan is useful when causes other than stones are suspected, such as malignancy and chronic pancreatitis.[53,54] An MRCP is considered superior to US and CT for imaging the biliary tree and for detecting bile duct stones.[54,55] The sensitivities of EUS and MRCP for detecting bile duct stones are comparable.[56,57] However, the accuracy of MRCP for lesions and stones smaller than 6 mm is limited.[58] EUS is highly sensitive and specific for imaging the biliary tree and the pancreas to evaluate for obstructing stones, tumors, and cysts. In addition, fine-needle aspiration (FNA) may be performed during EUS for tissue diagnosis. EUS is the preferred diagnostic test for patients who have a low to moderate probability for bile duct stones, and is especially useful in patients in whom an ERCP would be risky and undesirable unless absolutely indicated. The noninvasive and less invasive tests (US, CT, MRCP, EUS) may be performed in a clinically stable patient with low or moderate likelihood of

Table 2
Comparison of sensitivity and specificity of the Tokyo Guidelines criteria and the Charcot triad

	Charcot Triad	Tokyo Guidelines Criteria
Sensitivity (%)	26	92
Specificity (%)	96	78

cholangitis; however, in a severely ill patient with high probability of cholangitis, it is prudent to proceed directly to ERCP. ERCP is the gold standard test for diagnosing biliary obstruction and infection, and also serves as a therapeutic modality by facilitating biliary drainage. It is also the most invasive of the modalities discussed earlier and therefore it is preferred when a therapeutic intervention is planned and not as a purely diagnostic modality for cholangitis.[46,49] **Table 3** lists all these modalities along with their advantages and disadvantages.

Management

Therapy for acute cholangitis is directed toward the 2 main causal components, biliary infection and biliary obstruction, with systemic antibiotics and biliary drainage procedures respectively. Early management includes rehydration with intravenous fluids, correction of electrolyte abnormalities, and initiation of antibiotic therapy. Patients with severe cholangitis should be monitored in the intensive care unit, because rapid deterioration of clinical condition with development of septic shock is common. Correction of coagulopathy is important to minimize the risk of procedure-related bleeding.

Table 3
Diagnostic modalities in acute cholangitis

	Advantages	Disadvantages
Transabdominal US	Easily available, noninvasive Excellent sensitivity for cholelithiasis and biliary dilatation	Poor sensitivity for choledocholithiasis and cause of obstruction
CT	Noninvasive Detects signs of inflammation High sensitivity to detect cause and location of obstruction	Purely diagnostic, no therapeutic capability or tissue acquisition Low sensitivity for detecting cholelithiasis Radiation risk, contrast media exposure
MRCP	Noninvasive, no radiation risk High sensitivity for detecting bile duct stones and cause of obstruction	Purely diagnostic, no therapeutic capability or tissue acquisition Poor sensitivity for small stones Expensive, limited availability Cannot be used in patients with metal implants
EUS	Excellent sensitivity for common bile duct stones and pancreatobiliary malignancy Tissue acquisition for diagnosis possible Less invasive than ERCP, may be combined with ERCP	Mostly diagnostic, limited therapeutic potential More invasive than other radiologic tests Operator dependent
ERCP	Gold standard for diagnosing stones, cholangitis Allows intervention and establishes biliary drainage, eg, stone removal, stenting	Invasive, risk of complications Operator dependent
PTC	Establishes biliary drainage High sensitivity to localize site of obstruction	Invasive, risk of complications higher than ERCP Operator dependent

Antibiotic Therapy

Empiric antibiotic therapy should be initiated immediately in all patients with cholangitis after drawing blood cultures. The choice of antimicrobial agent should be based on severity of illness, setting of infection (community acquired or hospital acquired), presence of underlying hepatobiliary disease, history of biliary instrumentation or surgery such as bilioenteric anastomosis, age and immune status of the patient, and local susceptibility patterns.[3,9,46] Hospital-acquired infections may be caused by multiple and/or resistant organisms such as *Pseudomonas*, methicillin-resistant *Staphylococcus aureus* (MRSA), or vancomycin-resistant *Enterococcus* (VRE).[9] Anaerobic bacteria are found more frequently in patients with older age, altered biliary anatomy, and severe disease.[3]

Different antibiotics vary in their ability to penetrate into bile[59]; however, this has not been proved to be of importance. In addition, most antibiotics do not achieve adequate biliary levels in the setting of biliary obstruction with raised intraductal pressure.[60–62] Therefore, although it is reasonable to favor antibiotics with high bile penetration, this should not be the deciding factor.

The traditional antibiotic regimen for cholangitis comprised a combination of an aminoglycoside and ampicillin. However, because of high rates of drug toxicity and emerging drug resistance,[63,64] these have largely been replaced by more efficacious regimens such as broad-spectrum penicillins, cephalosporins, and fluoroquinolones. Extended-spectrum penicillins, such as piperacillin, are effective against the common organisms causing cholangitis, including aerobic and anaerobic gram-negative bacilli, and *Enterococcus* species. Studies comparing extended spectrum penicillins with the ampicillin and aminoglycoside combination have found them to be equally effective or superior.[6,65] Fluoroquinolones have been found to be effective in multiple studies and ciprofloxacin alone may be adequate for treatment of cholangitis.[66,67] Regimens containing cephalosporins have also been compared favorably with the aminoglycoside and ampicillin combination[64]; however, the potential drawbacks of cephalosporins include poor anaerobic coverage and lack of efficacy against enterococci. Metronidazole should be considered in patients with suspected mixed and anaerobic infections, such as the elderly and those with surgically altered anatomy.[68]

The recommended treatment duration has traditionally been 7 to 10 days; however, evidence indicates that, once biliary drainage is achieved, antibiotic therapy is complimentary and, therefore, courses of 2 to 3 days have been proposed for mild cases and 5 to 7 days for moderate or severe cholangitis.[34,48,69,70] The first-choice regimen is usually a penicillin/β-lactamase inhibitor combination such as piperacillin/tazobactam or a third-generation/fourth-generation cephalosporin. If the first line of therapy is ineffective, the antibiotic may be switched to a fluoroquinolone or a carbapenem. If blood or biliary cultures are positive, antibiotic therapy should be changed to narrow-spectrum agents.

Biliary Drainage

Biliary drainage is the most important intervention in the management of acute cholangitis. The mortality of acute cholangitis may approach 100% in patients managed only conservatively.[71,72] Biliary obstruction promotes a persistent source of infection and also impairs the biliary penetration of antibiotics.[46,60–62] In addition, persistent obstruction causes painful jaundice and pruritis.[46]

Surgical drainage with open or laparoscopic bile duct exploration is now rarely performed in acute cholangitis. Surgery involves a high risk of complications, including a mortality of up to 40%.[34,73,74] In a landmark study comparing endoscopic and surgical biliary drainage in cholangitis, a 66% complication rate and 30% mortality were found in patients undergoing surgery compared with figures of 34% and 10% in patients undergoing endoscopic drainage.[75] In extreme circumstances, when other minimally invasive methods have failed, surgeons often opt to perform a choledochotomy and a T-tube placement to allow biliary decompression, followed by definitive surgery at a later date when the patient's condition is stable.

Endoscopic Biliary Drainage

Endoscopic decompression with ERCP is the best method to achieve biliary drainage and is the recommended first line of intervention. The success rate of ERCP is 98% and it has several advantages and lower complication rates compared with surgical and percutaneous drainage.[34,76] In centers without the expertise to perform ERCP, or in low-volume centers where an initial attempt at ERCP fails, rapid transfer of the patient to a high-volume ERCP center should be considered.

There are no evidence-based recommendations regarding the ideal timing of biliary drainage. The Tokyo Guidelines suggest that biliary drainage should be performed as soon as possible in patients with moderate to severe cholangitis.[9] The clinical condition of patients with acute cholangitis may deteriorate rapidly and, as such, biliary drainage should not be delayed beyond 48 hours. However, it is important to resuscitate even the sickest of patients to optimize their cardiopulmonary parameters before subjecting them to an invasive procedure requiring sedation. Studies have shown that patients with cholangitis who did not undergo biliary drainage within 3 days did markedly worse compared with those who had early drainage.[77] In addition, a retrospective study showed a reduction in length of hospital stay for patients with early biliary drainage compared with those with delayed drainage (median 1 vs 3 days).[78] It is therefore appropriate to perform biliary drainage within 24 hours in patients with severe cholangitis and within 48 hours for patients with mild to moderate cholangitis.

Biliary cannulation or access to the bile duct is the first step. Care must be taken not to inject excess contrast into the biliary tree, because this may further increase the biliary pressure and worsen bacteremia. Wire-guided cannulation or a combination of minimal contrast injection and wire-guided cannulation should be strongly considered. Following successful biliary cannulation, bile should ideally be aspirated via a syringe attached to the sphincterotome or biliary cannula to reduce biliary pressure before injecting the contrast. The aspirated bile should be sent for a Gram stain and culture.

Once biliary cannulation is achieved, there are several techniques to facilitate biliary decompression. These techniques are compared in **Table 4**. Indwelling biliary stents or nasobiliary catheters may be placed in the bile duct. Because most patients with cholangitis have underlying choledocholithiasis, it is tempting to remove bile duct stones at the time of biliary decompression because this removes the need for further endoscopic procedures. However, in unstable patients, it is often prudent to minimize procedure duration and to focus on achieving biliary drainage with a stent or nasobiliary catheter as a priority and perform sphincterotomy and stone removal at a later date once the patient is clinically stable.

Placement of a nasobiliary catheter at ERCP was historically the procedure of choice for endoscopic biliary drainage. A nasobiliary catheter allows active decompression by nasobiliary suction, and allows continuous monitoring and culture of bile drainage.[79,80] Although nasobiliary catheters may still be useful in cases of severe suppurative cholangitis, their use has decreased considerably in recent years because there are several disadvantages compared with indwelling biliary stents. Nasobiliary catheters tend to be uncomfortable for patients, require more nursing care, which in

Table 4
Various biliary drainage techniques via ERCP

	Appropriate Setting	Advantages	Disadvantages
Biliary stent without sphincterotomy	Moderate/severe cholangitis and/or coagulopathy	Low risk of complications (bleeding, pancreatitis, perforation)	Requires repeat ERCP Difficult to place larger stent
Biliary stent with sphincterotomy	Mild cholangitis, papillary stenosis, absence of coagulopathy	Allows larger stent placement	Higher risk of complications, including bleeding
Nasobiliary drain	Severe cholangitis requiring monitoring of drainage	Allows monitoring of drainage and continuous flushing Repeat ERCP not required for removal	Catheter may get kinked or dislodged Uncomfortable for patient, requires added nursing care
Sphincterotomy with stone removal	Mild cholangitis, small stones	Avoids need for repeat ERCP	Risk of bleeding
Sphincter dilation with stone removal	Coagulopathic, elderly patients	Allows stone removal with low risk of bleeding	Increased risk of pancreatitis
Self-expanding metal stent	Malignant unresectable obstruction	Longer duration of patency	Difficult to remove Complications can be problematic: migration, bleeding

turn increases medical expenses, may cause electrolyte disturbances because of external diversion of bile, and tend to get dislodged or kinked frequently.[81]

Indwelling biliary stents have similar efficacy but lower costs and are not associated with patient discomfort.[81–83] Therefore, stent placement has largely supplanted nasobiliary tube placement. There are several types of biliary stents and the choice of stent should be based on the cause of obstruction, whether or not a sphincterotomy is being performed, and how soon the next procedure is planned. Stents of larger diameter tend to stay patent longer than smaller diameter stents, and double-pigtail stents tend to migrate less compared with straight stents. Multiple stents may be placed to create numerous interstices through which bile may flow. Metal stents may be placed in patients with malignant biliary obstruction (**Fig. 1**). Patients with malignant biliary obstruction usually develop cholangitis only after previous biliary instrumentation has been performed. The efficacy of endoscopic drainage with ERCP in these patients is similar to those with benign obstruction caused by stones.[84]

A sphincterotomy may be performed to allow placement of a larger stent or to facilitate stone removal. The common complications of a sphincterotomy include bleeding, pancreatitis, and perforation. Ascending cholangitis is an independent risk factor for postsphincterotomy bleeding.[85] Studies comparing stent or nasobiliary drainage catheter placement with and without a sphincterotomy have shown comparable success rates of biliary drainage in both groups and increased risk of complications in the sphincterotomy group (11%–12% vs 2%–3%).[80,83,85] However, there is some evidence that a sphincterotomy reduces recurrence of cholangitis.[86] Therefore, sphincterotomy should be performed in carefully selected patients such as those with

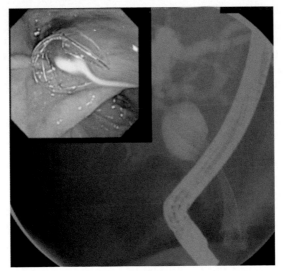

Fig. 1. Combined endoscopic and fluoroscopic image of a metallic biliary stent placed inside the bile duct of a patient with cholangitis caused by malignant biliary stricture, with drainage of pus evident at the ampulla.

mild cholangitis and choledocholithiasis or elderly patients in whom it is prudent to avoid multiple procedures. In all other patients, a stent-and-run approach is appropriate.

PTC

If ERCP fails, PTC with percutaneous biliary drain placement is the most commonly used second-line alternative for biliary drainage. PTC has a success rate of 90% in accessing and draining an obstructed biliary system.[87] The advantages of PTC are that the technique is readily available in most hospitals and can be performed with the use of a local anesthetic, which may have advantages in the unstable patient. There are no randomized studies comparing ERCP and PTC. However, PTC carries a higher complication rate compared with ERCP, with reports of morbidity and mortality as high as 80% and 15% respectively. Complications include pain at the drainage site, bile peritonitis, intraperitoneal hemorrhage, and hemobilia. In addition, patients undergoing PTC typically require longer hospitalization, and the presence of a percutaneous catheter is associated with increased patient discomfort.[80,88,89]

EUS-GUIDED BILIARY DRAINAGE/ROLE OF EUS

EUS-guided biliary drainage is becoming increasingly popular in recent years. It has been described in some cases in which biliary drainage via an ERCP is not possible. Common causes of ERCP failure include altered anatomy caused by prior surgeries, tumor involvement of the papilla, complex periampullary diverticula, papillary stenosis, and impacted stones. Two major EUS-guided biliary drainage techniques have been reported:

1. Rendezvous: the bile duct is punctured transgastrically/transduodenally under EUS guidance and a guidewire is advanced through the FNA needle into the bile duct

and through the papilla into the duodenum. This stage is followed by a standard ERCP as the guidewire is grasped and biliary access is obtained.
2. EUS-guided choledochoduodenostomy: the bile duct is punctured transduodenally, under EUS guidance from the duodenal bulb and a guidewire is advanced into the biliary tree. The track is widened using a needle knife or a balloon dilator and a stent (plastic or metal) is advanced transduodenally into the bile duct over the wire.

A recent review of EUS-guided biliary drainage has reported an 80% success rate (36/45) for the rendezvous method and a 4% complication rate.[90] The complications are essentially the same as for standard ERCP-guided biliary drainage. EUS-guided choledochoduodenostomy has a 94% success rate with 15% complication rate, including bile peritonitis and pneumoperitoneum.[90] EUS-guided hepaticogastrostomy has also been described in a few cases.[91]

These procedures have shown promising results; however, until definitive data are available, their use should be restricted to facilities with extensive experience in therapeutic EUS and only when drainage attempts via ERCP are unsuccessful.

TIMING OF CHOLECYSTECTOMY

There is substantial evidence that early cholecystectomy should be performed in patients with choledocholithiasis after their bile ducts have been cleared by ERCP, because these patients have a high risk of recurrent attacks.[92,93] However, surgical intervention in a patient with acute cholangitis carries significant morbidity and mortality.[73–75] Therefore, the gall bladder should be removed electively after the patient has recovered from the infection.

PARASITIC INFECTIONS OF THE BILIARY TRACT

Parasitic infestation of the biliary tree is a common cause of biliary obstruction for people in tropical countries. This infestation predisposes patients to serious complications such as bacterial cholangitis and cholangiocarcinoma,[42] necessitating accurate diagnosis and effective therapy. Most endemic areas have populations with a low socioeconomic status, inadequate sanitation, and poor hygiene.[94] These infections are not common in the United States; however, they may be encountered in the large immigrant population from these endemic areas as well as in travelers to endemic areas. The most common biliary parasites are listed in **Table 1**.

Ascaris lumbricoides, the roundworm, is the most common parasite infecting the human gastrointestinal tract. Roundworms normally reside in the jejunum, are actively motile, and can frequently traverse the papilla to enter the bile duct and cause biliary obstruction.[95] Fascioliasis is a zoonotic helminthiasis caused by the liver flukes *Fasciola hepatica* and *Fasciola gigantica.* Patients with fascioliasis may present with acute hepatitis or a chronic biliary tract infection.[96] *Clonorchis sinensis* infection is acquired by eating raw or uncooked fish, and can cause complications such as cholelithiasis, intrahepatic stones, recurrent pyogenic cholangitis, cirrhosis, pancreatitis, and cholangiocarcinoma.[97] Other parasites closely related to *C sinensis* include *Opisthorchis viverrini, Opisthorchis felineus,* and *Dicrocoelium dendriticum.*

Microscopic diagnosis is considered the gold standard. Eggs may be found in the stool, biliary aspirate, and duodenal aspirate.[94] Macroscopic diagnosis may be achieved by recovering the adult worm. Serologic tests are largely supplementary and considerable antigen cross reactivity exists among some parasites. Imaging studies such as abdominal US, CT scan, and MRCP may show biliary ductal dilatation, duct wall thickening, and occasionally an adult worm. ERCP can also be used to diagnose parasitic infections, but it should be reserved for cases in which therapy is anticipated.

Efficacy of pharmacologic agents varies with worm burden and presence of a mixed infection.[94] Stool ova and parasites may be periodically tested to determine success of treatment. ERCP is indicated in patients with failure of pharmacologic therapy and persistent worm infestation in the biliary tree, and in patients with acute cholangitis requiring urgent biliary drainage.[98] Extraction of parasites at ERCP has a high success rate and is frequently achieved in the initial attempt.[98]

RECURRENT PYOGENIC CHOLANGITIS

Primary hepatic lithiasis, recurrent pyogenic cholangitis, and oriental cholangiohepatitis are terms used interchangeably to describe the pathologic, clinical, and epidemiologic aspects of the same disease entity. Recurrent pyogenic cholangitis is characterized by the presence of intrahepatic stones and recurrent attacks of cholangitis.[99] The term oriental cholangiohepatitis was coined because of the high incidence of the disease in southeast Asia; however, because of immigration trends, it is now frequently encountered in the United States.

The etiopathogenesis of this condition is unclear but a strong association has been described with parasitic infections such as *A lumbricoides* and *C sinensis*, poor nutritional status, and lower socioeconomic status.[99,100] It has been hypothesized that chronic parasitic infections contribute to the inflammatory and fibrotic changes found in the bile duct walls that eventually result in stricturing, bile stasis, and stone formation.[100] The intrahepatic stones are typically pigmented and consist of calcium bilirubinate.

The most common clinical presentation consists of right upper quadrant abdominal pain, fever, and jaundice. Patients typically have a history of multiple similar episodes in the past. Laboratory tests may show moderately abnormal liver function tests and an increased white cell count. Imaging studies such as abdominal US, CT scan, and MRI/MRCP may show dilatation of intrahepatic bile ducts, duct wall thickening, intrahepatic stones, biliary strictures, and occasionally hepatic abscesses.

Key aspects of management include stone removal and biliary drainage.[101] ERCP is effective in draining the extrahepatic biliary tree and in removing distal stones; however, accessing the intrahepatic bile ducts is frequently difficult because of the presence of strictures and fibrosed angulated bile ducts.[102] Surgical resection is often a feasible option in patients with disease limited to the left lobe of the liver and creates a reduced risk of recurrent stones and cholangitis. In high-risk surgical candidates and patients with extensive stone disease, percutaneous transhepatic drainage and stone removal is often effective.[103] Long-term sequelae of recurrent pyogenic cholangitis include progression to secondary biliary cirrhosis (7%–10%)[104] and development of cholangiocarcinoma (2%–10%).[100]

AIDS CHOLANGIOPATHY

AIDS cholangiopathy is a form of sclerosing cholangitis that is thought to result from infection of the biliary tree by opportunistic pathogens and that is characterized by specific patterns of cholangiographic abnormalities.[105]

Infection of the biliary tree with *Cryptosporidium* was first described in patients with AIDS in 1983.[106] *Cryptosporidium* and cytomegalovirus (CMV) are the most common causative organisms in AIDS cholangiopathy. Other implicated pathogens include microsporidia, *Giardia*, *Cyclospora*, *Mycobacterium avium intracellulare*, *Isospora*, and *Encephalitozoon*.[44]

The most common presentation includes right upper quadrant or epigastric abdominal pain and abnormal liver tests in a cholestatic pattern. Other symptoms include fever, chills, and nausea.[44] Jaundice is characteristically uncommon. The most frequent laboratory abnormalities are an increased ALP and a CD4 lymphocyte count less than 100/ μL. Serum levels of transaminases may be modestly increased and serum bilirubin is usually normal or slightly increased.[44]

The initial imaging test of choice is an abdominal US, which is sensitive in detecting biliary ductal dilatation and duct wall thickening. A CT scan is superior in detecting intrahepatic ductal abnormalities but less sensitive for imaging the extrahepatic biliary tree. An ERCP is the gold standard test for diagnosing AIDS cholangiopathy and the following distinct cholangiographic patterns have been described: (1) sclerosing cholangitis and papillary stenosis, (2) sclerosing cholangitis alone, (3) papillary stenosis alone, and (4) long extrahepatic biliary strictures with or without intrahepatic disease.[105]

Antimicrobial therapy directed against opportunistic infections has been mostly ineffective. Endoscopic sphincterotomy performed during ERCP has been the mainstay of therapy in patients with papillary stenosis, and most patients achieve some degree of pain resolution and variable improvement in liver chemistry.[44,105] Occasional case reports describe endoscopic balloon dilatation and/or stent placement for biliary strictures associated with AIDS cholangiopathy.[107]

The incidence of biliary infections and AIDS cholangiopathy has decreased significantly with the advent of highly active antiretroviral (HAART) therapy.[108] HAART restores the immune system and results in clinical and histologic response against opportunistic infections. As a consequence, AIDS cholangiopathy is rarely encountered in the Western world today.

SUMMARY

Infection of the biliary tract or cholangitis is a potentially life-threatening systemic disease that results from a combination of bile duct obstruction and infection. Choledocholithiasis is the most common cause of acute cholangitis. Other important causes include benign and malignant bile duct strictures, instrumentation or surgery involving the biliary tree, and rare causes including infection with hepatobiliary parasites, AIDS cholangiopathy, and recurrent pyogenic cholangitis. Several mechanisms have been proposed to contribute to the pathogenesis of cholangitis, including bacterial ascension from the small bowel (ascending cholangitis), bacterial translocation through the bowel wall followed by hematogenous seeding, and bacterial contamination of portal blood. The most common organisms responsible for cholangitis are enteric gram-negative bacteria including E coli and Klebsiella, and gram-positive bacteria such as enterococci. Infection with multiple bacteria and anaerobic organisms is common in elderly patients and those with abnormal postsurgical biliary anatomy.

In the absence of established diagnostic criteria, a combination of clinical features, laboratory tests and imaging studies are used to accurately diagnose acute cholangitis. An ERCP is the gold standard test for diagnosing cholangitis and also offers definitive therapy by providing biliary drainage. Less invasive diagnostic tests are often used in clinically stable patients with unclear diagnoses. These tests include abdominal US, CT scan, MRCP, and EUS. Initial management of patients with cholangitis includes obtaining intravenous access, hemodynamic resuscitation, correction of electrolyte abnormalities, and initiating antibiotic therapy. Definitive treatment of cholangitis is directed at resolving biliary obstruction and infection. An ERCP is the first-line intervention for achieving biliary drainage and should be performed urgently in a clinically unstable patient with severe cholangitis and within 24 to 48 hours in a patient with mild to moderate cholangitis. During an ERCP, different techniques may be used to facilitate biliary drainage, including placement of a biliary stent or a nasobiliary drain with or without a sphincterotomy. These interventions are individualized based on the cause and severity of cholangitis and other patient characteristics. Second-line techniques for biliary drainage may be undertaken if ERCP fails or is technically impossible; these include PTC, EUS-guided biliary drainage, and surgical drainage. Common empiric antibiotics for cholangitis include extended-spectrum penicillins and fluoroquinolones.

REFERENCES

1. Charcot M. De la fievre hepatique symptomatique. Comparison avec la fievre uroseptique. Lecons sur les maladies du foie des voies biliares et des reins. [Of symptomatic hepatic fever. Comparison with uroseptic fever. Lessons on diseases of the liver, biliary tract and kidneys]. Paris: Bourneville et Sevestre; 1877. p. 176–85.
2. Hanau LH, Steigbigel NH. Cholangitis: pathogenesis, diagnosis, and treatment. Curr Clin Top Infect Dis 1995;15:153–78.
3. Hanau LH, Steigbigel NH. Acute (ascending) cholangitis. Infect Dis Clin North Am 2000;14(3):521–46.
4. Andrew DJ, Johnson SE. Acute suppurative cholangitis, a medical and surgical emergency. A review of ten years experience emphasizing early recognition. Am J Gastroenterol 1970;54(2):141–54.
5. Shimada H, Nakagawara G, Kobayashi M, et al. Pathogenesis and clinical features of acute cholangitis accompanied by shock. Jpn J Surg 1984;14(4):269–77.
6. Thompson JE Jr, Pitt HA, Doty JE, et al. Broad spectrum penicillin as an adequate therapy for acute cholangitis. Surg Gynecol Obstet 1990;171(4):275–82.
7. Tai DI, Shen FH, Liaw YF. Abnormal pre-drainage serum creatinine as a prognostic indicator in acute cholangitis. Hepatogastroenterology 1992;39(1):47–50.
8. Tokyo Guidelines for the management of acute cholangitis and cholecystitis. Proceedings of a consensus meeting, April 2006, Tokyo, Japan. J Hepatobiliary Pancreat Surg 2007;14(1):1–121.
9. Kiriyama S, Takada T, Strasberg SM, et al. New diagnostic criteria and severity assessment of acute cholangitis in revised Tokyo Guidelines. J Hepatobiliary Pancreat Sci 2012;19(5):548–56.
10. Csendes A, Sepúlveda A, Burdiles P, et al. Common bile duct pressure in patients with common bile duct stones with or without acute suppurative cholangitis. Arch Surg 1988;123(6):697–9.
11. Lygidakis NJ, Brummelkamp WH. The significance of intrabiliary pressure in acute cholangitis. Surg Gynecol Obstet 1985;161(5):465–9.
12. Lygidakis NJ. Incidence of bile infection in patients with choledocholithiasis. Am J Gastroenterol 1982;77(1):12–7.
13. Raper SE, Barker ME, Jones AL, et al. Anatomic correlates of bacterial cholangiovenous reflux. Surgery 1989;105(3):352–9.
14. Sung JY, Costerton JW, Shaffer EA. Defense system in the biliary tract against bacterial infection. Dig Dis Sci 1992;37(5):689–96.
15. Scott AJ. Bacteria and disease of the biliary tract. Gut 1971;12(6):487–92.
16. Csendes A, Fernandez M, Uribe P. Bacteriology of the gallbladder bile in normal subjects. Am J Surg 1975;129(6):629–31.

17. Carpenter HA. Bacterial and parasitic cholangitis. Mayo Clin Proc 1998;73(5): 473–8.
18. Cetta F. The route of infection in patients with bactibilia. World J Surg 1983;7(4): 562.
19. Dineen P. The importance of the route of infection in experimental biliary tract obstruction. Surg Gynecol Obstet 1964;119:1001–8.
20. Anderson RE, Priestley JT. Observations on the bacteriology of choledochal bile. Ann Surg 1951;133(4):486–9.
21. Scott AJ, Khan GA. Origin of bacteria in bileduct bile. Lancet 1967;2(7520): 790–2.
22. Elkeles G, Mirizzi PL. A study of the bacteriology of the common bile duct in comparison with the other extrahepatic segments of the biliary tract. Ann Surg 1942;116(3):360–6.
23. Flemma RJ, Flint LM, Osterhout S, et al. Bacteriologic studies of biliary tract infection. Ann Surg 1967;166(4):563–72.
24. Devière J, Motte S, Dumonceau JM, et al. Septicemia after endoscopic retrograde cholangiopancreatography. Endoscopy 1990;22(2):72–5.
25. Sung JY, Shaffer EA, Olson ME, et al. Bacterial invasion of the biliary system by way of the portal-venous system. Hepatology 1991;14(2):313–7.
26. Jiang WG, Puntis MC. Immune dysfunction in patients with obstructive jaundice, mediators and implications for treatments. HPB Surg 1997;10(3):129–42.
27. Kalser MH, Cohen R, Arteaga I, et al. Normal viral and bacterial flora of the human small and large intestine. N Engl J Med 1966;274(10):558–63 contd.
28. Plaut AG, Gorbach SL, Nahas L, et al. Studies of intestinal microflora. 3. The microbial flora of human small intestinal mucosa and fluids. Gastroenterology 1967;53(6):868–73.
29. Ding JW, Andersson R, Soltesz V, et al. Obstructive jaundice impairs reticuloendothelial function and promotes bacterial translocation in the rat. J Surg Res 1994;57(2):238–45.
30. Clements WD, Parks R, Erwin P, et al. Role of the gut in the pathophysiology of extrahepatic biliary obstruction. Gut 1996;39(4):587–93.
31. Shands JW, Chun PW. The dispersion of Gram-negative lipopolysaccharide by deoxycholate. J Biol Chem 1980;225:1221–6.
32. Clements WD, McCaigue M, Erwin P, et al. Biliary decompression promotes Kupffer cell recovery in obstructive jaundice. Gut 1996;38(6):925–31.
33. Huang T, Bass JA, Williams RD. The significance of biliary pressure in cholangitis. Arch Surg 1969;98(5):629–32.
34. Kinney TP. Management of ascending cholangitis. Gastrointest Endosc Clin N Am 2007;17(2):289–306, vi.
35. Tazuma S. Gallstone disease: epidemiology, pathogenesis, and classification of biliary stones (common bile duct and intrahepatic). Best Pract Res Clin Gastroenterol 2006;20(6):1075–83.
36. Kaufman HS, Magnuson TH, Lillemoe KD, et al. The role of bacteria in gallbladder and common duct stone formation. Ann Surg 1989;209(5):584–91 [discussion: 591–2].
37. Cetta FM. Bile infection documented as initial event in the pathogenesis of brown pigment biliary stones. Hepatology 1986;6(3):482–9.
38. Csendes A, Mitru N, Maluenda F, et al. Counts of bacteria and pyocites of choledochal bile in controls and in patients with gallstones or common bile duct stones with or without acute cholangitis. Hepatogastroenterology 1996;43(10): 800–6.

39. Lewis RT, Goodall RG, Marien B, et al. Biliary bacteria, antibiotic use, and wound infection in surgery of the gallbladder and common bile duct. Arch Surg 1987; 122(1):44–7.
40. Shimada K, Noro T, Inamatsu T, et al. Bacteriology of acute obstructive suppurative cholangitis of the aged. J Clin Microbiol 1981;14(5):522–6.
41. Shimada K, Inamatsu T, Yamashiro M. Anaerobic bacteria in biliary disease in elderly patients. J Infect Dis 1977;135(5):850–4.
42. Rana SS, Bhasin DK, Nanda M, et al. Parasitic infestations of the biliary tract. Curr Gastroenterol Rep 2007;9(2):156–64.
43. Gupta E, Chakravarti A. Viral infections of the biliary tract. Saudi J Gastroenterol 2008;14(3):158–60.
44. Yusuf TE, Baron TH. AIDS cholangiopathy. Curr Treat Options Gastroenterol 2004;7(2):111–7.
45. Wig JD, Singh K, Chawla YK, et al. Cholangitis due to candidiasis of the extrahepatic biliary tract. HPB Surg 1998;11(1):51–4.
46. Mosler P. Diagnosis and management of acute cholangitis. Curr Gastroenterol Rep 2011;13(2):166–72.
47. Anciaux ML, Pelletier G, Attali P, et al. Prospective study of clinical and biochemical features of symptomatic choledocholithiasis. Dig Dis Sci 1986;31(5):449–53.
48. Qureshi WA. Approach to the patient who has suspected acute bacterial cholangitis. Gastroenterol Clin North Am 2006;35(2):409–23.
49. Attasaranya S, Fogel EL, Lehman GA. Choledocholithiasis, ascending cholangitis, and gallstone pancreatitis. Med Clin North Am 2008;92(4):925–60.
50. Einstein DM, Lapin SA, Ralls PW, et al. The insensitivity of sonography in the detection of choledocholithiasis. AJR Am J Roentgenol 1984;142(4):725.
51. Pasanen PA, Partanen KP, Pikkarainen PH, et al. A comparison of ultrasound, computed tomography, and endoscopic retrograde cholangiopancreatography in the differential diagnosis of benign and malignant jaundice and cholestasis. Eur J Surg 1993;159(1):23.
52. Varghese JC, Liddell RP, Farrell MA, et al. Diagnostic accuracy of magnetic resonance cholangiopancreatography and ultrasound compared with direct cholangiography in the detection of choledocholithiasis. Clin Radiol 2000; 55:25.
53. Soto JA, Alvarez O, Munera F, et al. Diagnosing bile duct stones: comparison of unenhanced helical CT, oral contrast-enhanced CT cholangiography, and MR cholangiography. Am J Roentgenol 2000;175(4):1127.
54. Tseng CW, Chen CC, Chen TS, et al. Can computed tomography with coronal reconstruction improve the diagnosis of choledocholithiasis. J Gastroenterol Hepatol 2008;23(10):1586.
55. Moon JH, Cho YD, Cha SW, et al. The detection of bile duct stones in suspected biliary pancreatitis: comparison of MRCP, ERCP, and intraductal US. Am J Gastroenterol 2005;100(5):1051.
56. Verma D, Kapadia A, Eisen GM, et al. EUS vs MRCP for detection of choledocholithiasis. Gastrointest Endosc 2006;64(2):248.
57. Ledro-Cano D. Suspected choledocholithiasis: endoscopic ultrasound or magnetic resonance cholangio-pancreatography? A systematic review. Eur J Gastroenterol Hepatol 2007;19(11):1007.
58. Zidi SH, Prat F, Le Guen O, et al. Use of magnetic resonance cholangiography in the diagnosis of choledocholithiasis: prospective comparison with a reference imaging method. Gut 1999;44(1):118.

59. Nagar H, Berger SA. The excretion of antibiotics by the biliary tract. Surg Gynecol Obstet 1984;158:601–7.
60. Schoenfield LJ. Biliary excretion of antibiotics. N Engl J Med 1971;284:1213–4.
61. Van Delden OM, Van Leeuwen DJ, Jansen PL, et al. Biliary excretion of ceftriaxone into non-stagnant and stagnant bile. J Antimicrob Chemother 1994;33: 193–4.
62. Van Den Hazel SJ, De Vries XH, Speelman P, et al. Biliary excretion of ciprofloxacin and piperacillin in the obstructed biliary tract. Antimicrob Agents Chemother 1996;40:2658–60.
63. Desai TK, Tsang TK. Aminoglycoside nephrotoxicity in obstructive jaundice. Am J Med 1988;85:47–50.
64. Bergeron MG, Mendelson J, Harding GK, et al. Cefoperazone compared with ampicillin plus tobramycin for severe biliary tract infections. Antimicrob Agents Chemother 1988;32:1231–6.
65. Gerecht WB, Henry NK, Hoffman WW, et al. Prospective randomized comparison of mezlocillin therapy alone with combined ampicillin and gentamicin therapy for patients with cholangitis. Arch Intern Med 1989;149:1279–84.
66. Sung JJY, Lyon DJ, Suen R, et al. Intravenous ciprofloxacin as treatment for patients with acute suppurative cholangitis: a randomized controlled clinical trial. J Antimicrob Chemother 1995;35:855–64.
67. Karachalios GN, Nasiopoulou DD, Bourlinou PK, et al. Treatment of acute biliary tract infections with ofloxacin: a randomized controlled clinical trial. Int J Clin Pharmacol Ther 1996;34:555–7.
68. Baker AR, Neoptolemos JP, Carr-Locke DL, et al. Sump syndrome following choledocho-duodenostomy and its endoscopic treatment. Br J Surg 1985;72: 433.
69. Van lent AU, Bartelsman JF, Tytgat GN, et al. Duration of antibiotic therapy for cholangitis after successful endoscopic drainage of biliary tract. Gastrointest Endosc 2002;55:518.
70. Westphal JF, Brogard JM. Biliary tract infections: a guide to treatment. Drugs 1999;57:81.
71. Welch JP, Donaldson GA. The urgency of diagnosis and surgical treatment of acute suppurative cholangitis. Am J Surg 1976;131(5):527–32.
72. O'Connor MJ, Schwartz ML, McQuarrie DG, et al. Acute bacterial cholangitis: an analysis of clinical manifestation. Arch Surg 1982;117(4):437–41.
73. Lai EC, Tam PC, Paterson IA, et al. Emergency surgery for severe acute cholangitis. The high risk patients. Ann Surg 1990;211:55.
74. Boey JH, Way LW. Acute cholangitis. Ann Surg 1980;191:264.
75. Lai EC, Mok FP, Tan ES, et al. Endoscopic biliary drainage for severe acute cholangitis. N Engl J Med 1992;326:1582.
76. Cohen S, Bacon BR, Berlin JA, et al. National Institutes of Health State-of-the-Science Conference Statement: ERCP for diagnosis and therapy, January 14–16, 2002. Gastrointest Endosc 2002;56(6):803–9.
77. Boender J, Nix GA, de Ridder MA, et al. Endoscopic sphincterotomy and biliary drainage in patients with cholangitis due to common bile duct stones. Am J Gastroenterol 1995;90(2):233–8.
78. Chak A, Cooper GS, Lloyd Lt, et al. Effectiveness of ERCP in cholangitis: a community-based study. Gastrointest Endosc 2000;52(4):484–9.
79. Goenka MK, Bhasin DK, Kochhar R, et al. Endoscopic nasobiliary drainage in the management of acute cholangitis: an experience in 143 patients. Diagn Ther Endosc 1997;3(3):161–70.

80. Sugiyama M, Atomi Y. The benefits of endoscopic nasobiliary drainage without sphincterotomy for acute cholangitis. Am J Gastroenterol 1998;93(11):2065–8.
81. Lee DW, Chan AC, Lam YH, et al. Biliary decompression by nasobiliary catheter or biliary stent in acute suppurative cholangitis: a prospective randomized trial. Gastrointest Endosc 2002;56(3):361–5.
82. Sharma BC, Kumar R, Agarwal N, et al. Endoscopic biliary drainage by nasobiliary drain or by stent placement in patients with acute cholangitis. Endoscopy 2005;37(5):439–43.
83. Kumar R, Sharma BC, Singh J, et al. Endoscopic biliary drainage for severe acute cholangitis in biliary obstruction as a result of malignant and benign diseases. J Gastroenterol Hepatol 2004;19(9):994–7.
84. Freeman ML, Nelson DB, Sherman S, et al. Complications of endoscopic biliary sphincterotomy. N Engl J Med 1996;335(13):909–18.
85. Hui CK, Lai KC, Wong WM, et al. A randomized controlled trial of endoscopic sphincterotomy in acute cholangitis without common bile duct stones. Gut 2002;51:245.
86. Lee SH, Hwang JH, Yang KY, et al. Does endoscopic sphincterotomy reduce the recurrence rate of cholangitis in patients with cholangitis and suspected of a common bile duct stone not detected by ERCP? Gastrointest Endosc 2008; 67(1):51–7.
87. Joseph PK, Bizer LS, Sprayregen SS, et al. Percutaneous transhepatic biliary drainage. Results and complications in 81 patients. JAMA 1986;255(20): 2763–7.
88. Pessa ME, Hawkins IF, Vogel SB. The treatment of acute cholangitis. Percutaneous transhepatic biliary drainage before definitive therapy. Ann Surg 1987; 205(4):389–92.
89. Takada T, Yasuda H, Hanyu F. Technique and management of percutaneous transhepatic cholangial drainage for treating an obstructive jaundice. Hepatogastroenterology 1995;42(4):317–22.
90. Tarantino I. Endoscopic ultrasound guided biliary drainage. World J Gastrointest Endosc 2012;4(7):306.
91. Burmester E, Niehaus J, Leineweber T, et al. EUS-cholangio-drainage of the bile duct; report of 4 cases. Gastrointest Endosc 2003;57:246–51.
92. Lau JY, Leow CK, Fung TM, et al. Cholecystectomy or gallbladder in situ after endoscopic sphincterotomy and bile duct stone removal in Chinese patients. Gastroenterology 2006;130(1):96–103.
93. Sarli L, Iusco D, Sgobba G, et al. Gallstone cholangitis: a 10-year experience of combined endoscopic and laparoscopic treatment. Surg Endosc 2002;16(6): 975–80.
94. Khandelwal N, Shaw J, Jain MK. Biliary parasites: diagnostic and therapeutic strategies. Curr Treat Options Gastroenterol 2008;11(2):85–95.
95. Khusroo MS. Ascariasis. Gastroenterol Clin North Am 1996;25:553–77.
96. Aksoy DY, Kerimoğlu U, Oto A, et al. *Fasciola hepatica* infection: clinical and computerized tomographic findings of ten patients. Turk J Gastroenterol 2006; 17(1):40–5.
97. Rim HJ. Clonorchiasis: an update. J Helminthol 2005;79:269–81.
98. Shah OJ, Zargar SA, Robbani I. Biliary ascariasis: a review. World J Surg 2006; 30:1500–6.
99. Tsui WM, Lam PW, Lee WK, et al. Primary hepatolithiasis, recurrent pyogenic cholangitis, and oriental cholangiohepatitis: a tale of 3 countries. Adv Anat Pathol 2011;18(4):318–28.

100. Nguyen T, Powell A, Daugherty T. Recurrent pyogenic cholangitis. Dig Dis Sci 2010;55(1):8–10.
101. Mori T, Sugiyama M, Atomi Y. Management of intrahepatic stones. Best Pract Res Clin Gastroenterol 2006;20:1117–37.
102. Lam SK, Wong KP, Chan PK, et al. Recurrent pyogenic cholangitis: a study of endoscopic retrograde cholangiography. Gastroenterology 1978;74:1196–203.
103. Huang MH, Chen CH, Yang JC, et al. Long-term outcome of percutaneous transhepatic cholangioscopic lithotomy for hepatolithiasis. Am J Gastroenterol 2003;98:2589–90.
104. Jeng KS, Shih SL, Chiang HJ, et al. Secondary biliary cirrhosis. A limiting factor in the treatment of hepatolithiasis. Arch Surg 1989;124:1301–5.
105. Cello JP. Acquired immunodeficiency syndrome cholangiopathy: spectrum of disease. Am J Med 1989;86(5):539–46.
106. Guarda LA, Stein SA, Cleary KA, et al. Human cryptosporidiosis in the acquired immune deficiency syndrome. Arch Pathol Lab Med 1983;107(11):562–6.
107. Cordero E, López-Cortés LF, Belda O, et al. Acquired immunodeficiency syndrome-related cryptosporidial cholangitis: resolution with endobiliary prosthesis insertion. Gastrointest Endosc 2001;53(4):534–5.
108. Moore RD, Chaisson RE. Natural history of HIV infection in the era of combination antiretroviral therapy. AIDS 1999;13(14):1933–42.

Difficult Biliary Access at ERCP

Yan G. Bakman, MD, Martin L. Freeman, MD*

KEYWORDS

- Biliary access • Biliary cannulation • Advanced cannulation techniques
- Precut sphincterotomy • Advanced ERCP

KEY POINTS

- Multiple devices aid cannulation, including rotatable and steerable sphincterotomes and ultratapered cannulas, any of which can incorporate wire-guided techniques.
- Pancreatic duct guidewire or stent-assisted biliary access is increasingly used in advanced techniques.
- Pancreatic stent placement is often required to reduce risk of post-ERCP pancreatitis in difficult access.
- Precut biliary sphincterotomy and transpancreatic septotomy are generally considered only when prior are not feasible or successful.

INTRODUCTION

Establishing biliary access during endoscopic retrograde cholangiopancreatography (ERCP) requires deep cannulation and guidewire access, and is a prerequisite to successful biliary therapy. Achieving such access can be a challenge for experts and novices, and many accessories and techniques have been developed to aid biliary cannulation. Success at biliary cannulation can be enhanced by using such devices as papillotomies, guidewires, cannulas, and precut papillotomes. Similar techniques can also be applied to pancreatic access, which then allows instrumentation and protective stenting of the pancreatic duct. Some endoscopists may be unfamiliar with some of the newer devices and techniques. Many of these techniques can be successfully applied, and disagreement as to the most appropriate technique may exist even among experts. This is further amplified by lack of comparative data available to generalize various techniques outside of centers where such studies are

Financial Relationships: YGB has no financial relationships to disclose. MLF has done limited consulting for Cook Endoscopy and Boston Scientific.
Division of Gastroenterology, Hepatology and Nutrition, University of Minnesota, MMC 36, 406 Harvard Street Southeast, Minneapolis, MN 55455, USA
* Corresponding author. Division of Gastroenterology, Hepatology and Nutrition, University of Minnesota, MMC 36, 406 Harvard Street Southeast, Minneapolis, MN 55455.
E-mail address: freem020@umn.edu

performed. Inferences about relative safety and efficacy of one technique over another are limited because complications can depend on patients' susceptibility as much as the specific technique used by the endoscopist.[1,2] In this article judgment is avoided as to which method is preferable, and mention of any specific manufacturers is omitted because it is impossible to list them in entirety. A comprehensive list of devices for biliary cannulation and sphincterotomy was published in *Gastrointestinal Endoscopy* in 2010.[3]

DETERMINING THE SUCCESS OF CANNULATION

The clinical success of a procedure is determined by the balance between clinical efficacy, technical success, and adverse events.[4,5] Reported complications are highly variable because of differences in definition and rates of detection. Complications are most widely defined by consensus criteria established in 1991, which incorporate interventions and duration of hospital stay.[6] The rates of complications are determined by patient characteristics as much as by the technical aspects of the procedure.[1,4,7,8] Younger patients, those without obstructive jaundice, and patients with sphincter of Oddi dysfunction are known to be at higher risk for complications, although expeditious cannulation and pancreatic stents are protective.

Success rates at biliary cannulation can be difficult to measure because the procedure is performed for a variety of indications, at different centers, and by endoscopists with various levels of expertise. The decision to use various techniques, such as precut sphincterotomy, can be influenced by the patient's anatomy and the relationship between the frequency of its application and the total number of cannulation attempts. In addition, failed precut sphincterotomy requiring repeat procedures has not been consistently defined as failed cannulation.

Expert endoscopists are expected to be successful at biliary access in 95% to 100% of attempts, a goal that is supported by the literature. Community success rates should exceed 90%.[9] Trainees are deemed competent to perform endoscopic procedures independently when a success rate of 80% to 90% is achieved.[5,10–12] A direct association between the case volume, local expertise, endoscopic training, and practice setting has been demonstrated in multiple studies.[4,13,14] ERCP is a technically demanding procedure with many levels of complexity. A five-point scale, which was later revised to three points, has been proposed to describe the difficulty of the procedure.[5,15,16] The rates of technical success are inversely proportional to the difficulty of the procedure even at expert centers.[16] Given the potential risks, a possibility of failure, and limited success in some settings, ERCP should only be considered when therapeutic intervention is necessary. The advent of modern, noninvasive, or minimally invasive imaging modalities, such as Magnetic resonance cholangiopancreatography and endoscopic ultrasound, in combination with careful clinical assessment should help limit ERCP to patients in whom the need for intervention is almost certain.[5,10,13,17]

WHAT MAKES A CANNULATION DIFFICULT?

There are many reasons for difficult cannulation (**Box 1**). In some cases, the papilla may be flat and small. One example is sphincter of Oddi dysfunction. Although the anatomy is preserved, cannulation may be challenging because the sphincter is often stenotic. The papilla can be difficult to locate in the setting of tumor infiltration of the papilla or the duodenum, or pancreatitis that causes duodenal edema and distortion. Adequate duodenoscope positioning may be challenging in a patient with a large duodenum where the papilla has to be approached from a cephalad or distant

> **Box 1**
> **Possible causes of difficult cannulation**
>
> Small papilla
>
> Normal anatomy with stenotic sphincters
>
> Difficult (cephalad or distant) approach to papilla
>
> Tortuous ("elephantine") papilla
>
> Intradiverticular or peridiverticular papilla
>
> Malignant infiltration or distortion of papilla
>
> Duodenal edema or distortion caused by pancreatitis, tumor, and so forth
>
> Surgically altered anatomy (Billroth II, Roux-en-Y)
>
> Poorly controlled patient sedation or anesthesia
>
> "Bad day" for the endoscopist

position. Intradivertiucular or peridiverticular papillas are other well-known causes for difficult cannulation. Patients with surgically altered anatomy, such as post–Billroth II or post–Roux-en-Y, present particular challenges because the papilla is approached either from the opposite direction or using a forward-viewing endoscope that lacks the advantage of an elevator. Patient cooperation is essential when maneuvers as precise as biliary cannulation are attempted. Nurse-administered sedation or monitored anesthesia care can make bile duct access much more challenging and result in failed cannulation in up to 5% of cases.[7] Finally, the endoscopist may just be having a "bad day." Involving a colleague or postponing a procedure for a different day (if feasible) can be the best approach.

DEVICES AND TECHNIQUES FOR ENDOSCOPIC BILE DUCT ACCESS

Principle approaches to cannulation and difficult bile duct access techniques are shown in **Box 2**. Visual illustrations are also available from several online resources, including the DAVE project (http://daveproject.org). ASGE DVD learning library (http://www.asge.org/ell_list.aspx) contains a number of video resources available for purchase. In particular, ASGE DV035: Biliary Access Techniques for ERCP: From Basic to Advanced has been developed by the corresponding author and Dr Kapil Gupta, and presents a comprehensive overview of biliary access techniques ranging from basic to very advanced. All of the issues presented in this article are addressed in a video format.

Standard and newer techniques for accessing the bile duct are shown in **Figs. 1–13**. Most catheters used for ERCP are 5F to 7F in diameter and can accept guidewires up to 0.035 in in diameter. Simultaneous use of a guidewire and contrast injection can be accomplished through a triple-lumen catheter or a side arm adaptor. 5-4-3F ultratapered catheters are often used for biliary and pancreatic access through small or stenotic papillas, but require the use of smaller guidewires, such as 0.018 in. Standard catheters have never been compared with ultratapered cannulas in head-to-head studies. Regular cannulas with or without guidewires can be difficult to use because the angle of approach cannot be varied. Standard papillotomes are widely used for cannulation. This device can be bowed up to vary the vertical angle of approach and engage the papilla. The bow can then be relaxed to achieve deep cannulation

Box 2
Principle ERCP biliary cannulation techniques

Standard techniques

    Catheters

    Standard

    Ultratapered (5F-4F-3F)

    Steerable (swing tip) catheter

Papillotomes

    Single lumen or multilumen

    Rotatable

Guidewire cannulation in conjunction with catheters and papillotomes

    Standard

    Nitinol

    Hybrid

    Hydrophilic

Placement of pancreatic guidewire or stent to assist biliary cannulation

Precut "access" papillotomy

    Needle-knife

        Freehand starting at orifice

        Freehand "fistulotomy" starting above orifice

        Over pancreatic stent

    Traction papillotome

    Papillary roof incision

    Transpancreatic (pancreatic sphincterotomy)

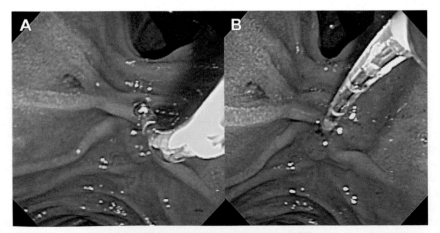

Fig. 1. Swing tip cannula flexed upward (*A*) and downward (*B*).

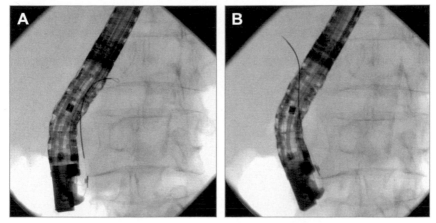

Fig. 2. Guidewire cannulation showing wire in pancreatic duct (*A*) and bile duct (*B*).

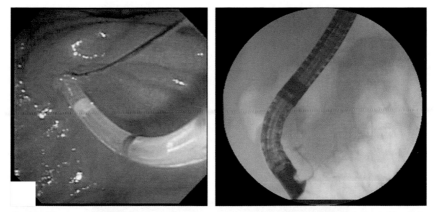

Fig. 3. Papillotome with flexed papillotome entering bile duct with puckered distal duct.

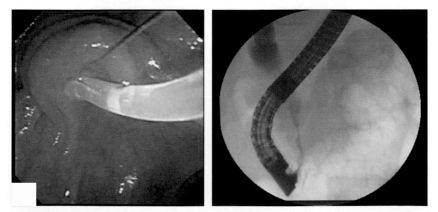

Fig. 4. Relaxation of the bow to achieve straightened alignment with the distal bile duct.

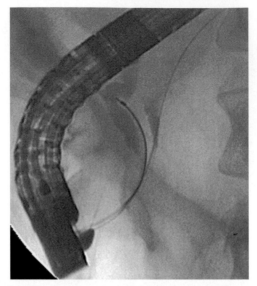

Fig. 5. Fluoroscopic view of dual wire cannulation (biliary and pancreatic guidewires).

of the bile duct (see **Figs. 3** and **4**).[18] A randomized trial comparing the success of biliary access using a sphincterotome with that of a regular cannula[19] found, in 100 patients, that a sphincterotome without a guidewire was successful in 84% using a sphincterotome compared with 62% using a standard cannula (*P*<.05). Crossover to the sphincterotome resulted in a cannulation rate of 94%. There was no difference in the rate of complications. These findings were confirmed in another randomized trial in which biliary cannulation was successful in 97% of patients using a sphincterotome

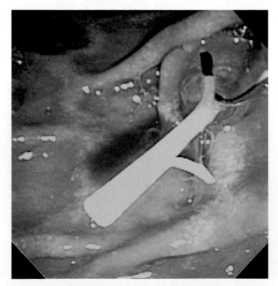

Fig. 6. Pancreatic stent inserted with biliary wire still in place.

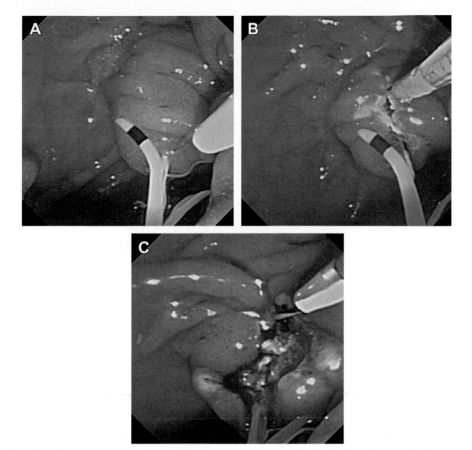

Fig. 7. (A) Needle knife precut papillotomy over pancreatic stent. (B) Extent of the incision (C) after deep cannulation of bile duct with extension of sphincterotomy.

compared with 67% using a standard catheter (P = .09). The use of a sphincterotome was associated with fewer cannulation attempts and shorter cannulation times. The study was not powered to assess for complications.[20] Swing tip is a cannula that can be flexed upward and downward, the latter particularly valuable in unusual anatomy, such as Billroth II or distorted intradiverticular papilla (see **Fig. 1**).[21] Standard cannula, sphincterotome, and a steerable catheter (swing tip) were prospectively compared in a randomized trial of 312 patients. End points included deep cannulation and time to cholangiography, number of pancreatic injections, number of attempts, and success of the procedure. Both the sphincterotome and the steerable catheter were superior to regular cannula (88% and 84%, respectively, vs 75%; P = .038). Successful cannulation using a sphincterotome or a steerable catheter was achieved in 26% of patients when cannulation with a regular catheter failed. The bile duct was successfully cannulated using advanced techniques (eg, precut) if all three methods failed. Although the study was not powered to assess for overall complications, pancreatitis occurred in 5.3% of patients.[22] The angle of approach to the papilla varies with biliary anatomy, endoscopes, and consistency in device manufacturing. The ability to change the angle of approach by rotating the sphincterotome has therefore been a long time goal. Manual grooming of the sphincterotome has been shown to

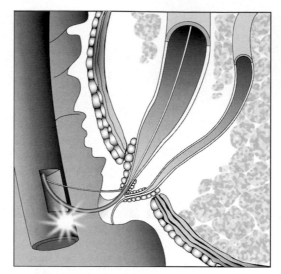

Fig. 8. Guidewire cannulation.

be effective in this setting, but is time consuming and imprecise.[23] Rotatable papillo-tomes are widely used now, which allow the endoscopist to match of the angle of approach of the papillotome to the specific course of the bile duct within the papilla. These devices may improve cannulation in surgically altered anatomy, distorted and peridiverticular papillas, or unusual angulation of the bile duct.

Guidewire cannulation is a popular and well-studied technique (see **Figs. 2** and **8**). There are two basic approaches to guidewire cannulation. In the first approach, the papilla is entered using only the guidewire. The second variant involves engaging the papillary orifice with the catheter or papillotome and then advancing the wire. In either technique, the wire is advanced without contrast, and then withdrawn and

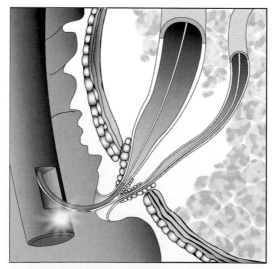

Fig. 9. Dual wire cannulation (pancreatic wire followed by biliary wire).

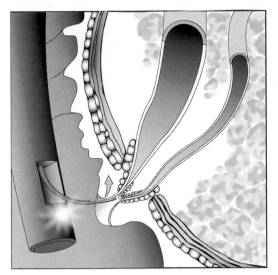

Fig. 10. Needle knife precut starting at orifice.

reoriented if it seems to be entering the pancreatic duct (see **Fig. 2**). If the wire is thought to be in the bile duct, a papillotome is advanced over the guidewire and contrast is injected in a usual fashion. This approach can be difficult because it is not always clear whether the wire has entered the duct of interest, despite passing the wire fairly deeply. Injection of minimal amount of contrast can clarify the exact location of the wire.

Complications can occur with guidewire cannulation, such as intramural dissection, pancreatic duct perforation, and creation of false passages. These complications can be minimized by using a soft-tip wire and extra care when passing the wire into the pancreatic duct. Despite great hope for the guidewire cannnulation technique to be

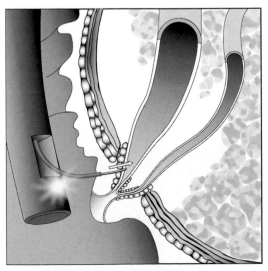

Fig. 11. Needle knife fistulotomy.

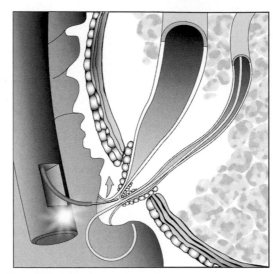

Fig. 12. Needle knife papillotomy over pancreatic stent.

a panacea, a recent large multicenter randomized trial of papillotome versus cannula, with and without primary guidewire technique, failed to show any difference in cannulation success rates or post-ERCP pancreatitis; the only difference with guidewire cannulation was shorter fluoroscopy times and more rapid cannulation.[24] Another study did not show reduction in post-ERCP pancreatitis with guidewire cannulation.[25] These studies are in contrast to earlier studies showing significant reduction in the risk of pancreatitis using a combination of guidewire and papillotome compared with papillotome alone.[26] In a randomized controlled study of 400 patients, the rate of pancreatitis was significantly reduced in the guidewire-papillotome versus papillotome alone groups (0% vs 4%; $P<.05$). There was no significant difference in cannulation rates

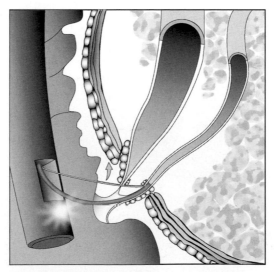

Fig. 13. Transpancreatic sphincterotomy as precut.

(98.5% vs 97.5%, respectively). It was postulated that the reduction in the rate of pancreatitis was secondary to reduced need for contrast injection. A combination of the two techniques is most commonly used in practice, wherein a small contrast injection is used to outline the duct, and definitive access and deep cannulation is performed over a guidewire. Although this approach has not been formally evaluated, it may help avoid guidewire dissection or perforation of the pancreatic side branches.

PANCREATIC DUCT ACCESS TO FACILITATE BILIARY ACCESS: GUIDEWIRE, CATHETER, OR STENT?

Using pancreatic duct techniques to facilitate biliary cannulation is becoming increasingly popular (see **Figs. 5** and **9**). An advantage of this approach is that a pancreatic duct stent can be placed to reduce the likelihood of pancreatitis in the setting of difficult biliary cannulation. Variations involve placing a catheter, guidewire, or stent in the pancreatic duct to aid biliary access. More advanced applications of this technique, such as placing a pancreatic stent followed by needle knife precut or a transpancreatic precut sphincterotomy, are discussed in the next section. Placement of a guidewire deep into the pancreatic duct can facilitate biliary access through a variety of mechanisms. The wire can stabilize scope position, anchor and straighten the pancreatic duct or the common channel, open a stenotic papilla and lift it toward the working channel of the duodenoscope, and separate the biliary and pancreatic orifices. Importantly, this technique facilitates draining the pancreatic duct and allows placing a pancreatic stent if necessary. The initial descriptions of this technique were in case reports of patients with surgically altered anatomy and in the setting of a tortuous common channel.[27,28] The efficacy and safety of biliary cannulation after pancreatic duct wire placement was assessed in a randomized trial of 53 patients in whom biliary cannulation failed after 10 minutes. The patients were then randomized to further attempts using biliary techniques versus pancreatic duct wire placement followed by repeat attempts at biliary cannulation. Successful cannulation was achieved in 93% when using the pancreatic wire, compared with 58% in the standard biliary techniques group (P<.05). No differences in pancreatitis were observed, although the amylase tended to be higher when using pancreatic duct access technique.[29] Efficacy of more than 90% was reported in recent randomized trials using "double-wire technique."[30] Another group using pancreatic wire-assisted biliary cannulation in 32% of all ERCPs requiring biliary access reported no difference in complications when compared with easy conventional cannulation (mild pancreatitis in 7.8% and 8.3%, respectively).[31]

Concerns regarding the safety of pancreatic guidewire-assisted biliary cannulation have been raised.[32,33] Substantial data exist to support using prophylactic pancreatic duct stenting to reduce the incidence of post-ERCP pancreatitis in high-risk patients, such as those with sphincter of Oddi dysfunction or difficult cannulation.[34,35] Deep passage of a wire into the pancreatic duct also seems to be a risk factor for pancreatitis, possibly because of a potential for ductal side branches perforation and failure to place a pancreatic guidewire deep in the pancreatic duct, which may occur in as many as 5% to 10% of procedures, especially if performed by less-experienced endoscopists.[34,35] One study reported substantial risk of pancreatitis in high-risk patients when manipulating a pancreatic duct without subsequent prophylactic stent placement.[36] Several factors, such as unusual pancreatic duct morphology (small caliber, tortuous duct, ansa pancreaticus), can make placement of a guidewire in the pancreatic duct difficult, and occasionally result in inability to place a prophylactic pancreatic stent. Virtually universal success at wire placement deep in the pancreatic duct has been reported using a modified technique with a 0.018-in nitinol-tipped wire.[36] This technique can then be followed by placement of a small (3F or 4F catheter) prophy- lactic pancreatic stent in patients deemed to be high risk for post-ERCP pancreatitis. The efficacy of prophylactic pancreatic stents when using double-wire technique has been assessed in a randomized trial, with a 10-fold reduction in the rate of pancreatitis (23%–2.3%).[30] A variant of a "double wire" technique involves initial placement of a pancreatic duct stent, which then allows deflection of a cannula or guidewire into the bile duct. A randomized trial has been conducted demonstrating higher rates of biliary cannulation (91% using pancreatic stent vs 67% using "double-wire" tech- nique) (see **Fig. 7**). However, more precut sphincterotomies were required with this technique (26% vs 10%, respectively). Overall complication rates were similar.[37] In a retrospective cohort study by the same group, successful biliary access over a previ- ously placed pancreatic stent was achieved in 93% of patients, most of whom did not require precut sphincterotomy.[38]

PRECUT (ACCESS) PAPILLOTOMY

Precut papillotomy can be accomplished by a variety of techniques, the success and complications of which heavily depend on technique-related factors and the risk profile and anatomic variations of the patient. In particular, the skill of the endoscopist, the indication for the procedure, and the use of pancreatic stents all influence the outcome of this procedure.

Free-hand needle knife is the most commonly applied technique, in which the inci- sion is made starting at the orifice and extended cephalad for a variable distance (see **Figs. 7** and **10**). The success and safety of this technique can be improved by loading the needle knife with upward traction of the endoscope, somewhat different than the traditional technique in which a sweeping motion of the needle knife is made using an elevator. Not unlike many other ERCP maneuvers, the procedure should be performed with the duodenoscope in a short position, which optimizes control of the catheter. Practice movements with the monofilament wire out of the catheter, but not touching the mucosa, can help direct the cut in the appropriate direction. Performing a fistulot- omy (see **Fig. 11**), which involves puncturing the papilla away from the orifice and then cutting either in a cephalad direction or toward the orifice, is a variation of the standard technique described previously, and is particularly suitable for large papillas. This vari- ation of the standard technique is theoretically safer because it avoids thermal injury to the pancreatic orifice.

Placing a pancreatic stent immediately preceding attempting needle knife papillot- omy can be very useful in preventing post-ERCP pancreatitis (see **Fig. 12**) after a precut papillotomy is performed, especially if this technique is used after multiple unsuccessful attempts at biliary cannulation using standard devices.[34,35] A pancreatic stent in this setting can serve not only to protect the pancreatic sphincter from thermal injury and maintain drainage, but also to provide guidance as to the anatomic direction to the location and direction of the bile duct.

The decision to use a precut technique relies on a variety of factors. For example, one group reported that this technique was more necessary in unusual or distorted anatomy of the papilla, such as in the case of duodenal stenosis or malignancy. Patients with bile duct stones rarely required a precut.[39] Precut sphincterotomy can also be performed using a specialized short-nosed traction sphincterotome. In this technique, a specialized short-nosed papillotome is wedged into the common channel and a cut is made in the direction of the common bile duct. This results in what is known as "papillary roof incision."[40] The application of this technique to 123 patients in whom biliary access had initially failed resulted in cannulation of 100%. A more common technique, known as "transpancreatic precut sphincterotomy," involves intentional seating of a standard papillotome into the pancreatic duct and making a transseptal incision to access the bile duct (see **Fig. 11**).[41–43]

The efficacy of precutting techniques has been assessed in several reports in which these techniques were performed in 4% to 38% of all cannulation or sphincterotome attempts. A total of 35% to 96% were effective in achieving immediate access. Clear definitions of success are important because obtaining biliary access during the initial procedure is the only valid outcome. A repeat attempt at cannulation at another time may have been successful with or without a precut sphincterotomy. As long as the major papilla is accessible, biliary access with or without precutting can be achieved by expert endoscopists in approximately 99% of cases.

Precut sphincterotomy is associated with higher rates of complications than standard biliary cannulation and traction sphincterotomy. The rate of complications has been reported to range between 2% and 34% based on a meta-analysis and a few multivariate analyses.[1,2,44,45] Severe post-ERCP pancreatitis occurs more commonly when precut sphincterotomy is performed without a protective pancreatic stent.[2,7,45] Bleeding and perforations are significantly more common.[46–50]

Only a limited body of data exists comparing specific precut techniques.[10,46,49,51–53] In a randomized study of 153 patients with choledocholithiasis, conventional needle knife precut sphincterotomy was compared with fistulotomy starting above the orifice.[47] The rates of initial cannulation success were similar; however, there was a lower risk of pancreatitis in the fistulotomy group (0% vs 8%), possibly because the pancreatic orifice is relatively spared with this technique, but there was no difference in overall complications. Despite the potential improved safety profile of a fistulotomy, the technique may not be feasible in patients with small papillas or in those at high risk for post-ERCP pancreatitis. Another study of the two precut sphincterotomy techniques found no difference between the success or complication rates whether starting at or above the orifice.[48]

The safety and efficacy of transpancreatic precut have been addressed in multiple studies. Although two initial reports of the transpancreatic technique from single centers suggested relative safety of this technique,[41,42] less favorable results were found in a subsequent large trial from Japan.[46] Relatively high success rates (85%) of transpancreatic precut were reported in a prospective series of 116 patients.[49] Although the complication rates were low, and the complications were of moderate severity (12%), two perforations were reported. In a randomized trial, transpancreatic precut was found to have higher biliary cannulation rates (100% vs 77%) and lower rates of complications (4% vs 18%) than needle-knife papillotomy.[50] This study is difficult to interpret, not only because prophylactic pancreatic stents were not always placed, but also because they may have been of larger caliber (5F–7F catheter) rather than the currently favored 3F to 4F catheter stents.[2] Such large-caliber stents may have caused pancreatitis themselves, and could interfere with biliary cannulation. Given conflicting data, caution should be advised against routine implementation of transpancreatic precut. Although this technique may be relatively safe in low-risk patients (eg, those with obstructive jaundice), performing a partial pancreatic sphincterotomy without placing a prophylactic pancreatic stent can be hazardous, especially in higher-risk patients. Thus in general, whenever possible, it is advisable to place a prophylactic stent after using this technique.

The discussion of the efficacy and complications of precut sphincterotomy is inherently hindered by the fact that these techniques are typically performed in cases where initial cannulation attempts have failed when using standard devices. As such, it is possible that the higher rates of pancreatitis could be caused by initial cannulation attempts rather than the precut. In a meta-analysis of six trials, a total of 966 patients were randomized to either persistent cannulation attempts or precut sphincterotomy.[51] Although the overall rate of complications (pancreatitis, bleeding, cholangitis, and perforation) was not different, pancreatitis developed in significantly fewer patients in the precut group (3% vs 5%).

In general, the decision to perform a precut should be made with caution, especially in the setting of altered anatomy, small or intradiverticular papilla, and deformed duodenum. Sufficient experience with the technique is mandatory before attempting a precut sphincterotomy. A pancreatic stent should be placed in most cases, unless there is a very prominent papillary bulge or if the patient has pancreas divisum.

INTRADIVERTICULAR PAPILLA

The ampulla may be located anywhere in or on the rim of a diverticulum. Such alterations in anatomy present a particular challenge for biliary cannulation. The rates of successful cannulation for intradiverticular papilla range from similar to less than that for patients without diverticula.[52–57] These reports have described several techniques for biliary access in an intradiverticular papilla. The fundamental principle of these techniques is to expose the papillary orifice and align the ducts in preparation for cannulation. This can be accomplished by balloon dilation of diverticular rim, passing two devices through one channel, everting the diverticulum using biopsy forceps, saline injection to lift the papilla, or endoscopic clipping of the papillary rim to expose the biliary orifice. The papilla can also be everted by placing a device in the common channel, or preferably by placing a guidewire or stent in the pancreatic duct. The most practical device to begin with is a steerable papillotome which allows orientation of access in the direction of the bile duct, which in turn run in an unusual direction inside the diverticulum. If the pancreatic is accessed first, a guidewire can be placed deeply into that duct and then used to evert the papilla, thus facilitating bile duct cannulation with the double-wire technique. In extreme cases where the papilla is entirely intradiverticular and pointing downward, a swing-tip steerable catheter allows caudal direction of the catheter (see **Fig. 1**).

WHAT TO DO WHEN CANNULATION FAILS

ERCP is a highly technical procedure, and as such can occasionally fail even in expert hands. An endoscopist can try a different technique, such as precut sphincterotomy, continue to attempt cannulation using the same technique, or request assistance from a colleague. The procedure can be postponed if the indication is not urgent, because

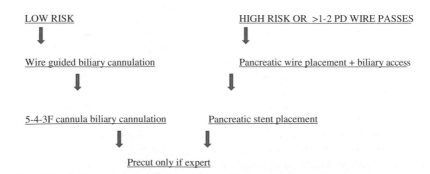

Fig. 14. Difficult biliary cannulation based on risk for post-ERCP pancreatitis.

an endoscopist may have more success at another time. Asking for assistance from a more experienced colleague may increase cannulation rates. In some reports this approach can result in a cannulation rate as high as 87%, although a significant number of patients still may require needle-knife papillotomy.[58] If the procedure is urgent, or multiple attempts by different local endoscopists fail, temporary percutaneous drainage can be performed. Whenever feasible, the preferred option is referral to an expert center where greater expertise is available. Expert tertiary centers have reported successful cannulation at ERCP in more than 95% of cases in which bile duct access failed elsewhere; in one series advanced techniques were used in 50% of cases with complications in less than 13%.[59] If ERCP fails at advanced centers, alternative techniques, such as endoscopic ultrasound–guided bile duct access are usually available. **Fig. 14** shows an algorithm for difficult cannulation under most circumstances.

REFERENCES

1. Freeman ML, DiSario JA, Nelson DB, et al. Risk factors for post-ERCP pancreatitis: a prospective multicenter study. Gastrointest Endosc 2001;54:425–34.
2. Freeman ML. Prevention of post-ERCP pancreatitis: a comprehensive review. Gastrointest Endosc 2004;59:845–64.
3. Kethu SR, Adler DG, Conway JD, et al. ERCP cannulation and sphincterotomy devices. Gastrointest Endosc 2010;71:435–45.
4. Freeman ML. Complications of endoscopic retrograde cholangiopancreatography: avoidance and management. Gastrointest Endosc Clin N Am 2012;22:567–86.
5. Cotton P. Income and outcome metrics for the objective evaluation of ERCP and alternative methods. Gastrointest Endosc 2002;56(Suppl 6):S283–90.
6. Cotton PB, Lehman G, Vennes J, et al. Endoscopic sphincterotomy complications and their management: an attempt at consensus. Gastrointest Endosc 1991;37:383–93.
7. Freeman ML, Nelson DB, Sherman S, et al. Complications of endoscopic sphincterotomy. N Engl J Med 1996;335:909–18.
8. Vandervoort J, Soetikno RM, Tham TC, et al. Risk factors for complications after performance of ERCP. Gastrointest Endosc 2002;56:652–6.
9. Colton JB, Curran CC. Quality indicators, including complications, of ERCP in a community setting: a prospective study. Gastrointest Endosc 2009;70:457–67.
10. Lehman GA. What are the determinants of success in utilization of ERCP in the setting of pancreatic and biliary diseases? Gastrointest Endosc 2002;56(Suppl 6):S291–3.
11. Principles of training in gastrointestinal endoscopy. From the ASGE, American Society for Gastrointestinal Endoscopy. Gastrointest Endosc 1999;49:845–53.
12. Kowalski T, Kanchana T. Perceptions of gastroenterology fellows regarding ERCP competency training. Gastrointest Endosc 2003;58:345–9.
13. Petersen BT. ERCP outcomes: defining the operators, experience, and environments. Gastrointest Endosc 2002;55:953–8.
14. Guda NM, Freeman ML. Are you safe for your patients? how many ERCPs should you be doing? Endoscopy 2008;40:675–6.
15. Schutz SM, Abbott RM. Grading ERCPs by degree of difficulty: a new concept to produce more meaningful outcome data. Gastrointest Endosc 2000;51:535–9.
16. Schutz SM. Grading the degree of difficulty of ERCP procedures. Gastroenterol Hepatol 2011;7:674–6.

17. NIH state-of-the-science statement on endoscopic retrograde cholangiopancrea-tography (ERCP) for diagnosis and therapy. NIH Consens State Sci Statements 2002;19:1–26.
18. Rossos PG, Kortan P, Haber G. Selective common bile duct canulation can be simplified by the use of a standard papillotome. Gastrointest Endosc 1993;39: 67–9.
19. Schwacha H, Allgaier HP, Deibert P, et al. A sphincterotome-based technique for selective transpapillary common bile duct cannulation. Gastrointest Endosc 2000;52:387–91.
20. Cortas GA, Mehta SN, Abraham NS, et al. Selective cannulation of the common bile duct: a prospective randomized trial comparing standard catheters with sphincterotomes. Gastrointest Endosc 1999;50:775–9.
21. Igarashi Y, Tada T, Shimura J, et al. A new cannula with a flexible tip (Swing Tip) may improve the success rate of endoscopic retrograde cholangiopancreatogra-phy. Endoscopy 2002;34:628–31.
22. Laasch HU, Tringali A, Wilbraham L, et al. Comparison of standard and steerable catheters for bile duct cannulation in ERCP. Endoscopy 2003;35:669–74.
23. Seibert DG. Consistent improvement in sphincterotome orientation with manual grooming. Gastrointest Endosc 1995;42:325–9.
24. Kawakami H, Maguchi H, Mukai T, et al. A multicenter, prospective, randomized study of selective bile duct cannulation performed by multiple endoscopists: the BIDMEN study. Gastrointest Endosc 2012;75:362–72.
25. Mariani A, Giussani A, Di Leo M, et al. Guidewire biliary cannulation does not reduce post-ERCP pancreatitis compared with the contrast injection technique in low-risk and high-risk patients. Gastrointest Endosc 2012;75:339–46.
26. Lella F, Bagnolo F, Colombo E, et al. A simple way of avoiding post-ERCP pancre-atitis. Gastrointest Endosc 2004;59:830–4.
27. Gotoh Y, Tamada K, Tomiyama T, et al. A new method for deep cannulation of the bile duct by straightening the pancreatic duct. Gastrointest Endosc 2001;53:820–2.
28. Dumonceau JM, Devière J, Cremer M. A new method of achieving deep cannu-lation of the common bile duct during endoscopic retrograde cholangiopancrea-tography. Endoscopy 1998;30:S80.
29. Maeda S, Hayashi H, Hosokawa O, et al. Prospective randomized pilot trial of selective biliary cannulation using pancreatic guide-wire placement. Endoscopy 2003;35:721–4.
30. Ito K, Fujita N, Noda Y, et al. Can pancreatic duct stenting prevent post-ERCP pancreatitis in patients who undergo pancreatic duct guidewire placement for achieving selective biliary cannulation? A prospective randomized controlled trial. J Gastroenterol 2010;45:1183–91.
31. Gyokeres T, Duhl J, Varasanyi M, et al. Double guide wire placement for endo-scopic pancreaticobiliary procedures. Endoscopy 2003;35:95–6.
32. Gonzalez LY, Abreu L, Calleja JL, et al. Selective biliary cannulation using pancre-atic guide-wire placement: further evidence needed to support the use of an already known technique [letter]. Endoscopy 2004;36:457.
33. Devière J. Using the pancreas for common bile duct cannulation? Endoscopy 2003;35:750–1.
34. Freeman ML. Pancreatic stents for prevention of post-ERCP pancreatitis: for everyday practice or for experts only? Gastrointest Endosc 2010;71:940–4.
35. Freeman ML. Pancreatic stents for prevention of post-endoscopic retrograde cholangiopancreatography pancreatitis. Clin Gastroenterol Hepatol 2007;5: 1354–65.

36. Freeman ML, Overby C, Qi D. Pancreatic stent insertion: consequences of failure and results of a modified technique to maximize success. Gastrointest Endosc 2004;59:8–14.
37. Cote GA, Mullady DK, Jonnalagadda SS, et al. Use of a pancreatic duct stent or guidewire facilitates bile duct access with low rates of precut sphincterotomy: a randomized clinical trial. Dig Dis Sci 2012;57:3271–8.
38. Cote GA, Ansstas M, Pawa R, et al. Difficult biliary cannulation: use of physician-controlled wire-guided cannulation over a pancreatic duct stent to reduce the rate of precut sphincterotomy. Gastrointest Endosc 2010;71:275–9.
39. Linder S, Söderlund C. Factors influencing the use of precut technique at endoscopic sphincterotomy. Hepatogastroenterology 2007;54:2192–7.
40. Binmoeller KF, Seifert H, Gerke H, et al. Papillary roof incision using the Erlangen-type precut papillotome to achieve selective bile duct cannulation. Gastrointest Endosc 1996;44:689–95.
41. Goff JS. Long-term experience with the transpancreatic sphincter pre-cut approach to biliary sphincterotomy. Gastrointest Endosc 1999;50:642–5.
42. Weber A, Roesch T, Pointer S, et al. Transpancreatic precut sphincterotomy for cannulation of inaccessible common bile duct: a safe and successful technique. Pancreas 2008;36:187–91.
43. Kapetanos D, Kokozidis G, Christodoulou D, et al. Case series of transpancreatic septotomy as precutting technique for difficult bile duct cannulation. Endoscopy 2007;39:802–6.
44. Loperfido S, Angelini G, Benedetti G, et al. Major early complications from diagnostic and therapeutic ERCP: a prospective multicenter study. Gastrointest Endosc 1998;48:1–10.
45. Masci E, Mariani A, Curioni S, et al. Risk factors for pancreatitis following endoscopic retrograde cholangiopancreatography: a meta-analysis. Endoscopy 2003;35:830–4.
46. Akashi R, Kiyozumi T, Jinnouchi K, et al. Pancreatic sphincter precutting to gain selective access to the common bile duct: a series of 172 patients. Endoscopy 2004;36:405–10.
47. Mavrogiannis C, Liatsos C, Romanos A, et al. Needle-knife fistulotomy versus needle-knife precut papillotomy for the treatment of common bile duct stones. Gastrointest Endosc 1999;50:334–9.
48. Kaffes AJ, Sriram PV, Rao G, et al. Early institution of pre-cutting for difficult biliary cannulation: a prospective study comparing conventional vs. a modified technique. Gastrointest Endosc 2005;62:669–74.
49. Kahaleh M, Tokar J, Mullick T, et al. Prospective evaluation of pancreatic sphincterotomy as a precut technique for biliary cannulation. Clin Gastroenterol Hepatol 2004;2:971–7.
50. Catalano MF, Linder JD, Geenen JE. Endoscopic transpancreatic papillary septotomy for inaccessible obstructed bile ducts: comparison with standard pre-cut papillotomy. Gastrointest Endosc 2004;60:557–61.
51. Cennamo V, Fuccio L, Zagari RM, et al. Can early precut implementation reduce endoscopic retrograde cholangiopancreatography-related complication risk? Meta-analysis of randomized controlled trials. Endoscopy 2010;42:381–8.
52. Chang-Chien CS. Do juxtapapillary diverticula of the duodenum interfere with cannulation at endoscopic retrograde cholangiopancreatography? A prospective study. Gastrointest Endosc 1987;33:298–300.
53. Batra SC, Trowers E, Dayemo K, et al. Novel approach to ampullary cannulation. Gastrointest Endosc 1996;44:360–1.

54. Fujita N, Noda Y, Kobayashi G, et al. ERCP for intradiverticular papilla: two-devices-in-one-channel method. Gastrointest Endosc 1998;48:517–20.
55. Sherman S, Hawes RH, Lehman GA. A new approach to performing endoscopic sphincterotomy in the setting of a juxtapapillary duodenal diverticulum. Gastrointest Endosc 1991;37:353–5.
56. Tantau M, Person B, Burtin P, et al. Duodenal diverticula and ERCP: a new trick. Endoscopy 1996;28:326.
57. Tóth E, Lindström E, Fork FT. An alternative approach to the inaccessible intradiverticular papilla. Endoscopy 1999;31:554–6.
58. Ramirez FC, Dennert B, Sanowski RA. Success of repeat ERCP by the same endoscopist. Gastrointest Endosc 1999;45:58–61.
59. Choudari CP, Sherman S, Fogel EL, et al. Success of ERCP at a referral center after previously unsuccessful attempt. Gastrointest Endosc 2000;52:478–83.

Choledochoscopy/ Cholangioscopy

Isaac Raijman, MD[a,b,c],*

KEYWORDS

- Cholangioscopy • Choledochoscopy • Biliary tract disease
- Endoscopic retrograde cholangiopancreatography

KEY POINTS

- Cholangioscopy provides direct assessment of the biliary epithelium.
- Cholangioscopy allows for targeted tissue acquisition.
- Cholangioscopy allows for targeted therapy, such as lithotripsy.

INTRODUCTION

Miniature endoscopes that can be introduced into the bile duct through the duodeno-scope during endoscopic retrograde cholangiopancreatography (ERCP) were developed to allow nonsurgical management of difficult biliary stones. The direct visualization enabled by these cholangioscopes of the biliary epithelium provides additional data in the assessment of biliary strictures. Cholangioscopy/choledocho-scopy has been available for four decades.[1,2] The original cholangioscopes lacked the refinement that was accomplished several years later[3] and that continues to improve to this day. Cholangioscopy allows assessment of the biliary lumen, biliary epithelium, targeted tissue acquisition, targeted therapy, and wire guidance.[3–6]

ERCP is a common procedure performed on a daily basis for various purposes, the most common of which is biliary stone management.[7] In some patients with biliary stone disease, standard methods or mechanical lithotripsy may not allow for complete stone removal because of size, shape, location, or stricture association. In these patients, direct stone visualization and fragmentation is the only endoscopic alternative to ensure ductal clearance. Biliary strictures can be determined during ERCP, but specific cause may elude blind biopsies and may not be possible by just radiographic appearance. Direct characterization of the mucosa within and around the stricture along with directed biopsies significantly increases the diagnostic accuracy. In addition, extension of the mucosal involvement can be assessed only by direct visualization.[3–6]

[a] Digestive Associates of Houston, 6620 Main Street, Suite 1510, Houston, TX 77030, USA; [b] Baylor College of Medicine, One Baylor Plaza, Room 176B, Houston, TX 77030, USA; [c] University of Texas Health Science Center in Houston, 6410 Fannin Street, Houston, TX 77030, USA Texas, USA
* Digestive Associates Houston, 6620 Main Street, Suite 1510, Houston, TX 77030.
E-mail address: iraijman@dahpa.com

Gastrointest Endoscopy Clin N Am 23 (2013) 237–249
http://dx.doi.org/10.1016/j.giec.2013.01.004
1052-5157/13/$ – see front matter © 2013 Elsevier Inc. All rights reserved.

AVAILABLE CHOLANGIOSCOPES

Peroral cholangioscopes are divided into two main systems: dual-operator mother-daughter systems; and single-operator catheter-based slim or ultraslim standard endoscopes. The mother-daughter systems (Olympus America, Center Valley, PA; Pentax, Orangeburg, NY) include a choledochoscope that is introduced through the therapeutic channel of the duodenoscope. These choledochoscopes vary in outer diameter from 2.4 to 3.4 mm. The 3.1- and 3.4-mm choledochoscopes have a 1.2-mm working channel. These endoscopes are mostly fiberoptic, without a separate irrigation channel. They have a two-way tip deflection and require two endoscopists.[8] Video cholangioscopes with narrow-band imaging capacity have also been used, but they are not widely available.[9,10]

The catheter-based or single-operator system is known as Spyglass (Boston Scientific, Natick, MA).[11–13] This system comprises a disposable 10 F, 230-cm long catheter with four lumens: two for irrigation (0.6 mm each); one for the optical fiber (0.9 mm); and one for instrumentation (caliber of 1.2 mm). The optical fiber is a 0.77-mm, 6000-pixel fiberoptic bundle that is introduced through the catheter allowing for visualization. The optical fiber is 231 cm long and provides a 70-degree field of view. This reusable fiber can be used numerous times (up to 20 in some instances). However, visualization deteriorates with further use of the fiber. The catheter has a four-way tip deflection much like a regular endoscope. In addition, because the channels are independent, simultaneous instrumentation and irrigation are possible. The irrigation port is attached to a water pump activated by a pedal controlled by the endoscopist. The SpyGlass tip movement is accomplished not only by the Spyscope access catheter itself but also by the movements of the duodenoscope and the movements of the endoscopist. The combination of these maneuvers allows for literally infinite possibilities. Limitations to the system are primarily dictated by the size of the duct investigated, sharp and angulated strictures, and anatomic variations of any cause that do not allow for proper duodenoscope position.

Slim or ultraslim upper endoscopes can be used for cholangioscopy in patients with dilated bile ducts only.[8] Routine straight-view endoscope use for cholangioscopy was first described in 1977.[14] Advantages of this system are better imaging and larger working channels. Only a single operator is needed. This type of cholangioscopy can be performed by direct introduction of the scope into the bile duct or by using commercially available devices that help anchor the endoscope into the bile duct. Compared with other cholangioscopes, more complications using this system have been reported.[15–17]

PERFORMANCE OF CHOLANGIOSCOPY

The procedure is usually performed at the time of ERCP; however, cholangioscopy can also be performed percutaneously. The preparation and sedation for cholangioscopy are the same as for ERCP. In our unit, most of the procedures are performed under propofol (monitored anesthesia) with the head of the fluoroscopy table elevated approximately 30 degree to decrease the risk of aspiration. Patients receive prophylactic antibiotics. In some patients, especially those with strictures or those who are immunocompromised, antibiotics are continued for a few days after cholangioscopy.

In most patients, a biliary sphincterotomy is either performed or is already existent. A standard cholangiogram provides guidance to the site of the lesion or to define the stones. Excess contrast injection should be avoided because it may interfere with visual clarity. A guidewire aids in the passage of the choledochoscope. Choledochoscopy can be performed without a guidewire but the risk of damage to the choledochoscope increases, especially for the mother-daughter systems. When the choledochoscope is advanced out of the duodenoscope and into the bile duct, the duodenoscope elevator can be used with Spyglass, but should be limited or avoided with the mother-daughter systems to avoid choledochoscope damage.

When the choledochoscope is inside the bile duct, the guidewire is removed to allow for better irrigation, to permit suction of bile contrast debris, and to advance either therapeutic fibers or biopsy forceps. If the intent of choledochoscopy is to aid in the cannulation of a difficult proximal stricture, the wire is left in the choledochoscope and advanced through the stricture.

Cholangioscopy and fluoroscopy should be used throughout the procedure to more precisely determine the location of the lesion, because choledochoscopy alone is not accurate in intraductal locations. It is also important to systematically assess the bile duct to ensure that lesions are not missed and the entire biliary lumen is examined. There are times when too much movement is applied to the tip of the choledochoscope to find the lesions, especially at the beginning of the procedure. Patiently identifying the lumen and then moving the choledochoscope tip should avoid problems.

INDICATIONS FOR CHOLANGIOSCOPY

Indications for cholangioscopy are divided into therapeutic and diagnostic (**Table 1**). By far the two most common indications for cholangioscopy are management of difficult stones and assessment of indeterminate strictures. In our practice, 52% of all cholangioscopies are performed for management of difficult biliary stones, 35% are for assessment of indeterminate strictures, and 13% for other indications.

Bile Duct Stones

Choledocholithiasis, either in the extrahepatic or intrahepatic tree, affects approximately 10% to 20% of patients with cholelithiasis. In 10% of the patients, the gallbladder may not be involved. In approximately 10% of patients with bile duct stones, standard methods may not resolve the problem either because of the stone's location, size, or shape, or because of the presence of a stricture. Cholangioscopy was initially introduced for the management of difficult biliary tract stones.[4,6] Direct visualization of the stone allows for reduced bile duct injury and for differentiation among stone fragments, blood clots, air bubbles, and so forth.

Intraductal lithotripsy is performed by using either electrohydraulic lithotripsy (EHL) or pulsed laser.[18–25] The method chosen depends on availability and expertise. Current EHL and laser fibers can be advanced through the choledochoscopes,

Table 1		
Therapeutic and diagnostic indications for cholangioscopy		
Therapeutic		**Diagnostic**
Lithotripsy		Biliary strictures
Tumor ablation		Staging
Control of bleeding		Filling defects
Guidewire advancement		Ductal abnormalities
Reopening occluded metal stents		Choledochal cysts
		Tissue acquisition
		Confocal microscopy

although it tends to be relatively easier to advance the laser fiber. In our unit we use both devices, but favor laser for many reasons, such as its superior aiming beam, reduced feedback on firing, less likelihood of biliary epithelium damage, durability of the fiber during procedures that require extensive application, and less tendency for stones to bounce away from the fiber when activated. It is our observation that laser tends to produce smaller fragments and a faster lithotripsy compared with EHL. The most commonly used method is EHL because of its more widespread availability.

EHL, developed approximately four decades ago, was the first form of contact lithotripsy. EHL is performed by using a fiber that is connected to a power source (Autolith; Nortech, Northgate Technologies Inc. Elgin, IL, USA). The EHL fiber is 1.9 F catheter, 375 cm long. The tip of the fiber contains an open tip with two coaxially insulated electrodes (bipolar technology). When the power source is activated, a spark is generated within the electrodes, which under water (0.9% saline) produces high-voltage hydraulic pressure waves, or a rapidly expanding cavitation bubble that on collapse creates a secondary pressure wave (shock wave). The difference in acoustic impedance at the stone-saline interface causes energy release with ensuing lithotripsy. For the wave to hit the stone it is important for the tip of the fiber to be no more than 3 to 4 mm from the stone; otherwise, the wave may dissipate before reaching the target. The energy density is obtained by combining frequencies of 1 to 20 per second and voltage from 50 to 100. With EHL, the fluid media must contain electrolytes to conduct the hydraulic pressure waves. En face application achieves better results and avoids ductal wall injury (**Figs. 1–3**).

In the early experiences of Spyglass, EHL application and lithotripsy was successful in five of five patients with an acceptable safety profile.[13] In a study of 32 patients with difficult bile duct stones (intrahepatic in 8, extrahepatic in 18, both in 6, and associated with biliary strictures in 20), complete stone clearance was achieved with cholangioscopy and EHL in 81% and partial in 16%.[20] When stone clearance is achieved with cholangioscopy, stone recurrence is low.

In a series of 94 patients with difficult bile duct stones, most of them greater than 20 mm, and using the mother-daughter system with EHL, complete stone fragmentation was achieved in 66% of the patients, and partial fragmentation was achieved in 30%.[23] A significant number of patients (18%) had complications, with the most common being cholangitis and jaundice. In a study of 121 patients, 41 of who had

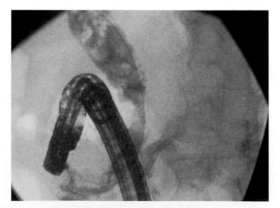

Fig. 1. Multiple bile duct stones associated with a stricture.

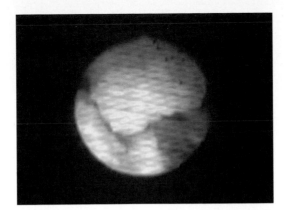

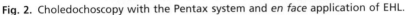

Fig. 2. Choledochoscopy with the Pentax system and *en face* application of EHL.

biliary stones, ductal clearance was achieved in 37 patients after one session and in the remaining 4 patients in two sessions. EHL and holmium laser were used.[25]

Pulsed laser lithotripsy, most commonly with the holmium neodymium:yttrium-aluminum-garnet laser, is performed in a similar fashion (**Figs. 4–6**).[22,23] The laser fibers are made of flexible quartz. We use the SlimLine SIS GI, 365 μm, 3 m long, end-fire fibers, with a maximum energy of 4 J, 100 W (Lumenis, Santa Clara, CA). The fiber emits an aiming beam that facilitates tip recognition and targeting. The fiber is connected to a laser (Versapulse P20; Lumenis) that is actuated by a pedal. The settings of the laser console are adjusted to produce an energy density (watts) that is the end product of frequency (hertz) multiplied by energy (joules). The laser is immediately absorbed within the fluid media (bile), producing a "vapor bubble" (a high-kinetic energy collection of ions and electrons). This bubble (plasma) expands quickly and produces a mechanical shockwave. The fiber must be within 2 to 4 mm of the stone to reach target. Laser can fragment the stone even when not *en face* application. However, if the fiber touches the stone, it will initially drill the stone before it causes fragmentation because there is no room for the vapor bubble to form.

In an international multicenter study of 66 patients with stone disease (out of a total of 297 patients being evaluated), the procedure was successful in 92%, complete stone clearance during the study session was 71%, and the complication rate was 6.1%.[22]

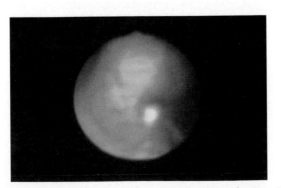

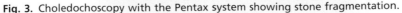

Fig. 3. Choledochoscopy with the Pentax system showing stone fragmentation.

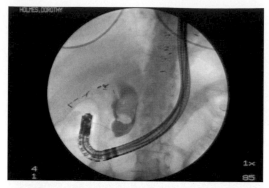

Fig. 4. Fluoroscopy revealing a giant bile duct stone with an associated suprapapillary stricture.

Bile Duct Strictures

Cholangioscopy provides valuable data used to evaluate indeterminate biliary strictures by providing direct assessment of the involved epithelium and the adjacent epithelium, and by providing direct visualization for biopsies. Cholangioscopy in addition to cholangiographic images obtained during ERCP increased the diagnostic yield from 78% to 85%, to 93% to 99% and the overall sensitivity from 58% to 100% (**Figs. 7 and 8**)[4,26]; In addition, cholangioscopy can assess the extent of the disease and identify synchronous lesions not seen during cholangiography. This is particularly important in distinguishing stones from neoplasia.[27] Fukuda and colleagues[4] used the combination of the presence of tumor vessels, easy oozing, and an irregular surface as the main criteria for malignancy.

Cholangioscopic characterization of a lesion is based on various factors: type of luminal narrowing, friability, vascularity, and mucosal changes. The presence of a tumor vessel (an irregular and tortuous vessel) by itself has a predictive value of 61% (see **Fig. 8**).[28] With the combination of the tumor vessel and cholangioscopy-guided biopsy, the diagnosis of malignancy was made in 39 (96%) of 41 patients. In strictures with tumor vessel present and negative biopsies, the most common form of cancer was infiltrative-type, which spreads more below the superficial epithelium and is

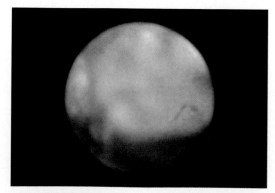

Fig. 5. Spyglass revealing the large stone.

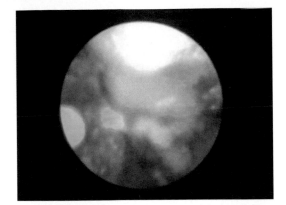

Fig. 6. Holmium laser application through Spyglass.

associated with significant desmoplastic tissue. Classifying malignancies into nodular, papillary, and infiltrative types based on visual characteristics was described.[29] In this classification, nodular cholangiocarcinoma produces luminal narrowing, usually short strictures and intense neovascularization. Papillary cholangiocarcinoma usually has little neovascularization, spreads superficially, has papillary mucosal projections, and may have associated mucus and sludge. Infiltrative cholangiocarcinoma produces subtle mucosal elevations, luminal narrowing, and little vascularization (**Figs. 9–11**).

In an early experience with Spyglass in the assessment of indeterminate strictures (22 patients), 20 patients had directed biopsy, with adequate specimens acquired in 19 patients. The sensitivities and specificities to diagnose malignant lesions were 71% and 100%, respectively.[13]

In a multicenter study of 297 patients, diagnostic cholangioscopy with the Spyglass system was performed in 86 patients without biopsy and in 140 patients with biopsy.[22] Tissue acquisition was possible in most of the patients (88%). In the final analysis of 95 patients, the overall sensitivity for malignancy was 78% for visual characteristics and 49% for directed biopsies. When the analysis was done for intrinsic biliary malignancy, the sensitivities were 84% and 66%, respectively. The specificities for visualization

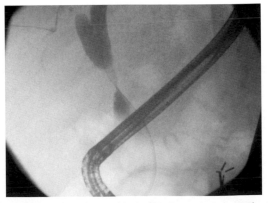

Fig. 7. Fluoroscopy revealing an indeterminate distal common hepatic stricture.

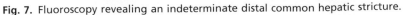

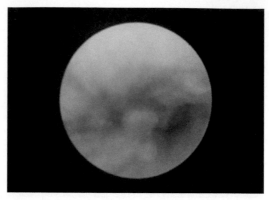

Fig. 8. Spyglass showing a tumor vessel in an indeterminate stricture with Spybite forceps revealing cholangiocarcinoma.

and directed biopsy were 82% and 98%, positive predictive values were 80% and 100%, and negative predictive values were 80% and 72%, respectively.

In a study of 121 patients, 25 with biliary strictures, the original diagnosis of the stricture was modified in 20 patients, confirmed to be malignant in almost 50% of the patients, and confirmed to be nonmalignant in 9 patients.[25] In a cohort of 18 patients, the overall sensitivity of cholangioscopy for detecting malignancy with or without biopsies had a sensitivity of 89%, specificity of 96%, positive predictive value of 89%, and negative predictive value of 96%.[30]

Primary sclerosing cholangitis (PSC) can be associated with dominant bile duct strictures, which can be malignant. Cholangiography alone cannot distinguish between malignant and benign strictures. In a study of 53 patients with primary sclerosing cholangitis and dominant strictures, cholangioscopy had sensitivity in diagnosing malignancy of 92% compared with 66% of cholangiography alone. Cholangioscopy was also superior for specificity (93% vs 51%); positive predictive value (79% vs 29%); and negative predictive value of (97% vs 84%) (**Figs. 12** and **13**).[31]

During tissue acquisition, three biopsies at a minimum are needed, which should be obtained from the exophytic tissue and from the margins of the lesion.[32] In our

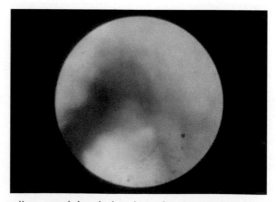

Fig. 9. Spyglass revealing a nodular cholangiocarcinoma.

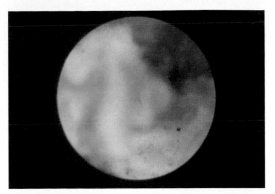

Fig. 10. Spyglass revealing an exophytic cholangiocarcinoma.

institution, we obtain a minimum of four biopsies per site of interest. The tissue is sent to pathology, where a cellblock is obtained.

OTHER INDICATIONS FOR CHOLANGIOSCOPY
Post Liver Transplantation

Patients after liver transplantation may be affected by biliary strictures, usually anastomotic. There are times when the stricture is related to a castlike stone that may not be recognized with cholangiography alone.[6,33] In addition, cholangioscopy can identify other lesions, such as ischemic or infectious ulcers (**Fig. 14**), and can distinguish blood clots from stones, scar tissue, and so forth. In our experience with 60 patients, additional data obtained with cholangioscopy altered the treatment in almost one-third of patients.[6]

Hemobilia

Cholangioscopy has been used in patients who were not able to be evaluated by other means: in one case a venous malformation was encountered in a patient with hereditary hemorrhagic telangiectasia.[34] A case of cytomegalovirus cholangiopathy was also reported.[35] We have detected metastatic breast cancer in one patient, metastatic colon cancer in another, and a pseudoaneurysm to the left hepatic artery in a third (**Fig. 15**).

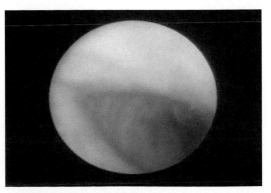
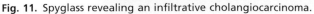

Fig. 11. Spyglass revealing an infiltrative cholangiocarcinoma.

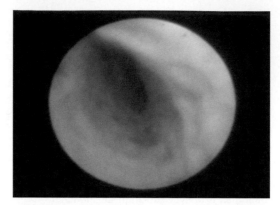

Fig. 12. Spyglass revealing scarring, luminal reduction, but no increased vascularity in a patient with noncomplicated PSC.

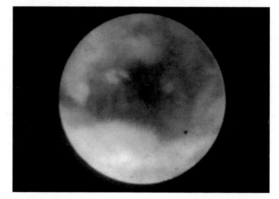

Fig. 13. Spyglass revealing exophytic mucosal protrusions, nodules, and increased vascularity in a patient with PSC complicated with cholangiocarcinoma.

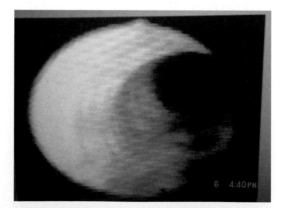

Fig. 14. Pentax choledochoscopy in a patient status post liver transplantation showing an anastomotic ulcer that showed fungal elements on biopsy.

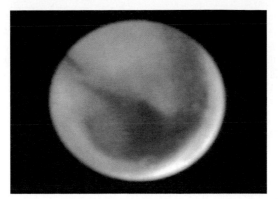

Fig. 15. Spyglass in a patient with hemobilia. Fresh blood is seen emanating from the main left hepatic duct. It was caused by a posttraumatic pseudoaneurysm.

Other Therapeutic Applications

Local treatment with photodynamic therapy,[36] argon plasma coagulation,[37] and brachytherapy[38] have been reported in patients with various biliary malignancies.

Staging Cholangiocarcinoma

Peroral cholangioscopy with narrow band imaging was successfully used in the preoperative assessment of cholangiocarcinoma, especially for papillary-type and mucin-producing cholangiocarcinoma, which have a greater risk of superficial spread.[39]

COMPLICATIONS OF CHOLANGIOSCOPY

Besides the potential complications of ERCP, there are risks associated with peroral cholangioscopy. Diagnostic cholangioscopy is quite safe; however, infection is the main risk, which is expected because the primary indication for performing cholangioscopy is the evaluation of patients with strictures. All patients should receive prophylactic antibiotics. Perforation is another risk of peroral cholangioscopy. During therapeutic cholangioscopy, the risk of bleeding or perforation increases mainly because of the use of lithotripsy, especially EHL. Direct contact of the bile duct wall during lithotripsy can cause bleeding, and excess or prolonged contact can potentially cause perforation. Therefore, if the stone is large and in contact with the bile duct wall the prolonged lithotripsy increases the potential for complications. In a study of 402 patients, the rate of cholangitis for cholangioscopy was 1% versus 0.2% for the ERCP group, the rate of pancreatitis was 2.2% versus 1.3%, and the rate of perforation was 1% versus 0.3%.

REFERENCES

1. Vennes JA, Silvis SE. Endoscopic visualization of bile and pancreatic ducts. Gastrointest Endosc 1972;18:149.
2. Rosch W, Koch H, Demling I. Per oral cholangioscopy. Endoscopy 1976;8:172–5.
3. Soda K, Shitou K, Yoshida Y, et al. Per oral cholangioscopy using a new fine-caliber flexible scope for detailed examination without papillotomy. Gastrointest Endosc 1996;43(3):233–8.

4. Fukuda Y, Tsuyuguchi T, Sakai Y, et al. Diagnostic utility of per oral cholangioscopy for various bile-duct lesions. Gastrointest Endosc 2005;62:374–82.
5. Nakajima M, Mukai H, Kawai K. Per oral cholangioscopy and pancreatoscopy. In: Sivak MV, editor. Gastrointest Endosc. 2nd edition. Philadelphia: WB Saunders; 2000. p. 1055–68.
6. Siddique I, Galati J, Ankoma-Sey V, et al. The role of choledochoscopy in the diagnosis and management of biliary tract diseases. Gastrointest Endosc 1999;50:67–73.
7. Cohen S, Bacon BR, Berlin JA, et al. National Institutes of Health State-of-the-Science Conference Statement: ERCP for diagnosis and therapy, January 14-16, 2002. Gastrointest Endosc 2002;56:803–9.
8. Nguyen NQ, Binmoeller KF, Shah JN. Cholangioscopy and pancreatoscopy. Gastrointest Endosc 2009;70:1200–10.
9. Itoi T, Neuhaus H, Chen YK. Diagnostic value of image-enhanced video cholangiopancreatoscopy. Gastrointest Endosc Clin N Am 2009;19:557–66.
10. Parsi MA, Stevens T, Collins J, et al. Utility of a prototype per oral video cholangioscopy system with narrow-band imaging for evaluation of biliary disorders. Gastrointest Endosc 2011;74:1148–51.
11. Chen YK. Preclinical characterization of the Spyglass per oral cholangiopancreatoscopy system for direct access, visualization and biopsy. Gastrointest Endosc 2007;65:303–11.
12. Farrell JJ, Bounds BC, Al-Shalabi S, et al. Single-operator duodenoscope-assisted cholangioscopy is an effective alternative in the management of choledocholithiasis not removed by conventional methods, including mechanical lithotripsy. Endoscopy 2005;37(6):542–7.
13. Chen YK, Pleskow DK. Spyglass single-operator per oral cholangiopancreatoscopy system for the diagnosis and therapy of bile duct disorders: a clinical feasibility study. Gastrointest Endosc 2007;65:832–41.
14. Urakami Y, Seifert E, Butke H. Per oral direct cholangioscopy (PODC) using routing straight-view endoscope: first report. Endoscopy 1977;9:27–30.
15. Moon JH, Ko BM, Choi HJ, et al. Direct peroral cholangioscopy using an ultraslim upper endoscope for the treatment of retained bile duct stones. Am J Gastroenterol 2009;104:2729–33.
16. Moon JH, Choi HJ, Ko BM. Therapeutic role of direct per-oral cholangioscopy using an ultra-slim upper endoscope. J Hepatobiliary Pancreat Sci 2011;18:350–6.
17. Parsi MA, Stevens T, Vargo JJ. Diagnostic and therapeutic direct per oral cholangioscopy using an intraductal-anchoring balloon. World J Gastroenterol 2012;18:3992–6.
18. Sievert CE Jr, Silvis SE. Evaluation of electrohydraulic lithotripsy as a means of gallstone fragmentation in a canine model. Gastrointest Endosc 1987;33:233–5.
19. Raijman I, Escalante Glorsky S. Electrohydraulic lithotripsy in the treatment of bile and pancreatic duct stones. In: Basow DS, editor. UpToDate. Waltham (MA): UpToDate; 2013.
20. Piraka C, Shah RJ, Awadallah NS, et al. Transpapillary cholangioscopy-directed lithotripsy in patients with difficult bile duct stones. Clin Gastroenterol Hepatol 2007;5:333 8.
21. Patel S, Rosenkranz L, Tarnasky P, et al. Holmium-YAG laser lithotripsy in the treatment of difficult biliary stones utilizing peroral single operator cholangioscopy (SpyGlass): a multi-center experience. Gastrointestinal Endoscopy 2009; 69:AB142.

22. Chen YK, Parsi MA, Binmoeller KF, et al. Single-operator cholangioscopy in patients requiring evaluation of bile duct disease or therapy of biliary stones. Gastrointest Endosc 2011;74:805–14.
23. Arya N, Nelles SE, Haber GB, et al. Electrohydraulic lithotripsy in 111 patients: a safe and effective therapy for difficult bile duct stones. Am J Gastroenterol 2004;99:2330–4.
24. Seelhoff A, Schumacher B, Neuhaus H. Review single operator cholangioscopic guided therapy of bile duct stones. J Hepatobiliary Pancreat Sci 2011;18:346–9.
25. Fishman DS, Tarnasky PR, Patel SN, et al. Management of pancreatobiliary disease using a new intra-ductal endoscope: the Texas experience. World J Gastroenterol 2009;15:1353–8.
26. Itoi T, Osanai M, Igarashi Y, et al. Diagnostic per oral video cholangioscopy is an accurate diagnostic tool for patients with bile duct lesions. Clin Gastroenterol Hepatol 2010;8:934–8.
27. Awadallah NS, Chen YK, Piraka C, et al. Is there a role for cholangioscopy in patients with primary sclerosing cholangitis? Am J Gastroenterol 2006;101:284.
28. Kim HJ, Kim MH, Lee SK, et al. Tumor vessel: a valuable cholangioscopic clue of malignant biliary stricture. Gastrointest Endosc 2000;52:635–8.
29. Seo DW, Lee SK, Yoo KS, et al. Cholangioscopic findings in bile duct tumors. Gastrointest Endosc 2000;52:630–4.
30. Shah RJ, Langer DA, Antillon MR, et al. Cholangioscopy and cholangioscopic forceps biopsy in patients with indeterminate pancreatobiliary pathology. Clin Gastroenterol Hepatol 2006;4:219–25.
31. Tischendorf JJ, Kruger M, Trautwein C, et al. Cholangioscopic characterization of dominant bile duct stenoses in patients with primary sclerosing cholangitis. Endoscopy 2006;38:665–9.
32. Tamada K, Kurihara K, Tomiyama T, et al. How many biopsies should be performed during percutaneous transhepatic cholangioscopy to diagnose biliary tract cancer? Gastrointest Endosc 1999;50:653–8.
33. Parsi MA, Guardino J, Vargo JJ. Per oral cholangioscopy-guided stricture therapy in living donor liver transplantation. Liver Transpl 2009;15:263–9.
34. Hayashi S, Baba Y, Ueno K, et al. Small arteriovenous malformation of the common bile duct causing hemobilia in a patient with hereditary hemorrhagic telangiectasia. Cardiovasc Intervent Radiol 2008;31:S131–4.
35. Prasad GA, Abraham SC, Baron TH, et al. Hemobilia caused by cytomegalovirus cholangiopathy. Am J Gastroenterol 2005;100:2592–5.
36. Talreja JP, Kahaleh M. Photodynamic therapy for cholangiocarcinoma. Gut Liver 2010;4:S62–6.
37. Park DH, Park BW, Lee HS, et al. Per oral direct cholangioscopic argon plasma coagulation by using an ultra-slim upper endoscope for recurrent hepatoma with intraductal tumor growth. Gastrointest Endosc 2007;66:201–3.
38. Lu XL, Itoi T, Kubota K. Cholangioscopy by using narrow-band imaging and transpapillary radiotherapy for mucin-producing bile duct tumor. Clin Gastroenterol Hepatol 2009;7:34–5.
39. Nimura Y. Staging cholangiocarcinoma by cholangioscopy. HPB 2008;10:113–5.

Modern Management of Common Bile Duct Stones

James Buxbaum, MD

KEYWORDS

- Cholangiopancreatography • Endoscopic retrograde • Common bile duct gallstones
- Biliary calculi • Lithotripsy • Sphincterotomy • Endoscopic • Balloon dilatation

KEY POINTS

- Given lack of efficacy relative to endoscopic retrograde cholangiography (ERCP), pharmacologic therapy for bile duct stones should be reserved for patients who are not candidates for therapeutic procedures.
- ERCP should be performed only if there is a high suspicion of bile duct stones; imaging studies for confirmation should be performed if there is intermediate suspicion, to minimize complications associated with ERCP.
- ERCP with sphincterotomy, mechanical lithotripsy, and stent placement may be used to remove most bile duct stones; biliary endoscopists should be adept at precut techniques and the removal of impacted baskets from the duct.
- Intraductal laser and electrohydraulic lithotripsy may be used to fragment most large bile duct stones, and their use will likely become more widespread with the introduction of single-operator cholangioscopes.
- Balloon dilatation after endoscopic sphincterotomy is an effective technique for removal of large bile duct stones.
- The approach to patients with concomitant bile duct stones and cholelithiasis depends on available laparoscopic surgical and biliary endoscopic expertise.

INTRODUCTION

Each year more than 210,000 Americans are hospitalized for acute pancreatitis, for which bile duct stones are the leading cause.[1] In addition, the acute increase in intraductal pressure by stone occlusion may drive bacteria into the bloodstream, resulting in septic cholangitis. Chronic obstruction may result in secondary biliary cirrhosis. It is imperative for gastroenterologists to understand the different formations of bile duct

Conflicts of interest: The author has nothing to disclose.
Division of Gastrointestinal and Liver Diseases, Keck School of Medicine, Los Angeles County Hospital, University of Southern California, D & T Building Room B4H100, 1983 Marengo Street, Los Angeles, CA 90033-1370, USA
E-mail address: jbuxbaum@usc.edu

Gastrointest Endoscopy Clin N Am 23 (2013) 251–275
http://dx.doi.org/10.1016/j.giec.2012.12.003   giendo.theclinics.com
1052-5157/13/$ – see front matter © 2013 Elsevier Inc. All rights reserved.

stones and the various medical treatments that are available. To minimize the compli-cations of endoscopic retrograde cholangiopancreatography (ERCP), it is critical to appropriately assess the risk of bile duct stones before intervention. Biliary endoscop-ists should be comfortable with the basic techniques of stone removal, including sphincterotomy, mechanical lithotripsy, and stent placement. It is also important to be aware of the advanced options, including laser and electrohydraulic stone frag-mentation, as well as papillary dilatation for problematic cases. Finally, the timing and need for ERCP in those who require a cholecystectomy is a consideration.

GENESIS AND PHARMACOLOGIC THERAPY FOR BILE DUCT STONES

Medical therapy for gallstone disease was championed particularly in the 1970s and early 1980s. Interest has waned since the introduction of laparoscopic cholecystec-tomy and ERCP, whereby stones in the gallbladder and bile duct may be removed with low morbidity. Medical therapy aims to correct the biochemical anomalies that cause cholesterol and pigment stone formation. More recently, there has been keen interest in addressing and treating stone disease as part of the metabolic syndrome.

Formation of Cholesterol Stones

Most bile duct stones in patients with a healthy biliary tree result from the migration of stones from the gallbladder into the ductal system. Between 10% and 20% of patients with symptomatic cholelithiasis harbor bile duct stones.[2] In the Western population, 80% of bile duct stones are cholesterol stones and 20% are pigment stones. The liver primarily eliminates cholesterol into the gut in the form of bile, which is aqueous. Hydrophobic cholesterol molecules are insoluble in this medium but are carried by phospholipids and bile salts that have both hydrophobic and hydrophilic moieties.[3] Increases in the levels of cholesterol or decreases in amounts of phospholipids or bile salts results in the supersaturation and precipitation of cholesterol from the bile mixture. Gallbladder stasis promotes the progression of cholesterol crystallization into stones, thus accounting for increased rates of cholesterol stone formation during fasting and pregnancy (**Fig. 1**A).

Choleretics

Administration of the bile salts ursodeoxycholic acid and chenodeoxycholic acid decreases the saturation of cholesterol in bile indirectly by increasing the secretion of phospholipids and bile salts, and by directly reducing the absolute cholesterol secretion.[4] Using bile salts to treat cholelithiasis yielded mediocre results.[5] In the National Cooperative Gallstone Study, which randomized 900 patients with radiolu-cent (cholesterol predominant) stones to placebo, 40% of patients had a complete or partial dissolution of gallbladder stones.[6] Controlled trials of ursodeoxycholic acid and chenodeoxycholic acid to treat bile duct stones consistently demonstrate modest efficacy with resolution of bile duct stones in, at most, 50% of patients.[7,8] Chenodeoxycholic acid also has potential hepatotoxicity, which limits its use. Several studies suggest that adding Rowachol, which is a mixture of vegetable oils (terpenes), moderately enhances the efficacy of bile salts in the dissolution of ductal stones.[9,10]

Nonetheless, clinical studies also revealed that a high percentage (25%–40%) of those undergoing medical therapy with bile salts and/or Rowachol develops complica-tions of bile duct stones requiring hospitalization and surgery.[7,11] Given the high efficacy of endoscopic and surgical stone removal, ursodeoxycholic acid and Rowa-chol should be reserved for the management of bile duct stones in special circum-stances, such as for patients who are too compromised to undergo intervention or

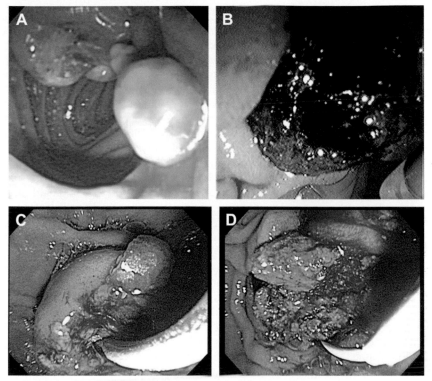

Fig. 1. Cholesterol stones (A) have a chalky yellow hue and mulberry appearance. Black pig-mented stones (B) are discrete and faceted in contrast to brown stones (C, D), which are soft and form casts.

have unusual disease patterns that will not respond to interventional techniques, such as hepatolithiasis related to cystic fibrosis or Caroli disease. The use of these agents in conjunction with endoscopic stenting is explored later in this article.

Solvents

The injection of solvents into the gallbladder to dissolve gallstones was first performed in the nineteenth century.[12] Thistle and colleagues[13] reported resolution of 90% of cases of gallbladder stones following infusion of the powerful solvent methyl-*tert*-butyl ether (MTBE) via a percutaneous transhepatic catheter. However, the results were less favorable when it was introduced by Di Padova and colleagues[14] into the bile duct to address choledocholithiasis. Complications, including peptic ulcer disease, somno-lence, and vomiting, were encountered. It was proposed that unlike the closed space of the gallbladder, the biliary tree allows leakage of the solvent into the duodenum, where direct injury and systemic absorption occurs. Although MTBE results in the complete dissolution of bile duct stones in 25% of cases, 58% developed complica-tions of abdominal pain, cholangitis, or lethargy. The somewhat milder solvent mono-octanoin has also been studied for dissolution of cholesterol bile duct stones in a large uncontrolled study of 343 patients.[15] It was helpful in 54% of cases, though definitely successful in only 26%; furthermore, 67% of patients developed side effects of pain, vomiting, and diarrhea. Solvent infusion into the bile duct has thus been limited by an adverse side-effect profile, and the approach has been largely abandoned in favor of more efficacious, better tolerated interventional methods.[16]

Formation and Treatment of Pigment Stones

Bile is also the medium for clearing senescent blood cells through the excretion of its by-product, bilirubin. Increased blood-cell destruction, as is seen in hemolytic anemia, overwhelms the liver's ability to conjugate bilirubin, which precipitates with calcium to form black pigment cells (**Fig. 1**B). Black stones are also seen in alcoholism, old age, and cirrhosis. Patients with damaged intrahepatic ducts from recurrent pyogenic cholangitis, which is thought to be due to prior parasitic injury as well as primary sclerosing cholangitis and ischemia, develop recurrent suppurative infections. Bacterial β-glucuronidase hydrolyzes conjugated bilirubin, which then complexes with calcium and mixes with sloughed epithelium and cholesterol crystals to form brown pigment stones (**Fig. 1**C, D). Given the composition of pigment stones, they do not respond well to cholesterol desaturation therapy with bile salts and dissolution with solvents. Addition of agents that chelate or complex with calcium found in pigment stones, such as ethylenediaminetetra-acetic acid, modestly improves efficacy.[17] However, a high rate of side effects of vomiting and diarrhea has limited their widespread use.

Relation to Metabolic Syndrome and Prevention

There has been recent interest in gallstones vis-à-vis the hypermetabolic syndrome. A high-fat diet results in high serum triglyceride levels and bile becomes oversaturated with exogenous cholesterol, which causes gallstones.[18] Studies have demonstrated that a high carbohydrate diet, a low high-density-lipoprotein level, and insulin sensitivity are also associated with gallstones.[19,20] The high rates of gallstone formation in Native Americans has been attributed to thrifty genes that favored survival for their ancestors during the last ice age.[21] Nonetheless, dietary and lifestyle factors still exert a potent influence.[22] The prevalence of symptomatic gallstones in Pima Indians, who consume a Western diet, exceeds 50%. However, in the genetically similar Tarahumara Indians, who do not consume a high-fat, high-starch diet and are extremely physically active, gallstones are very rare.[21] Therefore, the first step in the management of bile duct stones is to encourage patients to avoid high-fat, high-carbohydrate diets and a sedentary lifestyle.

Recent work has also demonstrated that using statins, which lower cholesterol by inhibiting the cholesterol synthetic enzyme 3-hydroxy-3-methylglutaryl coenzyme A reductase, is associated with less symptomatic gallstone disease.[23] The antihyperlipidemic ezetimibe, which prevents absorption of intestinal cholesterol, has also been shown to decrease biliary cholesterol saturation and crystallization in patients.[24] Animal models suggest that it may also lower biliary cholesterol secretion and improve gallbladder motility by preventing cholesterol absorption by smooth muscle cells.

CLINICAL APPROACH TO BILE DUCT STONES

In the contemporary era, most bile duct stones are removed by ERCP and concomitant gallbladder stones are removed by laparoscopic cholecystectomy. Although it is the least invasive approach, ERCP for the removal of bile duct stones is associated with complications in 8% to 10% of patients.[25] Thus it is critical that ERCP be used only for therapy and not diagnosis, which necessitates accurately assessing probability of bile duct stones.

Assessment of Probability of Bile Duct Stones

The transition from open cholecystectomy to laparoscopic approaches intensified interest in the preoperative predictors of choledocholithiasis. Removal of bile duct stones is straightforward during open cholecystectomy, but technically difficult to achieve laparoscopically.[26] Biochemical tests are the least invasive method of assessing the probability of bile duct stones: alanine aminotransferase, aspartate aminotransferase, bilirubin, and alkaline phosphatase are correlated with the presence of bile duct stones and if none are elevated, the likelihood is less than 3%.[27] However, the sensitivity and specificity of these individual laboratories are inadequate, and several groups have tried to identify combinations of biochemical tests that have a superior predictive capacity.[2,28–30] In the most widely cited study of the reliability of biochemical tests, Barkun and colleagues (**Fig. 2**) demonstrated that age older than 55 years, bilirubin level greater than 30 mmol/L (1.8 mg/dL), and bile duct dilatation greater than 6 mm best predicted common duct stones, with the probability being 92% if all are present.

However, even patients thought to have a high probability of bile duct stones on the basis of ductal dilatation on ultrasonography or liver-test anomalies have been found at ERCP not to have bile duct stones in more than two-thirds of cases.[31] Using removal of bile duct stones as the gold standard, magnetic resonance cholangiopancreatography

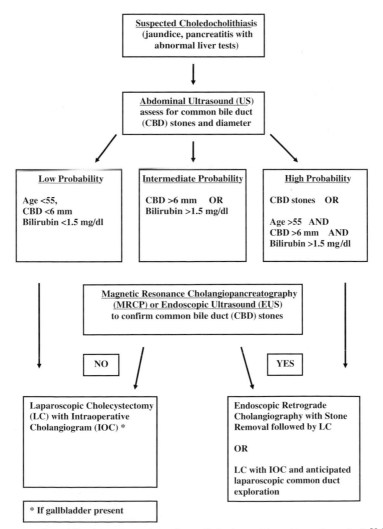

Fig. 2. Approach to bile duct stones based on clinical suspicion. (*Data from* Refs.[39,109,113])

(MRCP) was found to be equally specific but more sensitive than ultrasonography (93% vs 30%) for bile duct stones because the distal duct is often obscured from sonographic visualization by intervening bowel gas.[32] Studies have demonstrated that endoscopic ultrasonography (EUS), whereby the ultrasound probe is positioned immediately adjacent to the bile duct, has an accuracy and negative predictive value greater than 90% for choledocholithiasis.[25,33] Therefore, EUS and MRCP may be used to confirm or exclude bile duct stones with reasonable confidence (see **Fig. 2**).

Clinical Impact of Risk Stratification

Prospective studies have demonstrated that using MRCP and EUS to confirm or exclude bile duct stones minimizes complications in those with an intermediate probability of choledocholithiasis. Several groups have randomized patients with intermediate probability of bile duct stones to evaluation with ERCP or EUS followed by ERCP if stones are confirmed by endosonography.[34–37] These studies demonstrate that an EUS-based strategy avoids ERCP in 30% to 75% of patients.[35] Polkowski and colleagues[33,36] observed a trend toward more procedures in the EUS group compared with ERCP-based groups but significantly fewer complications; 8% versus 40%, driven by the much lower rate of adverse events in EUS (1.6%) compared with ERCP (12.5%). Nonetheless, EUS requires sedation and is associated with some, albeit low, procedural risk. Ainsworth and colleagues[38] compared the performance of EUS and ERCP in a group of 163 patients with suspected stones. The accuracies of EUS and MRCP for stone detection and their abilities to predict the necessity of therapeutic ERCP were equivalent.

An additional consideration is cost. Arguedes and colleagues[39] demonstrated, using a decision analysis model, that the most cost-effective strategy of managing gallstone pancreatitis was highly dependent on the probability of bile duct stones. Cholecystectomy with intraoperative cholangiography (IOC) was favored when the probability of bile duct stones was less than 10%, EUS when the probability was 10% to 50%, and ERCP when the probability was greater than 50%. In another prospective series of 463 patients managed with an EUS-based approach, ERCP was avoided in 216 patients, and the total cost was significantly less than it would have been if an ERCP-based approach had been used.[40]

ENDOSCOPIC REMOVAL OF BILE DUCT STONES

In the era of laparoscopic cholecystectomy, ERCP with sphincterotomy has achieved primacy in the management of bile duct stones. Sphincterotomy, mechanical lithotripsy, and stent placement are the fundamental techniques. If used appropriately, the biliary endoscopist may remove 80% to 90% of stones and may expect complications in fewer than 10% of cases.

Asymptomatic Stones

Patients who present with symptomatic bile duct stones have a greater than 50% chance of developing recurrent biliary pain, jaundice, or cholangitis; these complications are serious in 25% of cases.[41] Patients who have asymptomatic stones have a more benign clinical course. A large series of patients with cholelithiasis but minimal preoperative risk for bile duct stones were randomized to undergo IOC versus not to undergo IOC.[42] Unexpected stones were encountered in 12% of those who underwent IOC. The patients who were not randomized to IOC presumably had a similar frequency of an asymptomatic bile duct stone. Over the course of 3 years of follow-up, none of these patients developed biliary symptoms. In addition, spontaneous stone migration may be seen in approximately 20% of cases, particularly for small (<8 mm) stones.[43] Nevertheless, given the potential for serious complications, it is advised that bile duct stones are removed unless the patient's comorbidities make the procedure prohibitively high risk.[44]

Sphincterotomy

Although it was initially espoused only for patients who are poor candidates for surgery, with the advent of laparoscopic cholecystectomy endoscopic sphincterotomy has emerged as the primary modality for access to and removal of bile duct stones. In a classic study from the London Middlesex Hospital, sphincterotomy was used to manage biliary obstruction from suspected stones in 1000 consecutive patients and enabled successful endoscopic drainage in 985 (**Fig. 3**A).[45] Stones were confirmed in 797 patients and removed by balloon and basket sweep in 85% (**Fig. 3**B, C). In this initial report, sphincterotomy was complicated by bleeding in 4%, cholangitis in 2%, pancreatitis in 1%, and perforation in 1%. Subsequent large series have reported comparable complication rates for sphincterotomy for choledocholithiasis.[46–48] Large trials have demonstrated that the risk of sphincterotomy for bile duct stones (8.1%) is significantly lower than for other indications including dysfunction of sphincter of Oddi (20.4%), driven largely by the risk of pancreatitis.[46] In addition, sphincterotomy complications decrease with the increased experience of the endoscopist.[47]

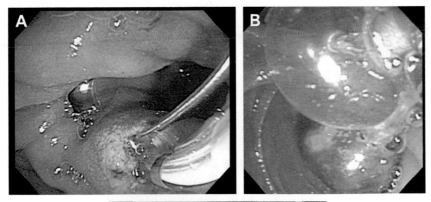

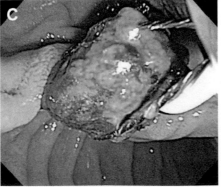

Fig. 3. After an adequate sphincterotomy (*A*) (note a juxtapapillary diverticulum), sweeps with extraction balloons (*B*) and dormia baskets (*C*) can be used to remove most bile duct stones.

Most perforations during stone removal are retroduodenal and, in contrast to free perforations, can be managed by conservative measures (see **Fig. 3**A, B).[49] Post-sphincterotomy bleeding can be controlled by injection of epinephrine, bipolar cautery, or argon plasma coagulation.[50] The placement of large stents may effectively tampo-nade bleeding and enable biliary drainage (see **Fig. 3**C). In some cases, it is necessary to extend the sphincterotomy during a subsequent procedure. It appears that there is a lower rate of pancreatitis but comparable rates of bleeding in such procedures in comparison with the initial sphincterotomy.[51] Some endoscopists have expressed concerns about the long-term effects of sphincterotomy, particularly for young patients. However, long-term follow-up data suggest that problems are unusual: subsequent biliary symptoms are seen in 12% to 13% and sphincter stenosis in 4% to 7%.[52,53] Furthermore, late biliary problems typically respond well to endoscopic treatment.[53]

Needle-Knife and Rendezvous Techniques

Sphincterotomy is classically performed using a catheter with a bowing wire (see **Fig. 3**A). After engagement of the biliary orifice, cutting is typically performed in the 11- to 12-o'clock direction along the axis of the duct (**Fig. 4**A). However, for challenging

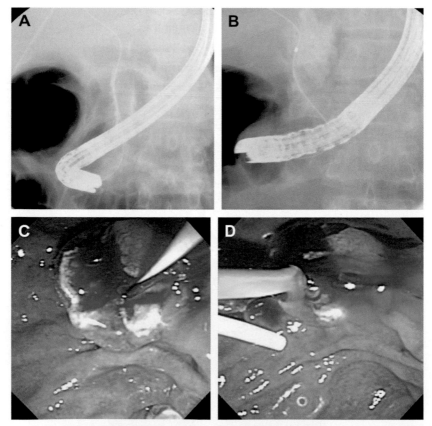

Fig. 4. Cholangiograms (*A, B*) demonstrate retroperitoneal leakage of contrast after sphinc-terotomy for bile duct stones. The patient responded to stent placement and conservative treatment. After sphincterotomy, hemorrhage occurred (*C*), but was controlled by place-ment of an Amsterdam type stent (*D*).

cases a needle knife may be used to unroof the bile duct and enable access. In a large series of 694 patients who underwent precut sphincterotomy for biliary access, Rabenstein and colleagues[46,48] demonstrated that the maneuver was successful in 85% of those who failed conventional access techniques. In contrast to prior work, they reported that complications of needle-knife papillotomy were not significantly higher than in conventional sphincterotomy (7.3% vs 6.8%). The investigators suggest that inexperienced operators and the delayed use of needle-knife techniques only after excessive failed attempts to access the bile duct account for the greater complication rates reported by other groups.

Patients who present with a crowning stone impacted in the papilla are particularly amenable to needle-knife excision, given the difficulty of advancing a sphincterotome into the meatus. Often the needle-knife excision will result in a prompt, satisfying expulsion of the biliary concretion (**Fig. 5**A, B).[54] In addition, in patients with situs anatomy, such as those who have undergone a Billroth II surgery, conventional sphincterotomes will not cut in the appropriate 5- to 6-o'clock direction; however, this may be accomplished using a needle knife (**Fig. 5**C). There are 2 approaches to needle-knife papillotomy. In the conventional approach, a cut in the direction of the bile duct is

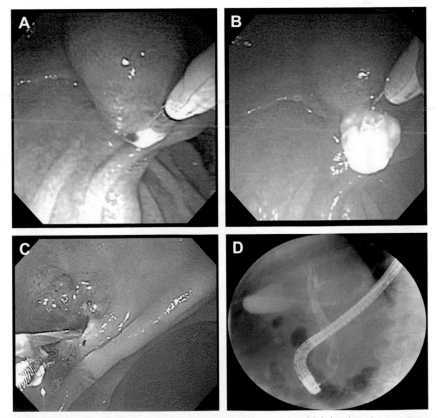

Fig. 5. A needle knife is used to unroof a crowning stone (*A*), which leads to its spontaneous expulsion (*B*). Needle-knife lithotripsy is used perform a sphincterotomy in a patient with inverted anatomy consequent to Roux-en-Y gastric bypass surgery (*C*). A percutaneously placed wire (*D*) is used to guide cannulation after an initial ERCP was unsuccessful because of failed cannulation.

made from the papillary meatus. In the fistulotomy approach, the papillary mound is incised and a cut made toward, but typically not to, the meatus. Randomized data suggest the fistulotomy approach is more likely to require subsequent mechanical lithotripsy but is less likely to cause pancreatitis.[55] Access may be achieved in those who fail precut techniques by rendezvous procedures whereby a wire is introduced percutaneously. Endoscopic cannulation can then be performed immediately adjacent to or over the percutaneous wire (**Fig. 5**D). Recently EUS has been used to introduce the guide wire in an anterograde fashion, enabling an entirely endoscopic rendezvous approach.[56]

Mechanical Lithotripsy

Mechanical lithotripsy is the favored technique to fragment and remove large stones with diameters that exceed the size of the maximal allowable sphincterotomy.[57] The stones are fractured between the basket and sheath covering the wire by closing the basket handle (**Fig. 6**A). Crushing very hard or large stones requires a coiled metal sleeve. This procedure is most easily performed by using an all-inclusive lithotripsy device, which contains a basket, plastic sheath, flexible metal coil sleeve, and an

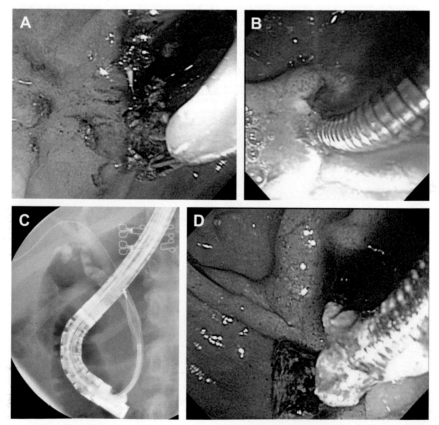

Fig. 6. A soft stone is crushed between a basket and standard sheath (*A*). Hard-pigment type stones required the use of an all-inclusive lithotripsy system. The flexible metal sleeve is introduced into the duct (*B*), and is used to crush the stone (*C*) and remove the hard fragments (*D*).

attachable cranking apparatus (**Fig. 6B–D**).[58] When aggressive mechanical lithotripsy is not anticipated and the stone and extraction basket become impacted together, an extraendoscopic lithotripter may be used (**Fig. 7**).[58]

The success of mechanical lithotripsy varies with stone size and papillary anatomy, but ranges from 84% to 99%.[57,59–62] Chang and colleagues[59] report that the risk of a single session of mechanical lithotripsy is comparable with sphincterotomy. However, if multiple sessions are necessary the rates of pancreatitis, bleeding, and cholangitis increase significantly. Complications unique to mechanical lithotripsy include basket impaction and malfunction.[63] If the impacted basket and stone cannot be freed by crushing the stone with the extraendoscopic lithotripter, a variety of maneuvers including sphincterotomy extension, stent placement, and stone fragmentation by extracorporeal shock-wave lithotripsy (ESWL) or laser lithotripsy may be used.[63–66] Bile duct exploration with removal of the stone and basket may also be performed surgically. Use of the extraendoscopic lithotripter may result in trauma to the mucosa of the gastric incisura, angle of the duodenum, and papilla by the exposed basket wires.[58]

Biliary Stent Placement

Another alternative for the management of more difficult cases is biliary stent placement. This technique was initially espoused for older patients with comorbidities.[67] Bergman and colleagues[68] reported on a cohort of 117 patients with median age of 80 years, all of whom underwent successful biliary drainage by stent placement. Complications

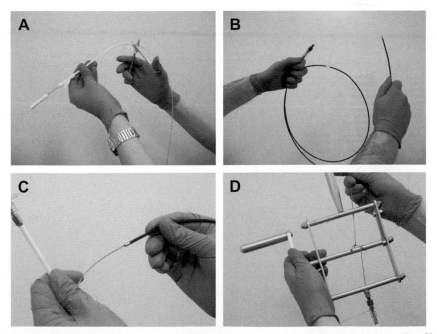

Fig. 7. The extraendoscopic emergency lithotripter is assembled by cutting the handle off of the dormia basket (*A*) and removing the plastic sheath. The back of the metal coil sleeve (*B*) is then attached to the cranking device, and the tip is fed over the exposed basket wire (*C*). As the metal coil sleeve is advanced toward the ampulla the wire emerges through the back and into the lithotripter, and is fastened to the cranking device (*D*), which is turned to crush the stone.

occurred in 10% of patients in whom stenting was used as a temporary measure before further endoscopic therapy or surgery. For those patients who received stents as permanent therapy, problems were unusual during the first year; however, complications associated with the stents, which were not routinely exchanged, exceeded 50% thereafter. Most importantly, 16% of the patients in this group died of infectious biliary complications. Several trials have randomized high-risk patients to aggressive ductal clearance versus long-term plastic stent placement, and the results are consistent with those of Bergman and colleagues.[69,70] Although the short-term morbidity attributable to the procedural complications was somewhat greater in clearance groups, the long-term morbidity was significantly higher in the stent groups because of high rates of cholangitis.

Although stents have fallen out of favor as destination therapy, recent work demonstrates that temporary stent placement facilitates stone removal.[71] Jain and colleagues[72] managed a series of patients with large stones by pigtail-stent placement. When the stents were removed 6 months later, there were no residual stones in half of the patients (**Fig. 8**). In a cohort of patients with large (>2 cm) or multiple (>3) stones, pigtail stents were placed and, when they were removed 2 months later, the stone burden in the group decreased by greater than 50% and clearance was achieved in 93%.[73] Given that the size reduction was more prominent in those with multiple rather than single stones, the mechanism of action was proposed to involve the friction between stents and stones. It is likely that multiple stents could further facilitate stone grinding and removal. Covered metal stents, which exert greater radial force, have been used with success in a single series of 36 patients, but have not been compared with plastic stents.[74]

There has been growing interest in administering oral choleretic medications in addition to stent placement for large stones after initial reports suggesting that they accelerate the dissolution of ductal stone.[75,76] Katsinelos and colleagues[77] randomized patients with challenging biliary stones to stent placement followed by treatment with ursodeoxycholic acid or stent placement followed by placebo. At 6 months, the patients were reassessed by ERCP; there was no difference in ductal clearance or stone burden between the 2 groups. The impact of adding a combination of Rowachol and terpene to inserting biliary stents has also been studied in a controlled trial, in which there was no significant difference in stone burden or successful duct clearance between those randomized to receive the choleretic regimen and those who did not receive the medications.[78]

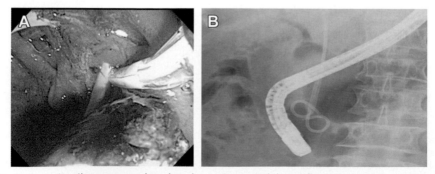

Fig. 8. Two pigtail stents are placed under endoscopic (*A*) and fluoroscopic (*B*) guidance to decompress an elderly patient with giant bile duct stones. The duct was cleared in a subsequent laser lithotripsy procedure.

ADVANCED ENDOSCOPIC TECHNIQUES FOR CHALLENGING BILE DUCT STONES

The management of difficult bile duct stones is a formidable challenge for the biliary endoscopist and has been the subject of extensive contemporary endoscopic research. Stone fragmentation may be accomplished by ESWL and intraductal methods of fragmentation, including electrohydraulic and laser lithotripsy. Intraductal treatment may be guided by fluoroscopy or choledochoscopy. Over the past decade, papillary balloon dilatation after endoscopic sphincterotomy has been introduced as a technique to address challenging stones.

Features of the Difficult Stone

Conventional techniques can fail because of features of the stone and papillary region. The most significant predictor of failed mechanical lithotripsy is the impaction of the stone in the bile duct, which prevents the opening of the lithotripsy basket and encircling of the stone (**Fig. 9**A).[57] Barrel-shaped and piston-shaped stones, as well as those that arise from the cystic duct takeoff, are difficult to manipulate (**Fig. 9**B, C). Perivaterian diverticulum (see **Fig. 3**A) and inverted papillary orientation, as is seen following Billroth II (**Fig. 11**A) or Roux-en-Y (see **Fig. 5**C) gastric bypass surgeries, make biliary access and sphincterotomy difficult. Finally, bile duct anomalies, including distal tapering or a sigmoid shape, also make stone removal challenging.[79]

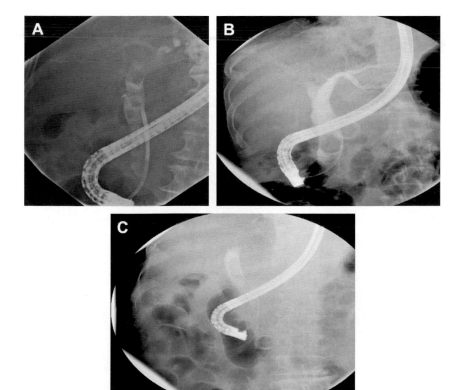

Fig. 9. Bile duct stones may be difficult to remove owing to impaction (*A*), large size (*B*), or piston shape (*C*), which limits manipulation of the mechanical basket.

Extracorporeal Shock-Wave Lithotripsy

ESWL was developed to address nephrolithiasis and is frequently used to manage calcified pancreatic duct stones. In classic ESWL, shock waves that are generated by electric discharges outside of the body are transmitted to the patient, who is submerged in a water bath. This approach has progressed from the original electrohydraulic designs, which required general anesthesia, to piezoelectric, electromagnetic, and focused electrohydraulic lithotripters, which use a fluid-filled cushion rather than a bath. Because modern lithotripters deliver focused shock waves, general anesthesia is unnecessary. Large series have demonstrated ductal clearance in patients with refractory stones from 83% to 100%, with complications reported in 6% to 9%.[80–84] Nevertheless, ESWL is typically guided by fluoroscopy; therefore, ERCP is required before the procedure to place a nasobiliary drain for the contrast agent, and also afterward to clear debris.[82]

Intraductal Shock-Wave Techniques

In electrohydraulic lithotripsy (EHL), a bipolar electrode probe is guided into the bile duct by either fluoroscopy or cholangioscopy.[70] High-voltage electric sparks discharged from the probe create a shock wave, and continuous irrigation with saline provides the medium for intraductal conduction. Cholangioscopic-guided and fluoroscopic-guided EHL have been used to clear bile duct stones in 77% to 90% of cases.[85,86] Complications occurred in 6% to 18%, mostly recurrent jaundice or cholangitis.

For the past 2 decades, lasers have also been used under fluoroscopic or cholangioscopic guidance to fragment large bile duct stones. Light-energy absorption from the surface of the stone creates an expanding plasma cloud, and the resulting mechanical shock wave fragments the stone (**Fig. 10**). A variety of lasers, including

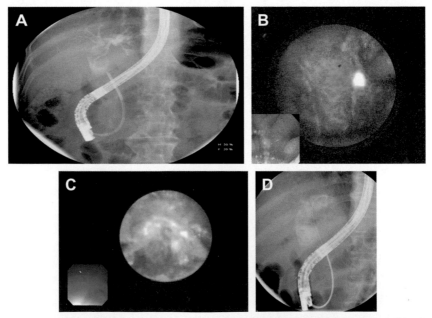

Fig. 10. The cholangioscope is advanced under endoscopic and fluoroscopic guidance to approach a very large stone (*A*). Under cholangioscopic guidance the laser is fired (*B*), and subsequent shock waves result in the fragmentation of the stone as seen by cholangioscopy (*C*) and fluoroscopy (*D*).

doubled-double-pulse neodymium:YAG (FREDDY), flashlamp-pumped pulse, alexandrite, and holmium have been used, with ductal clearance reported in 73% to 94% of patients. Complications have occurred in 0% to 9.6%, with cholangitis being the most frequent adverse event.[87–93] The rhodamine-6G flashlamp-pumped pulsed laser is notable in that the probe has the ability to differentiate scattered light from tissue versus stone, and it will automatically shut off if the former is sensed.[89,94]

Comparison of Advanced Fragmentation Techniques

Several controlled trials have compared ESWL with the intraductal methods of stone disruption. These studies suggest that the efficacy of ESWL is comparable with intracorporeal EHL and fluoroscopic-guided laser lithotripsy, although cholangioscopic-guided laser lithotripsy may be superior.[86,95,96] In addition, these trials have consistently shown that ESWL requires more procedures. Although not controlled, comparison of misdirected pulses in fluoroscopic- versus cholangioscopic-laser lithotripsy suggests that the latter strategy is more accurate and less likely to induce tissue injury.[89] Cholangioscopy may be performed through the papilla or percutaneously. However, when performed percutaneously, the resulting large biliocutaneous fistula is associated with bleeding and infection in 23% of cases, so the percutaneous approach should be reserved for exceptional cases of aberrant anatomy, strictures, and intrahepatic stones.[88]

During the past decade there have been significant developments in cholangioscopy. Early models required 2 expert endoscopists to drive mother-baby scopes that were awkward and fragile.[95] Recently, however, several single-operator cholangioscopes with improved durability and maneuverability have been introduced.[83,84] Preliminary studies indicate that they may be used to support intraductal laser and EHL, with favorable rates of ductal clearance.[83,97] In addition, long-length, ultraslim cholangioscopes, which are advanced directly through the mouth, have been used to perform laser lithotripsy and EHL.[90,93] Cholangioscopy is discussed further in a dedicated article elsewhere in this issue by Isaac and colleagues.

Papillary Balloon Dilatation Following Sphincterotomy

Recently the use of endoscopic balloon dilatation (EBD) has experienced a renaissance with the caveat that a sphincterotomy is first performed. EBD without sphincterotomy is viewed with caution, following the multicenter trial by Disario and colleagues.[98] In this study, the investigators randomized 238 patients with bile duct stones to EBD versus endoscopic sphincterotomy. Although the efficacy was equivalent, 97.4% for EBD compared with 92.5% for sphincterotomy, there were more complications in the EBD group (17.9% vs 3.3% in the sphincterotomy group), predominantly related to high rates of pancreatitis in the former group. There were 2 fatalities in the EBD group, both due to pancreatitis.

These results differed somewhat from a prior trial by Bergman and colleagues,[99] in which sphincterotomy and EBD had similar efficacy for stone removal and an equivalent modest rate of pancreatitis. Nonetheless, the population was much older in the Bergman trial (72 years compared with 47 years in the trial by Disario and colleagues), and the complication rates after EBD (18%) and endoscopic sphincterotomy (23%) were both high. A meta-analysis by Baron and Harewood[100] found that although the efficacy of both methods appeared equivalent, the rate of pancreatitis after EBD (7.4%) was significantly higher than the rate following sphincterotomy (4.3%). However, more bleeding was seen after endoscopic sphincterotomy (2%) than after EBD (0%). Given the risk of pancreatitis, EBD is no longer recommended for most stone cases, except those with a very high risk of hemorrhage, such as in cirrhotic patients with coagulapathy.[101]

A recently introduced approach is performing EBD immediately after sphincterotomy in patients not successfully treated with conventional techniques.[102] This method is promising in patients with large complex stones and those with narrow distal ducts.[79,102,103] In a multicenter study, EBD after sphincterotomy for bile duct stones achieved stone clearance in 95% of patients, and there were no episodes of pancreatitis.[104] The investigators postulated that the biliary sphincterotomy separates the biliary from the pancreatic orifice, and the subsequent force of dilatation is preferentially directed toward the sphincterotomy and away from the pancreatic duct. Experts also suggest that the risk of perforation can be minimized by placing two-thirds of the balloon in the bile duct and one-third outside, to dilate the papillary orifice and duct in a unidirectional manner.[103]

Stefanidis and colleagues[105] randomized patients to endoscopic sphincterotomy followed by mechanical lithotripsy or to sphincterotomy followed by EBD. The methods were equally effective for stone removal, both greater than 90%, but there were significantly more complications, primarily cholangitis, in the lithotripsy group. In addition, retrospective data suggest that endoscopic sphincterotomy combined with dilatation requires less mechanical lithotripsy, fluoroscopy time, and procedure time.[106] Endoscopic sphincterotomy followed by EBD is also particularly suited for patients in whom it is treacherous to perform a large sphincterotomy, such as those with diminutive papilla or inverted anatomy (see **Fig. 11**).[107] New devices, including

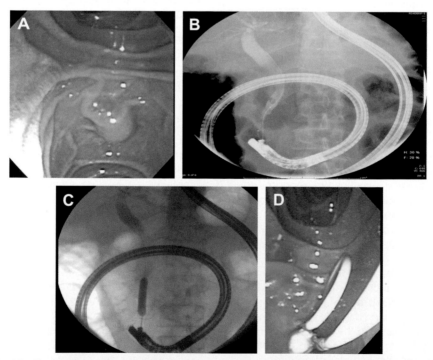

Fig. 11. Cholangiography was performed in a patient with an inverted papilla (*A*) after Billroth II surgery, revealing a ductal stone (*B*). Given the diminutive papilla and aberrant anatomy a small sphincterotomy was performed, and large balloon dilatation (*C*) facilitated stone removal (*D*).

a sphincterotome equipped with a large-diameter balloon, may further improve the efficiency of this method.[108]

APPROACH TO BILE DUCT STONES IN THE PATIENT WITH AN INTACT GALLBLADDER

The widespread introduction of ERCP and laparoscopic cholecystectomy has generated controversy regarding the best approach to patients with symptomatic bile duct stones and an intact gallbladder. Laparoscopic approaches to the bile duct are challenging and time consuming. Comparing the 2-stage approaches of ERCP along with laparoscopic cholecystectomy (**Fig. 12**) with laparoscopic cholecystectomy and laparoscopic common duct exploration (LCBDE) has been the subject of ongoing study and debate.

Laparoscopic Removal of Bile Duct Stones Versus ERCP

At the time of laparoscopic surgery, bile duct stones may be removed by the straightforward transcystic approach or by the technically demanding choledochotomy. In a recent series, Nathanson and colleagues[109] managed a cohort of 372 patients with choledocholithiasis who underwent laparoscopic cholecystectomy. Transcystic clearance was successful in 286. The remaining patients were randomized to either choledochotomy or postoperative ERCP. Operating time was greater in the cholecystectomy and choledochotomy group, 152.7 minutes, compared with the cholecystectomy-alone group, 102.8 minutes. However, when factoring in the ERCP time, the overall procedure time was similar in the 2 groups: 158.8 minutes for choledochotomy group compared with 147.9 minutes for the ERCP group.

Outcomes of Single Versus 2-Stage Approach to Simultaneous Choledocholithiasis and Cholelithiasis

Several trials have compared the clinical outcomes of the 2-stage approach with those of the single-stage strategy. Rogers and colleagues[110] randomized 122 patients to laparoscopic cholecystectomy plus LCBDE or to ERCP with sphincterotomy plus

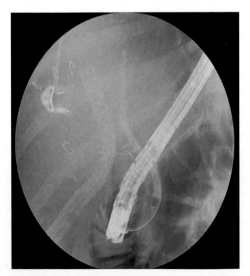

Fig. 12. A bile duct stone seen on ERCP after laparoscopic cholecystectomy.

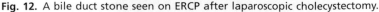

laparoscopic cholecystectomy. Although the techniques had equivalent efficacy and safety, the length of hospitalization was 2 days fewer for those who underwent the combined laparoscopic procedure. Rhodes and colleagues[111] randomized 427 patients with bile duct stones found on cholecystectomy to either laparoscopic exploration or postoperative ERCP. Consistent with the work of Rogers and colleagues, Rhodes and colleagues found that rates of ductal clearance and safety were comparable, but there was a longer median hospital stay (3.5 days) in the ERCP group, compared with 1 day in the LCBDE group. In both trials, patients with cholangitis and severe pancreatitis were excluded and proceeded directly to ERCP.

Recently, Lu and colleagues[112] performed a meta-analysis of 9 randomized trials that compared 2-stage ERCP and laparoscopic cholecystectomy with combined laparoscopic cholecystectomy and bile duct exploration. In the total group of 787 patients, the approaches were found to have equivalent efficacy and safety. The longer hospital stay seen in the ERCP group in the individual trials was not evident; however, significantly more procedures were required in the ERCP group than in the combined laparoscopic group. The problem with applicability of these data, however, is that most surgeons do not have the training to perform LCBDE.

Timing of ERCP in Relation to Laparoscopic Cholecystectomy

The timing of ERCP, either before or after the cholecystectomy, is debated. Some surgeons advocate preoperative ERCP so that surgery may be performed in patients who have undergone unsuccessful biliary endoscopy. In expert centers, operative removal of bile duct stones was required in 6.6% of patients who failed ERCP; however, additional operations were needed in 7.3% of those who underwent surgery to remove bile duct stones. Thus, additional procedures are unusual but may be required after unsuccessful ERCP or surgical removal of bile duct stones.[109] The optimal timing of ERCP and laparoscopic surgery is best guided by local availability and technical expertise.

SUMMARY

Bile duct stones are a source of significant morbidity, given their association with pancreatitis and cholangitis. Medical therapy for cholesterol and pigment bile duct stones aims to correct the biochemical aberrancies that lead to their formation. Hydrophilic bile salts and Rowachol decrease the biliary cholesterol supersaturation that underlies the formation of cholesterol stones. However, the modest efficacy of these agents relative to minimally invasive endoscopic and surgical interventions limits their use to exceptional circumstances. Significant side effects have limited the use of solvents for cholesterol stones and chelators for pigment stones. Lifestyle measures, such as avoidance of high-cholesterol and carbohydrate diets, and the future role of statins and ezetimibe are areas of active investigation in the prevention of gallstones.

Although accurate, ERCP is not recommended for the diagnosis of bile duct stones because of the significant risk of complications. Liver tests, clinical presentation, patient's age, and biliary dilatation can help stratify the probability of bile duct stones. Both EUS and MRCP may be used to confirm the presence of a bile duct stones in people with an intermediate probability of stones. Prospective studies indicate that using these technologies to confirm the need for ERCP in this group prevents complications and is likely a more cost-effective approach.

Removing bile duct stones is recommended for both symptomatic and asymptomatic stones, although asymptomatic stones may be observed in prohibitively high-risk patients. Endoscopic sphincterotomy followed by balloon and basket sweeps of the bile duct is successful in the majority of patients. Precut sphincterotomy and fistulotomy are important techniques that are best performed by an experienced endoscopist. For more difficult stones, mechanical lithotripsy is helpful, but the operator must be capable of managing basket and stone impaction. Stent placement is also useful for difficult cases. Temporary stent placement is very effective in achieving decompression and reducing stone size, and permanent stent therapy is associated with prohibitively high rates of cholangitis. There is insufficient evidence to recommend medical therapy as an adjunct to stent placement.

Certain stone, duct, and papillary features may cause widely available endoscopic techniques to be unsuccessful in removing the concrements. Advanced methods are required to remove large or odd-shaped stones as well as those in patients with narrow distal ducts and diminutive papillae. ESWL, intraductal laser, and electrohydraulic therapy may be used to fragment and remove difficult stones, although ESWL requires more procedures than do intraductal techniques. Expense and technical equipment have limited the use of these techniques to patients seen in specialized referral centers. However, a new generation of single-operator cholangioscopes will likely enable the more widespread use of fragmentation techniques. EBD alone is not recommended because of high rates of pancreatitis; however, balloon dilatation after sphincterotomy appears to be effective and safe.

In patients with bile duct stones and an intact gallbladder, both ERCP and laparoscopic common duct exploration are effective, although the latter approach requires fewer procedures. However, local availability and expertise in laparoscopic versus endoscopic techniques are currently the dominant factors that govern the management strategy at individual institutions.

ACKNOWLEDGMENTS

Special thanks are extended to Richard Molina, Kelvin Yeh, MD, and Arthur Yan, MD for assisting with figures.

REFERENCES

1. Fagenholz PJ, Castillo CF, Harris NS, et al. Increasing United States hospital admissions for acute pancreatitis, 1988-2003. Ann Epidemiol 2007;17(7):491–7.
2. Trondsen E, Edwin B, Reiertsen O, et al. Prediction of common bile duct stones prior to cholecystectomy: a prospective validation of a discriminant analysis function. Arch Surg 1998;133(2):162–6.
3. Paumgartner G, Sauerbruch T. Gallstones: pathogenesis. Lancet 1991;338(8775): 1117–21.
4. von Bergmann K, Epple-Gutsfeld M, Leiss O. Differences in the effects of chenodeoxycholic and ursodeoxycholic acid on biliary lipid secretion and bile acid synthesis in patients with gallstones. Gastroenterology 1984;87(1): 136–43.
5. Iser JH, Dowling H, Mok HY, et al. Chenodeoxycholic acid treatment of gallstones. A follow-up report and analysis of factors influencing response to therapy. N Engl J Med 1975;293(8):378–83.
6. Schoenfield LJ, Lachin JM. Chenodiol (chenodeoxycholic acid) for dissolution of gallstones: the National Cooperative Gallstone Study. A controlled trial of efficacy and safety. Ann Intern Med 1981;95(3):257–82.
7. Sue SO, Taub M, Pearlman BJ, et al. Treatment of choledocholithiasis with oral chenodeoxycholic acid. Surgery 1981;90(1):32–4.

8. Salvioli G, Salati R, Lugli R, et al. Medical treatment of biliary duct stones: effect of ursodeoxycholic acid administration. Gut 1983;24(7):609–14.

9. Ellis WR, Bell GD. Treatment of biliary duct stones with a terpene preparation. Br Med J (Clin Res Ed) 1981;282(6264):611.

10. Leiss O, von Bergmann K. Effect of Rowachol on biliary lipid secretion and serum lipids in normal volunteers. Gut 1985;26(1):32–7.

11. Somerville KW, Ellis WR, Whitten BH, et al. Stones in the common bile duct: experience with medical dissolution therapy. Postgrad Med J 1985;61(714):313–6.

12. Walker J. The removal of gallstones by ether solution. Lancet 1891;137:874–5.

13. Thistle JL, May GR, Bender CE, et al. Dissolution of cholesterol gallbladder stones by methyl tert-butyl ether administered by percutaneous transhepatic catheter. N Engl J Med 1989;320(10):633–9.

14. Di Padova C, Di Padova F, Montorsi W, et al. Methyl tert-butyl ether fails to dissolve retained radiolucent common bile duct stones. Gastroenterology 1986;91(5):1296–300.

15. Palmer KR, Hofmann AF. Intraductal mono-octanoin for the direct dissolution of bile duct stones: experience in 343 patients. Gut 1986;27(2):196–202.

16. Diaz D, Bories P, Ampelas M, et al. Methyl tert-butyl ether in the endoscopic treatment of common bile duct radiolucent stones in elderly patients with nasobiliary tube. Dig Dis Sci 1992;37(1):97–100.

17. Neoptolemos JP, Hofmann AF, Moossa AR. Chemical treatment of stones in the biliary tree. Br J Surg 1986;73(7):515–24.

18. Grunhage F, Lammert F. Gallstone disease. Pathogenesis of gallstones: a genetic perspective. Best Pract Res Clin Gastroenterol 2006;20(6):997–1015.

19. Tsai CJ, Leitzmann MF, Willett WC, et al. Glycemic load, glycemic index, and carbohydrate intake in relation to risk of cholecystectomy in women. Gastroenterology 2005;129(1):105–12.

20. Petitti DB, Friedman GD, Klatsky AL. Association of a history of gallbladder disease with a reduced concentration of high-density-lipoprotein cholesterol. N Engl J Med 1981;304(23):1396–8.

21. Carey MC, Paigen B. Epidemiology of the American Indians' burden and its likely genetic origins. Hepatology 2002;36(4 Pt 1):781–91.

22. Katsika D, Grjibovski A, Einarsson C, et al. Genetic and environmental influences on symptomatic gallstone disease: a Swedish study of 43,141 twin pairs. Hepatology 2005;41(5):1138–43.

23. Tsai CJ, Leitzmann MF, Willett WC, et al. Statin use and the risk of cholecystectomy in women. Gastroenterology 2009;136(5):1593–600.

24. Wang HH, Portincasa P, Mendez-Sanchez N, et al. Effect of ezetimibe on the prevention and dissolution of cholesterol gallstones. Gastroenterology 2008; 134(7):2101–10.

25. Prat F, Amouyal G, Amouyal P, et al. Prospective controlled study of endoscopic ultrasonography and endoscopic retrograde cholangiography in patients with suspected common-bileduct lithiasis. Lancet 1996;347(8994):75–9.

26. Cotton PB, Baillie J, Pappas TN, et al. Laparoscopic cholecystectomy and the biliary endoscopist. Gastrointest Endosc 1991;37(1):94–7.

27. Yang MH, Chen TH, Wang SE, et al. Biochemical predictors for absence of common bile duct stones in patients undergoing laparoscopic cholecystectomy. Surg Endosc 2008;22(7):1620–4.

28. Robertson GS, Jagger C, Johnson PR, et al. Selection criteria for preoperative endoscopic retrograde cholangiopancreatography in the laparoscopic era. Arch Surg 1996;131(1):89–94.

29. Del Santo P, Kazarian KK, Rogers JF, et al. Prediction of operative cholangiography in patients undergoing elective cholecystectomy with routine liver function chemistries. Surgery 1985;98(1):7–11.

30. Santucci L, Natalini G, Sarpi L, et al. Selective endoscopic retrograde cholangiography and preoperative bile duct stone removal in patients scheduled for laparoscopic cholecystectomy: a prospective study. Am J Gastroenterol 1996; 91(7):1326–30.

31. Tham TC, Lichtenstein DR, Vandervoort J, et al. Role of endoscopic retrograde cholangiopancreatography for suspected choledocholithiasis in patients undergoing laparoscopic cholecystectomy. Gastrointest Endosc 1998;47(1):50–6.

32. Laokpessi A, Bouillet P, Sautereau D, et al. Value of magnetic resonance cholangiography in the preoperative diagnosis of common bile duct stones. Am J Gastroenterol 2001;96(8):2354–9.

33. Canto MI, Chak A, Stellato T, et al. Endoscopic ultrasonography versus cholangiography for the diagnosis of choledocholithiasis. Gastrointest Endosc 1998; 47(6):439–48.

34. Karakan T, Cindoruk M, Alagozlu H, et al. EUS versus endoscopic retrograde cholangiography for patients with intermediate probability of bile duct stones: a prospective randomized trial. Gastrointest Endosc 2009;69(2):244–52.

35. Ang TL, Teo EK, Fock KM. Endosonography- vs. endoscopic retrograde cholangiopancreatography-based strategies in the evaluation of suspected common bile duct stones in patients with normal transabdominal imaging. Aliment Pharmacol Ther 2007;26(8):1163–70.

36. Polkowski M, Regula J, Tilszer A, et al. Endoscopic ultrasound versus endoscopic retrograde cholangiography for patients with intermediate probability of bile duct stones: a randomized trial comparing two management strategies. Endoscopy 2007;39(4):296–303.

37. Lee YT, Chan FK, Leung WK, et al. Comparison of EUS and ERCP in the investigation with suspected biliary obstruction caused by choledocholithiasis: a randomized study. Gastrointest Endosc 2008;67(4):660–8.

38. Ainsworth AP, Rafaelsen SR, Wamberg PA, et al. Is there a difference in diagnostic accuracy and clinical impact between endoscopic ultrasonography and magnetic resonance cholangiopancreatography? Endoscopy 2003;35(12):1029–32.

39. Arguedas MR, Dupont AW, Wilcox CM. Where do ERCP, endoscopic ultrasound, magnetic resonance cholangiopancreatography, and intraoperative cholangiography fit in the management of acute biliary pancreatitis? A decision analysis model. Am J Gastroenterol 2001;96(10):2892–9.

40. Buscarini E, Tansini P, Vallisa D, et al. EUS for suspected choledocholithiasis: do benefits outweigh costs? A prospective, controlled study. Gastrointest Endosc 2003;57(4):510–8.

41. Caddy GR, Kirby J, Kirk SJ, et al. Natural history of asymptomatic bile duct stones at time of cholecystectomy. Ulster Med J 2005;74(2):108–12.

42. Murison MS, Gartell PC, McGinn FP. Does selective peroperative cholangiography result in missed common bile duct stones? J R Coll Surg Edinb 1993; 38(4):220–4.

43. Frossard JL, Hadengue A, Amouyal G, et al. Choledocholithiasis: a prospective study of spontaneous common bile duct stone migration. Gastrointest Endosc 2000;51(2):175–9.

44. Caddy GR, Tham TC. Gallstone disease: symptoms, diagnosis and endoscopic management of common bile duct stones. Best Pract Res Clin Gastroenterol 2006;20(6):1085–101.

45. Vaira D, D'Anna L, Ainley C, et al. Endoscopic sphincterotomy in 1000 consecutive patients. Lancet 1989;2(8660):431–4.
46. Freeman ML, Nelson DB, Sherman S, et al. Complications of endoscopic biliary sphincterotomy. N Engl J Med 1996;335(13):909–18.
47. Lambert ME, Betts CD, Hill J, et al. Endoscopic sphincterotomy: the whole truth. Br J Surg 1991;78(4):473–6.
48. Rabenstein T, Ruppert T, Schneider HT, et al. Benefits and risks of needle-knife papillotomy. Gastrointest Endosc 1997;46(3):207–11.
49. Kayhan B, Akdogan M, Sahin B. ERCP subsequent to retroperitoneal perforation caused by endoscopic sphincterotomy. Gastrointest Endosc 2004;60(5):833–5.
50. Oviedo JA, Barrison A, Lichtenstein DR. Endoscopic argon plasma coagulation for refractory postsphincterotomy bleeding: report of two cases. Gastrointest Endosc 2003;58(1):148–51.
51. Mavrogiannis C, Liatsos C, Papanikolaou IS, et al. Safety of extension of a previous endoscopic sphincterotomy: a prospective study. Am J Gastroenterol 2003;98(1):72–6.
52. Hawes RH, Cotton PB, Vallon AG. Follow-up 6 to 11 years after duodenoscopic sphincterotomy for stones in patients with prior cholecystectomy. Gastroenterology 1990;98(4):1008–12.
53. Sugiyama M, Atomi Y. Risk factors predictive of late complications after endoscopic sphincterotomy for bile duct stones: long-term (more than 10 years) follow-up study. Am J Gastroenterol 2002;97(11):2763–7.
54. Leung JW, Banez VP, Chung SC. Precut (needle knife) papillotomy for impacted common bile duct stone at the ampulla. Am J Gastroenterol 1990;85(8):991–3.
55. Mavrogiannis C, Liatsos C, Romanos A, et al. Needle-knife fistulotomy versus needle-knife precut papillotomy for the treatment of common bile duct stones. Gastrointest Endosc 1999;50(3):334–9.
56. Shah JN, Marson F, Weilert F, et al. Single-operator, single-session EUS-guided anterograde cholangiopancreatography in failed ERCP or inaccessible papilla. Gastrointest Endosc 2012;75(1):56–64.
57. Garg PK, Tandon RK, Ahuja V, et al. Predictors of unsuccessful mechanical lithotripsy and endoscopic clearance of large bile duct stones. Gastrointest Endosc 2004;59(6):601–5.
58. Binmoeller KF, Schafer TW. Endoscopic management of bile duct stones. J Clin Gastroenterol 2001;32(2):106–18.
59. Chang WH, Chu CH, Wang TE, et al. Outcome of simple use of mechanical lithotripsy of difficult common bile duct stones. World J Gastroenterol 2005;11(4):593–6.
60. Cipolletta L, Costamagna G, Bianco MA, et al. Endoscopic mechanical lithotripsy of difficult common bile duct stones. Br J Surg 1997;84(10):1407–9.
61. Schneider MU, Matek W, Bauer R, et al. Mechanical lithotripsy of bile duct stones in 209 patients—effect of technical advances. Endoscopy 1988;20(5):248–53.
62. Hintze RE, Adler A, Veltzke W. Outcome of mechanical lithotripsy of bile duct stones in an unselected series of 704 patients. Hepatogastroenterology 1996; 43(9):473–6.
63. Thomas M, Howell DA, Carr-Locke D, et al. Mechanical lithotripsy of pancreatic and biliary stones: complications and available treatment options collected from expert centers. Am J Gastroenterol 2007;102(9):1896–902.
64. Sauter G, Sackmann M, Holl J, et al. Dormia baskets impacted in the bile duct: release by extracorporeal shock-wave lithotripsy. Endoscopy 1995; 27(5):384–7.

65. Ranjeev P, Goh K. Retrieval of an impacted Dormia basket and stone in situ using a novel method. Gastrointest Endosc 2000;51(4 Pt 1):504–6.
66. Hintze RE, Adler A, Veltzke W, et al. Management of traction wire fracture complicating mechanical basket lithotripsy. Endoscopy 1997;29(9):883–5.
67. Maxton DG, Tweedle DE, Martin DF. Retained common bile duct stones after endoscopic sphincterotomy: temporary and longterm treatment with biliary stenting. Gut 1995;36(3):446–9.
68. Bergman JJ, Rauws EA, Tijssen JG, et al. Biliary endoprostheses in elderly patients with endoscopically irretrievable common bile duct stones: report on 117 patients. Gastrointest Endosc 1995;42(3):195–201.
69. Chopra KB, Peters RA, O'Toole PA, et al. Randomised study of endoscopic biliary endoprosthesis versus duct clearance for bileduct stones in high-risk patients. Lancet 1996;348(9030):791–3.
70. Hui CK, Lai KC, Ng M, et al. Retained common bile duct stones: a comparison between biliary stenting and complete clearance of stones by electrohydraulic lithotripsy. Aliment Pharmacol Ther 2003;17(2):289–96.
71. Chan AC, Ng EK, Chung SC, et al. Common bile duct stones become smaller after endoscopic biliary stenting. Endoscopy 1998;30(4):356–9.
72. Jain SK, Stein R, Bhuva M, et al. Pigtail stents: an alternative in the treatment of difficult bile duct stones. Gastrointest Endosc 2000;52(4):490–3.
73. Horiuchi A, Nakayama Y, Kajiyama M, et al. Biliary stenting in the management of large or multiple common bile duct stones. Gastrointest Endosc 2010;71(7): 1200–1203.e2.
74. Cerefice M, Sauer B, Javaid M, et al. Complex biliary stones: treatment with removable self-expandable metal stents: a new approach (with videos). Gastrointest Endosc 2011;74(3):520–6.
75. Johnson GK, Geenen JE, Venu RP, et al. Treatment of non-extractable common bile duct stones with combination ursodeoxycholic acid plus endoprostheses. Gastrointest Endosc 1993;39(4):528–31.
76. Han J, Moon JH, Koo HC, et al. Effect of biliary stenting combined with ursodeoxycholic acid and terpene treatment on retained common bile duct stones in elderly patients: a multicenter study. Am J Gastroenterol 2009;104(10):2418–21.
77. Katsinelos P, Kountouras J, Paroutoglou G, et al. Combination of endoprostheses and oral ursodeoxycholic acid or placebo in the treatment of difficult to extract common bile duct stones. Dig Liver Dis 2008;40(6):453–9.
78. Lee TH, Han JH, Kim HJ, et al. Is the addition of choleretic agents in multiple double-pigtail biliary stents effective for difficult common bile duct stones in elderly patients? A prospective, multicenter study. Gastrointest Endosc 2011; 74(1):96–102.
79. Draganov PV, Evans W, Fazel A, et al. Large size balloon dilation of the ampulla after biliary sphincterotomy can facilitate endoscopic extraction of difficult bile duct stones. J Clin Gastroenterol 2009;43(8):782–6.
80. Ellis RD, Jenkins AP, Thompson RP, et al. Clearance of refractory bile duct stones with extracorporeal shockwave lithotripsy. Gut 2000;47(5):728–31.
81. Amplatz S, Piazzi L, Felder M, et al. Extracorporeal shock wave lithotripsy for clearance of refractory bile duct stones. Dig Liver Dis 2007;39(3):267–72.
82. Sackmann M, Holl J, Sauter GH, et al. Extracorporeal shock wave lithotripsy for clearance of bile duct stones resistant to endoscopic extraction. Gastrointest Endosc 2001;53(1):27–32.
83. Farrell JJ, Bounds BC, Al-Shalabi S, et al. Single-operator duodenoscope-assisted cholangioscopy is an effective alternative in the management of

choledocholithiasis not removed by conventional methods, including mechanical lithotripsy. Endoscopy 2005;37(6):542–7.

84. Chen YK, Pleskow DK. SpyGlass single-operator peroral cholangiopancreatoscopy system for the diagnosis and therapy of bile-duct disorders: a clinical feasibility study (with video). Gastrointest Endosc 2007;65(6):832–41.

85. Arya N, Nelles SE, Haber GB, et al. Electrohydraulic lithotripsy in 111 patients: a safe and effective therapy for difficult bile duct stones. Am J Gastroenterol 2004;99(12):2330–4.

86. Adamek HE, Buttmann A, Wessbecher R, et al. Clinical comparison of extracorporeal piezoelectric lithotripsy (EPL) and intracorporeal electrohydraulic lithotripsy (EHL) in difficult bile duct stones. A prospective randomized trial. Dig Dis Sci 1995;40(6):1185–92.

87. Cotton PB, Kozarek RA, Schapiro RH, et al. Endoscopic laser lithotripsy of large bile duct stones. Gastroenterology 1990;99(4):1128–33.

88. Neuhaus H, Hoffmann W, Zillinger C, et al. Laser lithotripsy of difficult bile duct stones under direct visual control. Gut 1993;34(3):415–21.

89. Ell C, Hochberger J, May A, et al. Laser lithotripsy of difficult bile duct stones by means of a rhodamine-6G laser and an integrated automatic stone-tissue detection system. Gastrointest Endosc 1993;39(6):755–62.

90. Kim HI, Moon JH, Choi HJ, et al. Holmium laser lithotripsy under direct peroral cholangioscopy by using an ultra-slim upper endoscope for patients with retained bile duct stones (with video). Gastrointest Endosc 2011;74(5):1127–32.

91. Kalaitzakis E, Webster GJ, Oppong KW, et al. Diagnostic and therapeutic utility of single-operator peroral cholangioscopy for indeterminate biliary lesions and bile duct stones. Eur J Gastroenterol Hepatol 2012;24(6):656–64.

92. Schreiber F, Gurakuqi GC, Trauner M. Endoscopic intracorporeal laser lithotripsy of difficult common bile duct stones with a stone-recognition pulsed dye laser system. Gastrointest Endosc 1995;42(5):416–9.

93. Moon JH, Ko BM, Choi HJ, et al. Direct peroral cholangioscopy using an ultra-slim upper endoscope for the treatment of retained bile duct stones. Am J Gastroenterol 2009;104(11):2729–33.

94. Neuhaus H, Hoffmann W, Gottlieb K, et al. Endoscopic lithotripsy of bile duct stones using a new laser with automatic stone recognition. Gastrointest Endosc 1994;40(6):708–15.

95. Neuhaus H, Zillinger C, Born P, et al. Randomized study of intracorporeal laser lithotripsy versus extracorporeal shock-wave lithotripsy for difficult bile duct stones. Gastrointest Endosc 1998;47(5):327–34.

96. Jakobs R, Adamek HE, Maier M, et al. Fluoroscopically guided laser lithotripsy versus extracorporeal shock wave lithotripsy for retained bile duct stones: a prospective randomised study. Gut 1997;40(5):678–82.

97. Chen YK, Parsi MA, Binmoeller KF, et al. Single-operator cholangioscopy in patients requiring evaluation of bile duct disease or therapy of biliary stones (with videos). Gastrointest Endosc 2011;74(4):805–14.

98. Disario JA, Freeman ML, Bjorkman DJ, et al. Endoscopic balloon dilation compared with sphincterotomy for extraction of bile duct stones. Gastroenterology 2004;127(5):1291–9.

99. Bergman JJ, Rauws EA, Fockens P, et al. Randomised trial of endoscopic balloon dilation versus endoscopic sphincterotomy for removal of bileduct stones. Lancet 1997;349(9059):1124–9.

100. Baron TH, Harewood GC. Endoscopic balloon dilation of the biliary sphincter compared to endoscopic biliary sphincterotomy for removal of common bile

duct stones during ERCP: a metaanalysis of randomized, controlled trials. Am J Gastroenterol 2004;99(8):1455–60.

101. Park DH, Kim MH, Lee SK, et al. Endoscopic sphincterotomy vs. endoscopic papillary balloon dilation for choledocholithiasis in patients with liver cirrhosis and coagulopathy. Gastrointest Endosc 2004;60(2):180–5.

102. Ersoz G, Tekesin O, Ozutemiz AO, et al. Biliary sphincterotomy plus dilation with a large balloon for bile duct stones that are difficult to extract. Gastrointest Endosc 2003;57(2):156–9.

103. Maydeo A, Bhandari S. Balloon sphincteroplasty for removing difficult bile duct stones. Endoscopy 2007;39(11):958–61.

104. Attasaranya S, Cheon YK, Vittal H, et al. Large-diameter biliary orifice balloon dilation to aid in endoscopic bile duct stone removal: a multicenter series. Gastrointest Endosc 2008;67(7):1046–52.

105. Stefanidis G, Viazis N, Pleskow D, et al. Large balloon dilation vs. mechanical lithotripsy for the management of large bile duct stones: a prospective randomized study. Am J Gastroenterol 2011;106(2):278–85.

106. Itoi T, Itokawa F, Sofuni A, et al. Endoscopic sphincterotomy combined with large balloon dilation can reduce the procedure time and fluoroscopy time for removal of large bile duct stones. Am J Gastroenterol 2009;104(3):560–5.

107. Choi CW, Choi JS, Kang DH, et al. Endoscopic papillary large balloon dilation in Billroth II gastrectomy patients with bile duct stones. J Gastroenterol Hepatol 2012;27(2):256–60.

108. Itoi T, Sofuni A, Itokawa F, et al. New large-diameter balloon-equipped sphincterotome for removal of large bile duct stones (with videos). Gastrointest Endosc 2010;72(4):825–30.

109. Nathanson LK, O'Rourke NA, Martin IJ, et al. Postoperative ERCP versus laparoscopic choledochotomy for clearance of selected bile duct calculi: a randomized trial. Ann Surg 2005;242(2):188–92.

110. Rogers SJ, Cello JP, Horn JK, et al. Prospective randomized trial of LC+LCBDE vs ERCP/S+LC for common bile duct stone disease. Arch Surg 2010;145(1): 28–33.

111. Rhodes M, Sussman L, Cohen L, et al. Randomised trial of laparoscopic exploration of common bile duct versus postoperative endoscopic retrograde cholangiography for common bile duct stones. Lancet 1998;351(9097):159–61.

112. Lu J, Cheng Y, Xiong XZ, et al. Two-stage vs single-stage management for concomitant gallstones and common bile duct stones. World J Gastroenterol 2012;18(24):3156–66.

113. Barkun AN, Barkun JS, Fried GM, et al. Useful predictors of bile duct stones in patients undergoing laparoscopic cholecystectomy. McGill Gallstone Treatment Group. Ann Surg 1994;220(1):32–9.

Endoscopic Evaluation of Bile Duct Strictures

Won Jae Yoon, MD, William R. Brugge, MD*

KEYWORDS

- Bile duct stricture • Endoscopic retrograde cholangiopancreatography
- Fluorescence in situ hybridization • Endoscopic ultrasonography
- Intraductal ultrasonography • Cholangioscopy
- Probe-based confocal laser endomicroscopy • Optical coherence tomography

KEY POINTS

- Cholangiographic impression with brush cytology and/or endobiliary forceps biopsy may offer high sensitivity and specificity.
- Advanced cytologic methods such as fluorescence in situ hybridization and digital image analysis offer modest improvement of sensitivity. These methods may be helpful in patients with presumed malignancy with negative cytology and histology.
- Endoscopic ultrasonography offers imaging of bile duct stricture, staging of lymph nodes, prediction of portal vein invasion, and fine-needle aspiration. Endoscopic retrograde cholangiopancreatography with intraductal ultrasonography may improve the diagnostic yield of bile duct strictures.
- Although conventional (percutaneous or mother-and-babyscope) cholangioscopy with or without biopsy shows impressive performance, it requires percutaneous biliary access with subsequent dilations or 2 endoscopists, with a long procedure time.
- Single-operator cholangioscopy enables peroral cholangioscopy without the need for 2 endoscopists.
- Probe-based confocal laser endomicroscopy and optical coherence tomography may provide in vivo histology. However, more evaluation and refinement is needed as regards their clinical utility.

INTRODUCTION

Bile duct strictures may result from various malignant and benign processes, and differentiating between a malignant and benign stricture is of paramount importance. However, this is not always easily achieved. Even after exhaustive workup, the definite diagnosis of the bile duct stricture may not be obtained. Bile duct strictures are

Conflict of interest: None.
Financial support: None.
Gastrointestinal Unit, Massachusetts General Hospital, Harvard Medical School, 55 Fruit Street, Boston, MA 02114, USA
* Corresponding author.
E-mail address: wbrugge@partners.org

considered indeterminate when cross-sectional imaging is unrevealing and pathology is nondiagnostic.[1,2] This review focuses on endoscopic evaluation of bile duct strictures.

ENDOSCOPIC RETROGRADE CHOLANGIOPANCREATOGRAPHY

Endoscopic retrograde cholangiopancreatography (ERCP) is certainly the most widely used endoscopic procedure in evaluating bile duct strictures.[1] Diagnostically, ERCP provides high-quality images of the bile ducts and enables tissue sampling.[1] Therapeutically, it provides means for biliary drainage (**Fig. 1**)[1] and ablative therapy, such as photodynamic therapy[3] or radiofrequency ablation.[4]

Cholangiographic appearance of the bile duct stricture alone is not adequate to differentiate malignant from benign strictures. Some suggested cholangiographic features of malignant bile duct strictures include a long stricture that is irregular or asymmetric in appearance (**Fig. 2**).[5] In one study, a stricture length of 14 mm or more predicted malignancy with a sensitivity of 78%, specificity of 75%, and log odds ratio of 11.23.[6] The transition zones of malignant bile duct strictures are usually abrupt (<1 cm), with a nodular or round shoulder.[5] Benign strictures tend to have a longer transition zone with a smooth, concentric narrowing (**Fig. 3**). The sensitivity, specificity, positive predictive value (PPV), negative predictive value (NPV), and accuracy of cholangiography (ERCP or percutaneous) in diagnosing malignancy are about 74% to 85%, 70% to 75%, 74% to 79%, 70% to 82%, and 72% to 80%, respectively.[6–8] The low accuracy rates of cholangiography in diagnosing malignancy have stimulated research in tissue acquisition and advanced imaging techniques.

Methods of tissue sampling during ERCP include intraductal bile aspiration cytology, cytopathologic analysis of retrieved plastic biliary stents, fine-needle aspiration (FNA) cytology, brush cytology (**Fig. 4**), and endobiliary forceps biopsy (**Fig. 5**).[9,10] Multimodal tissue sampling can improve the detection of cancer.[10] Brush cytology and endobiliary forceps biopsy are probably the most routinely used method of tissue sampling during ERCP. A review of tissue sampling techniques during ERCP published in 2002 revealed that the sensitivity, specificity, PPV, and NPV of brush cytology

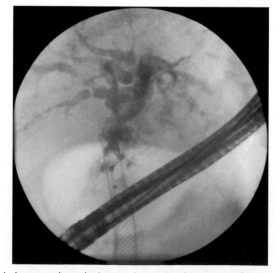

Fig. 1. Fluoroscopic image taken during endoscopic placement of a self-expandable metal stent for the palliation of malignant bile duct stricture.

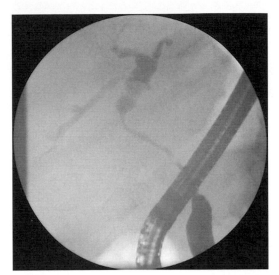

Fig. 2. Endoscopic retrograde cholangiography of a malignant bile duct stricture. Note the long stricture with irregular appearance.

for diagnosis of malignant bile duct stricture were 30% to 57%, 90% to 100%, 94% to 100%, and 8% to 62%, respectively.[10] The poor sensitivity of brush cytology is attributed to sampling error, low cellular yield, and/or misinterpretation of the specimen because of subtle differences between malignant and nonmalignant cells.[11,12] Primary sclerosing cholangitis adds more difficulty to the interpretation of the cytology specimens, as reactive cells may mimic malignant cells, thus lowering the specificity of cytology.[13–15] Various methods have been tested to increase the sensitivity of brush cytology, including stricture dilation and repeat brushing,[16] a novel (and longer)

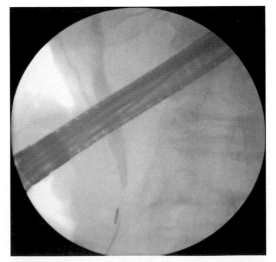

Fig. 3. An example of benign bile duct stricture: distal common bile duct stricture secondary to autoimmune pancreatitis. Note the smooth, concentric narrowing.

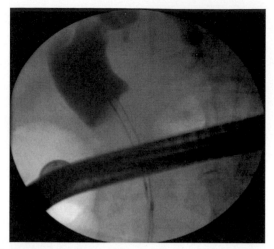

Fig. 4. Fluoroscopic image of brush cytology performed during ERCP.

cytology brush,[17] and a combination of stricture dilation, endoscopic needle aspiration, and brush cytology.[18] Of these techniques, repeat brushing seems to improve the rate of cancer detection.[19]

Endobiliary forceps biopsy of the bile duct has many advantages over brush cytology. The reported sensitivity, specificity, PPV, and NPV of endobiliary forceps biopsy for diagnosis of malignant bile duct stricture are 43% to 81%, 90% to 100%, 94% to 100%, and 31% to 75%, respectively.[10] Endobiliary forceps biopsy apparently offers a modestly improved sensitivity compared with brush cytology. Biliary sphincterotomy may be required to pass the forceps to the bile duct stricture.[1] However, passing the forceps along a guidewire without sphincterotomy is possible.[20,21]

Review of the literature shows that the highest overall tissue yield is achieved when at least 2 tissue-sampling methods are combined. Combining brush cytology with

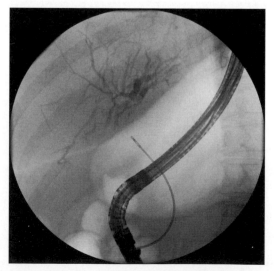

Fig. 5. Fluoroscopic image during an endobiliary forceps biopsy.

forceps biopsy increases the sensitivity for diagnosis of a malignant bile duct stricture up to 73.5%.[10,22] Although it can be argued that combining tissue-sampling methods may be more time consuming, one study reported that the mean time needed for brush cytology plus forceps biopsy was 11.7 minutes, with the mean duration of the entire procedure (ERCP, sphincterotomy, brush cytology, forceps biopsy, and biliary drainage) being 57.8 minutes.[22]

Because ERCP with cytology and/or endobiliary biopsy is usually performed after cross-sectional imaging, failure to obtain a diagnosis would render the bile duct stricture indeterminate. Because of the low sensitivity of the cytology, advanced cytologic methods, such as fluorescence in situ hybridization (FISH) and digital image analysis (DIA), have been used recently. FISH is a cytogenetic technique that detects and localizes the presence or absence of specific DNA sequences on chromosomes by using fluorescently labeled DNA probes. The DNA probes bind to the area of sequence complementarity on chromosomes.[23] FISH has been shown to detect malignancy in cytology specimens obtained from the bladder,[24] breast,[25] and lung.[26] DIA quantifies the microscopic images of a cell by digital conversion and computer analysis,[27] and can be used to quantify nuclear DNA content and evaluate nuclear features.

The first reports on the utility of FISH[28] and DIA[29] for the detection of malignant bile duct stricture were published in 2004. Kipp and colleagues[28] used fluorescently labeled probes to the centromeres of chromosomes 3, 7, and 17 and chromosomal band 9p21. Positivity for malignancy was defined as at least 5 cells exhibiting polysomy (gain of 2 or more chromosomes within a single cell). The sensitivity to detect malignancy was significantly higher for FISH (34%) than for routine cytology (15%). However, there was a tendency for FISH to have a lower specificity than routine cytology (91% vs 98%, $P = .06$).[28] Although this study was criticized for the unusual low sensitivity of routine cytology, it suggested that FISH may be a useful modality for detecting malignant bile duct strictures.[30] Baron and colleagues[29] compared the accuracy of DIA and routine cytology in 110 patients undergoing ERCP for bile duct strictures. The sensitivity, specificity, PPV, NPV, and accuracy of DIA for the detection of malignancy were 39.3%, 77.3%, 68.8%, 50.0%, and 56.0%, respectively. Compared with routine cytology, DIA demonstrated significantly higher sensitivity and lower specificity.[29] In a study that evaluated the diagnostic utility of routine cytology, FISH, and DIA in assessing pancreaticobiliary strictures, routine cytology demonstrated low sensitivity (4%–20%) but 100% specificity. When routine cytology was negative, FISH increased the sensitivity (35%–60%) when assessing for polysomy while maintaining the specificity of cytology. The sensitivity and specificity of DIA were intermediate in comparison with routine cytology and FISH.[31] In another study, the sensitivity/specificity of routine cytology, FISH (polysomy considered positive), and DIA were 15%/100%, 44%/98%, and 43%/92%, respectively.[32] DIA and FISH may be helpful in cases where the cytology and histology are both negative for malignancy. Levy and colleagues[33] demonstrated that in the subset of 21 patients with malignant bile duct strictures with negative cytology and histology, a diagnosis of malignancy was established by DIA, FISH, and composite DIA/FISH in 14%, 62%, and 67%, respectively. In this study the overall sensitivity, specificity, PPV, NPV, and accuracy of FISH (trisomy 7 considered benign) were 45%, 100%, 100%, 60%, and 70%, respectively. DIA showed an overall sensitivity, specificity, PPV, NPV, and accuracy of 38%, 95%, 90%, 56%, and 64%, respectively.[33] In a multivariable analysis of advanced cytologic methods for the evaluation of indeterminate pancreaticobiliary strictures, the sensitivity of polysomy FISH (42.9%) was higher than that of routine cytology (20.1%). FISH was independently associated with malignancy, whereas DIA was not.[34] Gonda and colleagues[35] recently reported that including the deletion of the 9p21 locus (p16) in the diagnostic criteria of FISH for malignant bile duct strictures can increase the sensitivity of FISH from 47% to 84% without compromising the specificity.

Similar to that of routine cytology, the specificity of FISH decreases in primary sclerosing cholangitis. Indeed, in a study that looked at the long-term outcome of 235 patients with primary sclerosing cholangitis with at least one FISH, the specificity of FISH polysomy was 88% and its sensitivity was 46%.[36]

ENDOSCOPIC ULTRASONOGRAPHY

Endoscopic ultrasonography (EUS) may be useful in the evaluation of bile duct strictures, as it readily visualizes the common bile duct. In addition, EUS offers the advantages of permitting FNA and lymph node staging, and predicting portal vein invasion. However, strictures of the common hepatic duct and hilar area are sometimes not visualized.[37]

In a meta-analysis of 9 studies (555 subjects) differentiating malignant from benign biliary obstruction, the estimated sensitivity and specificity of EUS without FNA were 78% and 84%, respectively.[38] In one study, EUS features associated with malignancy in patients with bile duct strictures were presence of a pancreatic mass, an irregular bile duct wall, or bile duct wall thickness of 3 mm or more.[39]

Review of the literature regarding the diagnostic performance of EUS-guided FNA (EUS-FNA) shows the reported sensitivity, specificity, PPV, NPV, and accuracy of 43% to 89%, 100%, 100%, 29% to 67%, and 70% to 91%, respectively.[39–47] Two studies showed that the sensitivities of EUS-FNA after negative or unsuccessful ERCP sampling were 68% to 89%.[42,47] One study showed that the sensitivity of EUS-FNA for distal cholangiocarcinoma was higher than that for proximal cholangiocarcinoma (81% vs 59%, P = .04).[47]

The possibility of tumor seeding during EUS-FNA in patients with suspected extrahepatic cholangiocarcinoma is a concern; this is more of an issue for proximal bile duct lesions, as the FNA needle traverses peritoneum and omental fat that will not be resected.[37] One report evaluated the incidence of peritoneal metastasis in patients who underwent transperitoneal FNA of hilar cholangiocarcinoma. Of 191 patients with localized, unresectable hilar cholangiocarcinoma who were scheduled for neoadjuvant chemoradiotherapy followed by liver transplantation, 16 patients underwent transperitoneal FNA biopsy (13 percutaneous and 3 EUS). Six patients had biopsies positive for adenocarcinoma, 5 (83%) of whom were found to have peritoneal metastasis at operative staging. Nine patients who underwent biopsies that did not demonstrate adenocarcinoma had no evidence of metastasis. One patient had an equivocal biopsy. Of 175 patients who did not undergo transperitoneal biopsy, 14 (8%) had peritoneal metastasis. Patients with a positive preoperative FNA were significantly more likely to have peritoneal metastasis than those who did not undergo transperitoneal biopsy (P = .0097). The report, however, did not state how many of the 3 patients who underwent EUS-FNA developed peritoneal metastasis.[48]

INTRADUCTAL ULTRASONOGRAPHY

Intraductal ultrasonography (IDUS) involves introducing a thin (2.0–3.1 mm), high-frequency (12–30 MHz) ultrasound probe into the bile duct under ERCP guidance, providing detailed visualization of the stricture wall within a radius of 2 cm from the probe. The normal bile duct wall is usually visualized as a 2-layer structure, the inner hypoechoic layer and the outer hyperechoic layer. Occasionally an interface echo is seen between the bile and the inner hypoechoic layer.[49]

IDUS features that are suggestive of malignancy include disruption of the normal bile duct structure on IDUS, presence of sessile tumor lesions, tumor size greater than 10 mm, evident hypoechoic infiltrating lesion, hypoechoic masses with irregular margins, heterogeneous echo-poor area invading surrounding tissue, and continuation of the main hypoechoic mass into adjacent structures.[50–54]

The reported sensitivity, specificity, PPV, NPV, and accuracy of IDUS for the diagnosis of malignant bile duct strictures are 83% to 91%, 50% to 92%, 92% to 96%, 67% to 100%, and 76% to 90%, respectively.[50,52,54,55] In one study, adding IDUS to ERCP/tissue sampling significantly increased the sensitivity, NPV, and accuracy from 48.4% to 90.3%, 64% to 90%, and 73.3% to 91.6%, respectively; however, although statistically insignificant, specificity and PPV decreased from 100% to 93.1% and 100% to 93.3%, respectively.[53]

CHOLANGIOSCOPY

Cholangioscopy, which can be done either percutaneously or perorally, enables direct visualization of the bile duct strictures using a cholangioscope (**Fig. 6**). Percutaneous cholangioscopy requires percutaneous biliary access (**Fig. 7**) and repeated subsequent dilatations to allow the insertion of the cholangioscope. Peroral cholangioscopy, traditionally done in mother-and-babyscope scope fashion (**Fig. 8**), requires 2 experienced biliary endoscopists and a long procedure time. Direct peroral cholangioscopy uses ultraslim pediatric or transnasal endoscopes for visualization of the bile duct.[56,57]

In 2000, Seo and colleagues[58] reported their experience of cholangioscopic evaluation of bile duct tumors. According to cholangioscopic findings, adenocarcinoma of the bile duct could be classified into nodular, papillary, and infiltrative types. The nodular types were characterized by the presence of nodular mass with an irregular mucosa and intense neovascularization. Numerous papillary mucosal projections were characteristic of the papillary type. The infiltrative type did not have a definite mass and the tumor appeared as a smooth, tapered narrowing of the lumen. Of note, the neovascularization was usually less intense than that of nodular types. A whitish mucosal discoloration and subtle elevations were visible on the margin of tumor vessels in infiltrative types.[58]

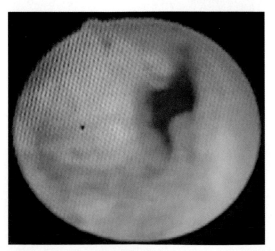

Fig. 6. Cholangioscopic finding of cholangiocarcinoma obstructing the bile duct.

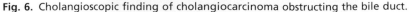

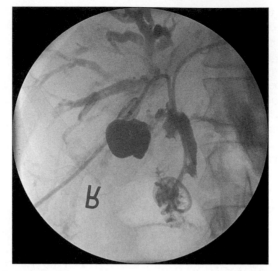

Fig. 7. Fluoroscopic image taken during percutaneous transhepatic biliary drainage. Such percutaneous biliary access, followed by tract dilation, is needed for percutaneous cholangioscopy.

The presence of tumor vessel (an irregularly dilated and tortuous vessel) in a bile duct stricture was reported to indicate the presence of malignancy. In a study of 63 patients with bile duct strictures, tumor vessels were present in 25 of 41 patients with malignant bile duct strictures. Of the 22 patients with benign bile duct strictures, none had tumor vessels. The sensitivity, specificity, PPV, and NPV of tumor vessels for the diagnosis of malignant bile duct stricture were 61%, 100%, 100%, and 57%, respectively. By combining the presence of tumor vessels with histopathologic evaluation of cholangioscopy-guided biopsies, the sensitivity and NPV increased to 96% and 91%, respectively.[59]

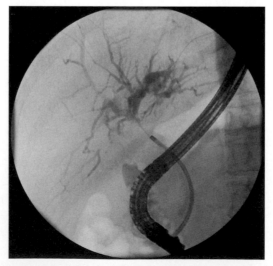

Fig. 8. Peroral cholangioscopy done in mother-and-babyscope fashion.

Peroral cholangioscopy may improve the low sensitivity of ERCP/tissue sampling. In a study of 97 patients who underwent peroral cholangioscopy for the diagnosis of biliary disorders, Fukuda and colleagues[60] reported that the addition of peroral cholangioscopy to ERCP/tissue sampling significantly increased the sensitivity (from 78.1% to 93.4%), NPV (from 68.6% to 100%), and accuracy (from 78.1% to 93.4%) in the diagnosis of malignant bile duct strictures. The addition of peroral cholangioscopy decreased the specificity and PPV without statistical significance.[60] In another study involving 62 patients with indeterminate pancreaticobiliary abnormality (72 examinations; 64 peroral and 8 percutaneous), cholangioscopy with or without biopsy resulted in sensitivity, specificity, PPV, and NPV of 89%, 96%, 89%, and 96%, respectively.[61]

Wire-guided direct cholangioscopy (SpyGlass Direct Visualization System; Microvasive Endoscopy, Boston Scientific, Natick, MA) was recently introduced, allowing single-operator cholangioscopy (SOC) and providing 4-way deflected steering with dedicated irrigation channels. The system comprises a reusable optical probe, a disposable access and delivery catheter, and a disposable biopsy forceps. The outer diameter of the access and delivery catheter is 10F, with a working channel 1.2 mm in diameter and 2 irrigation channels 0.6 mm in diameter.[62]

In a clinical feasibility study involving 35 patients, the procedural success rate of SOC was 91%. Twenty patients underwent SOC-directed biopsy, and the specimens from 19 (95%) patients were found to be adequate for histologic evaluation. The sensitivity and specificity of visual diagnosis to diagnose malignancy were 100% and 77%, respectively. SOC-directed biopsy demonstrated sensitivity and specificity of 71% and 100%, respectively.[63]

A prospective, single-arm, single-center study evaluating the role of SOC in the diagnosis of 36 patients with indeterminate bile duct lesions was reported in 2011. The sensitivity, specificity, PPV, NPV, and accuracy of visual diagnosis to diagnose malignancy were 95%, 79%, 88%, 92%, and 89%, respectively. SOC-directed biopsy showed sensitivity, specificity, PPV, NPV, and accuracy of 82%, 82%, 100%, 100%, and 82%, respectively.[64]

Subsequently, Chen and colleagues[65] reported the results of a multicenter, prospective, observational study that evaluated the utility of SOC in 297 patients requiring evaluation of bile duct disease or biliary stone therapy. The overall procedure success rate was 89%. Ninety-five patients with a final diagnosis (malignant or benign) had all the results of ERCP impression, SOC visual impression, and SOC-directed biopsy available. The sensitivity, specificity, PPV, NPV, and accuracy of each modality for the diagnosis of malignancy were as follows: ERCP impression 51%, 54%, 88%, 77%, and 53%; SOC impression 78%, 82%, 80%, 80%, and 80%; and SOC-directed biopsy 49%, 98%, 100%, 72%, and 75%.

PROBE-BASED CONFOCAL LASER ENDOMICROSCOPY

Confocal laser endomicroscopy (CLE) may provide high-resolution in vivo histology.[66] In CLE, the reflected fluorescence is collected through a small aperture after illuminating an area with a low-power argon blue laser (wavelength 488 nm). Only in-focus light is collected through the small aperture. A computer-based reconstruction of collected images generates high-resolution microscopic images. Probe-based CLE (pCLE) collects microscopic images of the mucosa at a fixed depth, whereas endoscope-based CLE collects microscopic images at multiple but limited depths from the surface.[67]

Fluorescent contrast agents are needed to appreciate cellular details. Intravenous fluorescein is used in most pCLEs.[68] Fluorescein has been shown to be safe, with no serious adverse events and mild adverse events occurring in 1.4% of patients. The commonly administered dose is 2.5 to 5 mL of 10% sodium fluorescein.[69] The pCLE probe can be introduced through the working channel of the duodenoscope during ERCP or that of a cholangioscope.[70]

The initial study by Meining and colleagues[71] evaluated pCLE for the detection of neoplasia in the bile duct. Fourteen patients underwent pCLE of bile duct stricture, which was introduced to the stricture via the accessory channel of a cholangioscope. By applying the pCLE patterns of (1) "dark-gray background without identification of mucosal structures but large white streaks resembling fluorescein-filled tortuous, dilated, and saccular vessels with inconsistent branching" and (2) "a reticular pattern of different gray scales or small dark-gray villous structures but no white streaks," the sensitivity, specificity, and accuracy for the detection of neoplasia were 83%, 88%, and 86%, respectively. For cholangioscopy-guided biopsy the respective values were 50%, 100%, and 79%.[71]

The Miami classification of pCLE findings in the pancreaticobiliary system for evaluation of indeterminate strictures was described as an abstract in 2010, after a consensus meeting.[72] The Miami classification was subsequently published in the form of a review article in 2011.[70] However, the article stated that "specific pCLE image interpretation criteria are under development" for biliary disease. The Miami criteria of pCLE for the prediction of neoplasia in the pancreaticobiliary system have been introduced in subsequent studies. Criteria suggestive of malignancy are (1) thick dark bands (>40 μm), (2) thick white bands (>20 μm), (3) dark clumps, (4) visualized epithelium (villi, glands), and (5) fluorescein leakage. The criteria suggestive of benign strictures are (1) thin dark (branching) bands and (2) thin white bands.[73,74]

A multicenter report of pCLE on the diagnosis of indeterminate pancreaticobiliary strictures reported that the sensitivity, specificity, PPV, NPV, and accuracy of pCLE were 98%, 67%, 71%, 97%, and 81%, respectively. The index pathology demonstrated sensitivity, specificity, PPV, NPV, and accuracy of 45% ($P<.001$ compared with pCLE), 100%, 100%, 69% ($P<.001$ compared with pCLE), and 75%, respectively. The accuracy for combination of ERCP and pCLE was higher than that of ERCP with tissue acquisition (90% vs 73%, $P = .001$).[73] In another report, the presence of irregular vessels, large black bands (>20 μm), and black clumps in pCLE enabled the prediction of neoplasia in bile duct stricture, which gave sensitivity, specificity, and accuracy of 83%, 75%, and 86%, respectively.[75] In the study that validated the Miami criteria, the single criterion that occurred most frequently in malignant cases was epithelial structures. The grouped criteria of "epithelial structures" or "thick white bands," or "thick, dark bands (>40 μm)" or "dark clumps" gave sensitivity, specificity, PPV, and NPV of 97%, 33%, 80%, and 80%, respectively. The interobserver variability was moderate for most criteria.[74]

One study reported that in pCLE of bile duct strictures, a normal reticular pattern without other potential markers of malignancy was observed in all patients without malignancy. Based on histologic evaluation of the rat common bile duct, the investigators suggested that this reticular pattern may correlate with lymphatic ductules.[76]

One of the issues of pCLE in the evaluation of bile duct strictures is interobserver variability. In one study, 6 observers at 5 institutions reviewed 25 de-identified pCLE video clips of indeterminate bile duct strictures. The video clips were interpreted based on Miami classification. Based on kappa statistic, the interobserver agreement for pCLE image interpretation ranged from poor to fair. The only variable that had fair interobserver agreement was the presence of dark bands (all observer κ = 0.3000, $P<.001$). The variable of final diagnosis demonstrated only slight interobserver agreement (all observer κ = 0.149, $P<.0001$).[77]

OPTICAL COHERENCE TOMOGRAPHY

Optical coherence tomography (OCT) uses infrared light to obtain high-resolution, cross-sectional, subsurface tomographic imaging. OCT is similar to ultrasound imaging, except that it uses infrared light. This method's imaging provides depth of penetration of 1 to 3 mm and lateral and axial spatial resolution of 10 μm.[78] OCT offers capabilities distinct from those of other imaging modalities: because the contrast in OCT is derived from light-scattering properties of the tissue, OCT does not require contrast agents or labeling. Also, OCT can obtain deeper images than optical microscopy, and the mechanical components of OCT can be miniaturized, making it possible to integrate OCT optics into small probes, thus enabling it to be used in conjunction to endoscopy. OCT is currently used in ophthalmology and interventional cardiology.[79]

In an ex vivo study comparing OCT images and histology of the common bile duct, OCT was able to obtain images to a depth of approximately 1 mm. From the surface of the duct, 3 layers were recognizable: a thin and regular hyporeflective layer, a larger intermediate hyperreflective layer, and an outer hyporeflective layer. Each layer corresponded with the single layer of epithelial cells, the connective-muscular layer surrounding the epithelium, and the connective tissue with muscular strips, respectively.[80]

Table 1
Summary of diagnostic performances of various endoscopic methods used to evaluate bile duct strictures

Method[Refs.]	Sensitivity (%)	Specificity (%)	PPV (%)	NPV (%)	Accuracy (%)
Cholangiography[6–8,a]	74–85	70–75	74–79	70–82	72–80
Brush cytology[10]	30–57	90–100	94–100	8–62	—
Endobiliary forceps biopsy[10]	43–81	90–100	94–100	31–75	—
FISH[28,31–34,b]	34–48[c]	91–100[c]	100[c]	60–88[c]	70[c]
DIA[29,31–34,b]	38–49	77–98	69–97	50–87	56–64
EUS without FNA[38]	78	84	—	—	—
EUS-guided FNA[39–47]	43–89	100	100	29–67	80–91
IDUS[50,52,54,55]	83–91	50–92	92–96	67–100	76–90
Cholangioscopy[d] with or without biopsy[59–61]	89–96	96–100	89–100	91–96	—
SOC impression[63–65]	78–100	77–82	80–88	80–92	80–89
SOC-guided biopsy[63–65]	49–82	82–100	100	72–100	75–82
pCLE[71,73–75]	83–98	33–88	71–80	80–97	81–86
OCT[83]	79	69	75	73	74

Abbreviations: DIA, digital image analysis; EUS, endoscopic ultrasonography; FISH, fluorescence in situ hybridization; FNA; fine-needle aspiration; IDUS, intraductal ultrasonography; NPV, negative predictive value; OCT, optical coherence tomography; pCLE, probe-based confocal laser endomicroscopy; PPV, positive predictive value; SOC, single-operator cholangioscopy.
  [a] Includes both endoscopic and percutaneous cholangiography.
  [b] Moreno Luna and colleagues[31] stratified the bile duct strictures as proximal or distal without primary sclerosing cholangitis, and strictures in patients with primary sclerosing cholangitis. The values of diagnostic performances for the 3 stratifications were reported separately. For each parameter, the highest value among the stratification was considered representative and selected for this table. For example, sensitivity of FISH polysomy for proximal, distal, and primary sclerosing cholangitis strictures was 31%, 48%, and 47%, respectively; 48% was selected for this table.
  [c] Only FISH trisomy considered malignant.
  [d] Does not include SOC.

The first in vivo application of OCT in the human bile duct was reported in 2001.[81] Subsequent study showed that OCT was able to visualize the epithelial morphology of papillary cholangiocarcinoma in vivo.[82]

Arvanitakis and colleagues[83] evaluated the ability of OCT to detect malignant bile duct strictures in 37 patients. The OCT criteria for malignancy were (1) unrecognizable layer architecture and (2) presence of large, nonreflective areas, which could be considered as tumor vessels. OCT was performed during ERCP on 35 patients. Ultimately, 19 patients had malignant bile duct strictures. The presence of at least 1 criterion was able to detect malignant bile duct stricture with sensitivity, specificity, PPV, NPV, and accuracy of 79%, 69%, 75%, 73%, and 74%, respectively. The presence of both criteria resulted in sensitivity, specificity, PPV, NPV, and accuracy of 53%, 100%, 100%, 64%, and 74%, respectively. The sensitivity of bile duct brushings and/or biopsy was 67%, which increased to 84% when pathology and at least 1 criterion were combined.[83]

SUMMARY

The diagnostic performances of the endoscopic methods reviewed in this article are summarized in **Table 1**. Only the values that were presented in the actual articles are listed.

ERCP with brush cytology and/or endobiliary forceps biopsy is undoubtedly the initial and most widely used method for the evaluation of bile duct strictures endoscopically. Combining cholangiographic impression with cytology and/or endobiliary forceps biopsy may offer sensitivity up to 85% and specificity up to 100%. Advanced cytologic methods, such as FISH or DIA, offer modest improvement of sensitivity. It seems that these methods may be helpful in patients with presumed malignancy with negative cytology and histology. EUS offers imaging of bile duct strictures, lymph node staging, prediction of portal vein invasion, and FNA. ERCP with IDUS may improve the diagnostic yield of bile duct strictures. Although conventional (percutaneous or mother-and-babyscope) cholangioscopy with or without biopsy shows impressive performance, it is hindered by the need for a percutaneous biliary access with subsequent dilations, or 2 endoscopists with a long procedure time. SOC may be a breakthrough in cholangioscopy, as it enables peroral cholangioscopy without the need for 2 endoscopists. pCLE and OCT may provide in vivo histology; however, both need more evaluation and refinement of their clinical utility.

REFERENCES

1. Petersen BT. Indeterminate biliary stricture. In: Baron TH, Kozarek R, Carr-Locke DL, editors. ERCP. Philadelphia: Elsevier Saunders; 2008. p. 313–25.
2. Khashab MA, Fockens P, Al-Haddad MA. Utility of EUS in patients with indeterminate biliary strictures and suspected extrahepatic cholangiocarcinoma (with videos). Gastrointest Endosc 2012;76:1024–33.
3. Zoepf T, Jakobs R, Arnold JC, et al. Palliation of nonresectable bile duct cancer: improved survival after photodynamic therapy. Am J Gastroenterol 2005;100: 2426–30.
4. Steel AW, Postgate AJ, Khorsandi S, et al. Endoscopically applied radiofrequency ablation appears to be safe in the treatment of malignant biliary obstruction. Gastrointest Endosc 2011;73:149–53.
5. Taylor AJ. Endoscopic retrograde cholangiopancreatography. In: Gore RM, Levine MS, editors. Textbook of gastrointestinal radiology. 3rd edition. Philadelphia: Elsevier Saunders; 2008. p. 1357–81.

6. Bain VG, Abraham N, Jhangri GS, et al. Prospective study of biliary strictures to determine the predictors of malignancy. Can J Gastroenterol 2000;14:397–402.
7. Rosch T, Meining A, Fruhmorgen S, et al. A prospective comparison of the diagnostic accuracy of ERCP, MRCP, CT, and EUS in biliary strictures. Gastrointest Endosc 2002;55:870–6.
8. Park MS, Kim TK, Kim KW, et al. Differentiation of extrahepatic bile duct cholangiocarcinoma from benign stricture: findings at MRCP versus ERCP. Radiology 2004;233:234–40.
9. De Bellis M, Sherman S, Fogel EL, et al. Tissue sampling at ERCP in suspected malignant biliary strictures (part 1). Gastrointest Endosc 2002;56:552–61.
10. de Bellis M, Sherman S, Fogel EL, et al. Tissue sampling at ERCP in suspected malignant biliary strictures (part 2). Gastrointest Endosc 2002;56:720–30.
11. Kocjan G, Smith AN. Bile duct brushings cytology: potential pitfalls in diagnosis. Diagn Cytopathol 1997;16:358–63.
12. Logrono R, Kurtycz DF, Molina CP, et al. Analysis of false-negative diagnoses on endoscopic brush cytology of biliary and pancreatic duct strictures: the experience at 2 university hospitals. Arch Pathol Lab Med 2000;124:387–92.
13. Ryan ME, Baldauf MC. Comparison of flow cytometry for DNA content and brush cytology for detection of malignancy in pancreaticobiliary strictures. Gastrointest Endosc 1994;40:133–9.
14. Ponsioen CY, Vrouenraets SM, van Milligen de Wit AW, et al. Value of brush cytology for dominant strictures in primary sclerosing cholangitis. Endoscopy 1999;31:305–9.
15. Harewood GC, Baron TH, Stadheim LM, et al. Prospective, blinded assessment of factors influencing the accuracy of biliary cytology interpretation. Am J Gastroenterol 2004;99:1464–9.
16. de Bellis M, Fogel EL, Sherman S, et al. Influence of stricture dilation and repeat brushing on the cancer detection rate of brush cytology in the evaluation of malignant biliary obstruction. Gastrointest Endosc 2003;58:176–82.
17. Fogel EL, deBellis M, McHenry L, et al. Effectiveness of a new long cytology brush in the evaluation of malignant biliary obstruction: a prospective study. Gastrointest Endosc 2006;63:71–7.
18. Farrell RJ, Jain AK, Brandwein SL, et al. The combination of stricture dilation, endoscopic needle aspiration, and biliary brushings significantly improves diagnostic yield from malignant bile duct strictures. Gastrointest Endosc 2001;54:587–94.
19. Barkun A, Liu J, Carpenter S, et al. Update on endoscopic tissue sampling devices. Gastrointest Endosc 2006;63:741–5.
20. Lin LF, Siauw CP, Ho KS, et al. Guidewire technique for endoscopic transpapillary procurement of bile duct biopsy specimens without endoscopic sphincterotomy. Gastrointest Endosc 2003;58:272–4.
21. Higashizawa T, Tamada K, Tomiyama T, et al. Biliary guidewire facilitates bile duct biopsy and endoscopic drainage. J Gastroenterol Hepatol 2002;17:332–6.
22. Kitajima Y, Ohara H, Nakazawa T, et al. Usefulness of transpapillary bile duct brushing cytology and forceps biopsy for improved diagnosis in patients with biliary strictures. J Gastroenterol Hepatol 2007;22:1615–20.
23. Brugge WR, Wallace MB. FISHing: new methods to improve the diagnostic sensitivity of fine needle aspiration cytology. Gastroenterology 2012;142:1055–7.
24. Kipp BR, Karnes RJ, Brankley SM, et al. Monitoring intravesical therapy for superficial bladder cancer using fluorescence in situ hybridization. J Urol 2005;173:401–4.

25. Gu M, Ghafari S, Zhao M. Fluorescence in situ hybridization for HER-2/neu amplification of breast carcinoma in archival fine needle aspiration biopsy specimens. Acta Cytol 2005;49:471–6.
26. Ylagan LR, Liu LH, Maluf HM. Endoscopic bile duct brushing of malignant pancreatic biliary strictures: retrospective study with comparison of conventional smear and ThinPrep techniques. Diagn Cytopathol 2003;28:196–204.
27. Sebo TJ. Digital image analysis. Mayo Clin Proc 1995;70:81–2.
28. Kipp BR, Stadheim LM, Halling SA, et al. A comparison of routine cytology and fluorescence in situ hybridization for the detection of malignant bile duct strictures. Am J Gastroenterol 2004;99:1675–81.
29. Baron TH, Harewood GC, Rumalla A, et al. A prospective comparison of digital image analysis and routine cytology for the identification of malignancy in biliary tract strictures. Clin Gastroenterol Hepatol 2004;2:214–9.
30. Wamsteker EJ, Anderson MA. Fluorescence in situ hybridization for the detection of malignant bile duct strictures: has FISH found a new pond? Am J Gastroenterol 2004;99:1682–3.
31. Moreno Luna LE, Kipp B, Halling KC, et al. Advanced cytologic techniques for the detection of malignant pancreatobiliary strictures. Gastroenterology 2006;131: 1064–72.
32. Barr Fritcher EG, Kipp BR, Slezak JM, et al. Correlating routine cytology, quantitative nuclear morphometry by digital image analysis, and genetic alterations by fluorescence in situ hybridization to assess the sensitivity of cytology for detecting pancreatobiliary tract malignancy. Am J Clin Pathol 2007;128:272–9.
33. Levy MJ, Baron TH, Clayton AC, et al. Prospective evaluation of advanced molecular markers and imaging techniques in patients with indeterminate bile duct strictures. Am J Gastroenterol 2008;103:1263–73.
34. Fritcher EG, Kipp BR, Halling KC, et al. A multivariable model using advanced cytologic methods for the evaluation of indeterminate pancreatobiliary strictures. Gastroenterology 2009;136:2180–6.
35. Gonda TA, Glick MP, Sethi A, et al. Polysomy and p16 deletion by fluorescence in situ hybridization in the diagnosis of indeterminate biliary strictures. Gastrointest Endosc 2012;75:74–9.
36. Bangarulingam SY, Bjornsson E, Enders F, et al. Long-term outcomes of positive fluorescence in situ hybridization tests in primary sclerosing cholangitis. Hepatology 2010;51:174–80.
37. Topazian M. Endoscopic ultrasonography in the evaluation of indeterminate biliary strictures. Clin Endosc 2012;45:328–30.
38. Garrow D, Miller S, Sinha D, et al. Endoscopic ultrasound: a meta-analysis of test performance in suspected biliary obstruction. Clin Gastroenterol Hepatol 2007;5: 616–23.
39. Lee JH, Salem R, Aslanian H, et al. Endoscopic ultrasound and fine-needle aspiration of unexplained bile duct strictures. Am J Gastroenterol 2004;99:1069–73.
40. Fritscher-Ravens A, Broering DC, Sriram PV, et al. EUS-guided fine-needle aspiration cytodiagnosis of hilar cholangiocarcinoma: a case series. Gastrointest Endosc 2000;52:534–40.
41. Eloubeidi MA, Chen VK, Jhala NC, et al. Endoscopic ultrasound-guided fine needle aspiration biopsy of suspected cholangiocarcinoma. Clin Gastroenterol Hepatol 2004;2:209–13.
42. Fritscher-Ravens A, Broering DC, Knoefel WT, et al. EUS-guided fine-needle aspiration of suspected hilar cholangiocarcinoma in potentially operable patients with negative brush cytology. Am J Gastroenterol 2004;99:45–51.

43. Byrne MF, Gerke H, Mitchell RM, et al. Yield of endoscopic ultrasound-guided fine-needle aspiration of bile duct lesions. Endoscopy 2004;36:715–9.
44. Rosch T, Hofrichter K, Frimberger E, et al. ERCP or EUS for tissue diagnosis of biliary strictures? A prospective comparative study. Gastrointest Endosc 2004; 60:390–6.
45. Meara RS, Jhala D, Eloubeidi MA, et al. Endoscopic ultrasound-guided FNA biopsy of bile duct and gallbladder: analysis of 53 cases. Cytopathology 2006;17:42–9.
46. DeWitt J, Misra VL, Leblanc JK, et al. EUS-guided FNA of proximal biliary strictures after negative ERCP brush cytology results. Gastrointest Endosc 2006;64:325–33.
47. Mohamadnejad M, DeWitt JM, Sherman S, et al. Role of EUS for preoperative evaluation of cholangiocarcinoma: a large single-center experience. Gastrointest Endosc 2011;73:71–8.
48. Heimbach JK, Sanchez W, Rosen CB, et al. Trans-peritoneal fine needle aspiration biopsy of hilar cholangiocarcinoma is associated with disease dissemination. HPB (Oxford) 2011;13:356–60.
49. Fujita N, Noda Y, Kobayashi G, et al. Intraductal ultrasonography (IDUS) for the diagnosis of biliopancreatic diseases. Best Pract Res Clin Gastroenterol 2009; 23:729–42.
50. Tamada K, Ueno N, Tomiyama T, et al. Characterization of biliary strictures using intraductal ultrasonography: comparison with percutaneous cholangioscopic biopsy. Gastrointest Endosc 1998;47:341–9.
51. Tamada K, Tomiyama T, Wada S, et al. Endoscopic transpapillary bile duct biopsy with the combination of intraductal ultrasonography in the diagnosis of biliary strictures. Gut 2002;50:326–31.
52. Vazquez-Sequeiros E, Baron TH, Clain JE, et al. Evaluation of indeterminate bile duct strictures by intraductal US. Gastrointest Endosc 2002;56:372–9.
53. Farrell RJ, Agarwal B, Brandwein SL, et al. Intraductal US is a useful adjunct to ERCP for distinguishing malignant from benign biliary strictures. Gastrointest Endosc 2002;56:681–7.
54. Stavropoulos S, Larghi A, Verna E, et al. Intraductal ultrasound for the evaluation of patients with biliary strictures and no abdominal mass on computed tomography. Endoscopy 2005;37:715–21.
55. Menzel J, Poremba C, Dietl KH, et al. Preoperative diagnosis of bile duct strictures—comparison of intraductal ultrasonography with conventional endosonography. Scand J Gastroenterol 2000;35:77–82.
56. Chin MW, Byrne MF. Update of cholangioscopy and biliary strictures. World J Gastroenterol 2011;17:3864–9.
57. Itoi T, Moon JH, Waxman I. Current status of direct peroral cholangioscopy. Dig Endosc 2011;23(Suppl 1):154–7.
58. Seo DW, Lee SK, Yoo KS, et al. Cholangioscopic findings in bile duct tumors. Gastrointest Endosc 2000;52:630–4.
59. Kim HJ, Kim MH, Lee SK, et al. Tumor vessel: a valuable cholangioscopic clue of malignant biliary stricture. Gastrointest Endosc 2000;52:635–8.
60. Fukuda Y, Tsuyuguchi T, Sakai Y, et al. Diagnostic utility of peroral cholangioscopy for various bile-duct lesions. Gastrointest Endosc 2005;62:374–82.
61. Shah RJ, Langer DA, Antillon MR, et al. Cholangioscopy and cholangioscopic forceps biopsy in patients with indeterminate pancreaticobiliary pathology. Clin Gastroenterol Hepatol 2006;4:219–25.
62. Chen YK. Preclinical characterization of the Spyglass peroral cholangiopancreatoscopy system for direct access, visualization, and biopsy. Gastrointest Endosc 2007;65:303–11.

63. Chen YK, Pleskow DK. SpyGlass single-operator peroral cholangiopancreato-scopy system for the diagnosis and therapy of bile-duct disorders: a clinical feasibility study (with video). Gastrointest Endosc 2007;65:832–41.

64. Ramchandani M, Reddy DN, Gupta R, et al. Role of single-operator peroral chol-angioscopy in the diagnosis of indeterminate biliary lesions: a single-center, prospective study. Gastrointest Endosc 2011;74:511–9.

65. Chen YK, Parsi MA, Binmoeller KF, et al. Single-operator cholangioscopy in patients requiring evaluation of bile duct disease or therapy of biliary stones (with videos). Gastrointest Endosc 2011;74:805–14.

66. Dunbar K, Canto M. Confocal endomicroscopy. Curr Opin Gastroenterol 2008;24:631–7.

67. Canto MI. Endomicroscopy of Barrett's esophagus. Gastroenterol Clin North Am 2010;39:759–69.

68. Wallace MB, Fockens P. Probe-based confocal laser endomicroscopy. Gastroen-terology 2009;136:1509–13.

69. Wallace MB, Meining A, Canto MI, et al. The safety of intravenous fluorescein for confocal laser endomicroscopy in the gastrointestinal tract. Aliment Pharmacol Ther 2010;31:548–52.

70. Wallace M, Lauwers GY, Chen Y, et al. Miami classification for probe-based confocal laser endomicroscopy. Endoscopy 2011;43:882–91.

71. Meining A, Frimberger E, Becker V, et al. Detection of cholangiocarcinoma in vivo using miniprobe-based confocal fluorescence microscopy. Clin Gastroenterol Hepatol 2008;6:1057–60.

72. Chen YK, Shah RJ, Pleskow DK, et al. Miami classification (MC) of probe-based laser endomicroscopy (pCLE) findings in the pancreaticobiliary (PB) system for evaluation of indeterminate strictures: interim results from an international multi-center registry. Gastrointest Endosc 2010;71:AB134.

73. Meining A, Chen YK, Pleskow D, et al. Direct visualization of indeterminate pan-creaticobiliary strictures with probe-based confocal laser endomicroscopy: a multicenter experience. Gastrointest Endosc 2011;74:961–8.

74. Meining A, Shah RJ, Slivka A, et al. Classification of probe-based confocal laser endomicroscopy findings in pancreaticobiliary strictures. Endoscopy 2012;44:251–7.

75. Giovannini M, Bories E, Monges G, et al. Results of a phase I-II study on intraduc-tal confocal microscopy (IDCM) in patients with common bile duct (CBD) stenosis. Surg Endosc 2011;25:2247–53.

76. Loeser CS, Robert ME, Mennone A, et al. Confocal endomicroscopic examination of malignant biliary strictures and histologic correlation with lymphatics. J Clin Gastroenterol 2011;45:246–52.

77. Talreja JP, Sethi A, Jamidar PA, et al. Interpretation of probe-based confocal laser endomicroscopy of indeterminate biliary strictures: is there any interobserver agreement? Dig Dis Sci 2012;57:3299–302.

78. Testoni PA, Mangiavillano B. Optical coherence tomography in detection of dysplasia and cancer of the gastrointestinal tract and bilio-pancreatic ductal system. World J Gastroenterol 2008;14:6444–52.

79. Vakoc BJ, Fukumura D, Jain RK, et al. Cancer imaging by optical coherence tomography: preclinical progress and clinical potential. Nat Rev Cancer 2012;12:363–8.

80. Testoni PA, Mariani A, Mangiavillano B, et al. Main pancreatic duct, common bile duct and sphincter of Oddi structure visualized by optical coherence tomog-raphy: an ex vivo study compared with histology. Dig Liver Dis 2006;38:409–14.

81. Seitz U, Freund J, Jaeckle S, et al. First in vivo optical coherence tomography in the human bile duct. Endoscopy 2001;33:1018–21.
82. Poneros JM, Tearney GJ, Shiskov M, et al. Optical coherence tomography of the biliary tree during ERCP. Gastrointest Endosc 2002;55:84–8.
83. Arvanitakis M, Hookey L, Tessier G, et al. Intraductal optical coherence tomography during endoscopic retrograde cholangiopancreatography for investigation of biliary strictures. Endoscopy 2009;41:696–701.

Endoscopic Management of Benign Bile Duct Strictures

Todd H. Baron Sr, MD, FASGE[a],*, Tomas DaVee, MD[b]

KEYWORDS

- ERCP • Biliary strictures • Liver transplant • Sclerosing cholangitis
- Autoimmune cholangiopathy • Pancreatitis • Biliary strictures • Endoscopic therapy

KEY POINTS

- This article discusses the diverse causes of benign biliary strictures, including strictures caused by postoperative adverse events, primary sclerosing cholangitis, chronic pancreatitis, ischemia, and autoimmune cholangiopathy.
- Endoscopic evaluation and treatment are the standard of practice, with specific management based on correctly identifying the underlying cause, characteristics, and location of the stricture(s). The relative merits of endoscopic retrograde cholangiopancreatography (ERCP) with dilation, plastic stents, and self-expandable metal stents are discussed.
- The most common therapy for benign biliary strictures involves ERCP with balloon dilation and placement of multiple plastic stents in a side-by-side fashion, followed by the periodic exchange of these stents for approximately 1 year to allow for expansion and remodeling of the stricture(s).
- The use of covered, self-expandable, removable metal stents for the treatment of benign biliary strictures is under investigation; clinical trials are underway to determine the best management approach.

INTRODUCTION

Benign biliary strictures (BBS) are rarely encountered in the general population and require coordinated care between medical, surgical, pathologic, and radiologic specialties for appropriate evaluation and management. Differentiation of BBS from malignant causes of biliary stricture and obstruction is not always straightforward, with malignant causes being more common. BBS have diverse causes, each with different natural histories and management strategies, most of which incorporate the use of endoscopic retrograde cholangiopancreatography (ERCP). The causes of BBS are shown in **Box 1**. Depending on the severity of the obstruction, the clinical presentation of a biliary stricture may vary from subclinical disease with mild increase

[a] Mayo Clinic, Division of Gastroenterology and Hepatology, 200 First Street, South West Rochester, MN, 55905, USA; [b] Stanford University Medical Center, Department of Internal Medicine, 300 Pasteur Drive, Lane 154, Stanford, CA, 94305, USA
* Corresponding author.
E-mail address: baron.todd@mayo.edu

Gastrointest Endoscopy Clin N Am 23 (2013) 295–311
http://dx.doi.org/10.1016/j.giec.2013.01.001
1052-5157/13/$ – see front matter © 2013 Elsevier Inc. All rights reserved.

Box 1
The POT-I3 classification system of BBS

Postoperative strictures

CCY: open or laparoscopic

Orthotopic liver transplant: deceased donor and living related donor transplants

Biliary-enteric anastomosis: hepaticojejunostomy, choledochojejunostomy, and pancreaticoduodenectomy (Whipple procedure)

ERCP: biliary sphincterotomy, dilation, and stenting

Percutaneous therapy for hepatocellular carcinoma: transcatheter arterial chemoembolization, radiofrequency ablation, percutaneous ethanol injection

Radiation therapy

Traumatic

Choledocholithiasis

Pancreatolithiasis

Mirizzi syndrome

Physical injury: motorized vehicle accident, blunt abdominal trauma

Ischemic

Hypotension

Hepatic artery thrombosis or stenosis

Prolonged transplant organ ischemia: warm and cold ischemic times

Portal biliopathy

Inflammatory

Chronic pancreatitis

Primary sclerosing cholangitis

Autoimmune cholangiopathy (immunoglobulin G4–associated cholangiopathy)

Vasculitis: systemic lupus erythematosus, antineutrophil cytoplasmic antibody –associated vasculitis, Behçet disease

Infectious

Recurrent pyogenic cholangitis

Parasitosis: *Ascaris lumbricoides*, *Clonorchis sinensis*, and *Opisthorchis viverrini*

Granulomatous: tuberculosis, histoplasmosis

Viral: cytomegalovirus, human immunodeficiency virus

Abbreviations: I3, Ischemic, Inflammatory and Infectious; PO, Postoperative strictures; T, Traumatic.

---

of liver function tests alone to complete biliary obstruction with resultant jaundice, with or without cholangitis. In some cases, symptoms may not develop until years after the initial insult, with delayed presentation mostly commonly seen with ischemic causes of bile duct injury. The most common cause of BBS in the Western world is surgical injury to the bile duct, particularly during cholecystectomy (CCY).[1] Inflammatory injuries to the biliary ducts are the second most common cause of BBS, and include diseases such as chronic pancreatitis, primary sclerosing cholangitis, and autoimmune cholangiopathy. Complete occlusion or transection of the common bile duct (CBD) generally requires surgical management.

CLASSIFICATION

There are 2 main classification systems used to evaluate biliary duct strictures. The Bismuth classification, which is most commonly used, is based on stricture location (**Table 1**). The Strasberg classification (**Table 2**) describes the anatomy and characteristics of the stricture.[2,3]

GENERAL PRINCIPLES OF ENDOSCOPIC THERAPY FOR BBS

ERCP has emerged as the therapeutic intervention of choice for managing biliary strictures, both benign and malignant. Selective cannulation of the CBD during ERCP is the prerequisite on which all diagnostic and therapeutic biliary procedures are based.[4]

Treatment of benign biliary strictures (not related to primary sclerosing cholangitis [PSC]) during ERCP involves the following steps:

1. Passing the endoscope (with native anatomy, a side-viewing endoscope) through the mouth and into the duodenum.
2. Aligning the sphincterotome so that the major duodenal papilla is at the 11 o'clock position.
3. Superficially cannulating the papilla is then followed by using a guidewire and/or contrast injection to visualize the course of the CBD and to allow selective biliary cannulation.
4. If selective biliary cannulation is difficult, experienced endoscopists may choose to perform a precut (access) sphincterotomy to facilitate cannulating the CBD.[4]
5. Obtaining a cholangiogram to estimate the diameter of the biliary ducts and the length of the stricture(s) by injecting contrast into the CBD under fluoroscopy.
6. Dilating the stricture by either balloon or bougie may be useful before stenting, and is required when placing multiple large-bore plastic stents (ie, 10 Fr).
7. Balloon dilation is performed using 4-mm to 12-mm diameter balloons advanced over a guidewire and across the stricture under fluoroscopic guidance. The balloon is maintained fully inflated for 30 to 60 seconds.
8. Inserting rigid plastic biliary stents side by side. Depending on the diameter of the stricture and distal bile duct diameters, 1 or 2 stents are initially placed.
9. During the next year of treatment, the patient returns every 3 to 4 months for periodic dilation and stent exchange and placement of additional stents up to a maximum of usually 5 or 6 (**Fig. 1**).

Table 1 Bismuth classification for BBS	
Bismuth Classification	**Location**
I	>2 cm distal to hepatic confluence
II	<2 cm distal to hepatic confluence
III	At the level of the hepatic confluence
IV	Involves the right or left hepatic duct
V	Extends into the left or right hepatic branch ducts

Table 2	
Strasberg classification for BBS	
Class	**Description**
A	Injury to small ducts in continuity with biliary system, with cystic duct leak
B	Injury to sectoral duct with consequent obstruction
C	Injury to sectoral duct with consequent bile leak from a duct not in continuity with biliary system
D	Injury lateral to extrahepatic ducts
E1	Stricture located >2 cm from bile duct confluence
E2	Stricture located <2 cm from bile duct confluence
E3	Stricture located at bile duct confluence
E4	Stricture involving right and left bile ducts
E5	Complete occlusion of all bile ducts

Placing multiple side-by-side, large-bore plastic stents has been shown to improve long-term outcomes of BBS compared with placing 1 or 2 stents alone.[5–7] The dilation of anastomotic strictures within the perioperative period (<30 days after surgery) carries a higher risk of perforation and resultant bile leak. In such cases, the strictures are dilated less aggressively using smaller balloons/bougies.[8,9] With regard to the stent exchange interval, inserting multiple plastic biliary stents for benign (nonhilar) strictures after 6 postoperative months, compared with exchange within 6 months, is associated with a low rate of symptomatic stent occlusion and a longer occlusion-free survival.[10]

USE OF A GUIDEWIRE

Accepted nomenclature in Europe and the United States regarding guidewires dictates that they are measured by inches.[11,12] Standard 0.035-inch guidewires are commonly used to traverse BBS. Traversing tight strictures may require specialized guidewires, such as those with an angulated tip, hydrophilic coating, or small diameter 0.021 inch and 0.018 inch. A stone extraction balloon may be inflated below the stricture while gently applying distal traction to help straighten the CBD and allow for guidewire passage. Hydrophilic guidewires can be exchanged for stiffer 0.035-inch wires, or a nonhydrophilic guidewire, to prevent loss of access during subsequent catheter exchange, dilation, and stenting maneuvers.[13] Additional options for traversing difficult biliary strictures include using angioplasty balloons mounted on 3-Fr catheters, using a steerable catheter with a 3.9-Fr to 4.9-Fr tapered tip, or using 7-Fr to 8.5-Fr screw-type devices (Soehendra stent extractor, Cook Endoscopy, Winston-Salem, NC).[14–17]

SELF-EXPANDING METAL STENTS FOR BBS

Metal stents have inherent properties that allow for an expansion diameter 3 times that of standard 10-Fr plastic stents. Moreover, self-expanding metal stents (SEMS) have the advantages of smaller predeployment delivery systems that do not require aggressive dilation before stent placement, and confer the additional advantage of not requiring several procedures to achieve the same result using multiple plastic stents. In the United States, no SEMS is currently approved for use in benign disease. The following 3 types of SEMS have been used for the treatment of BBS: uncovered, partially covered, and fully covered stents.

Beginning in 1991, uncovered SEMS were placed during ERCP and via percutaneous routes for managing BBS. The most common indications were in patients

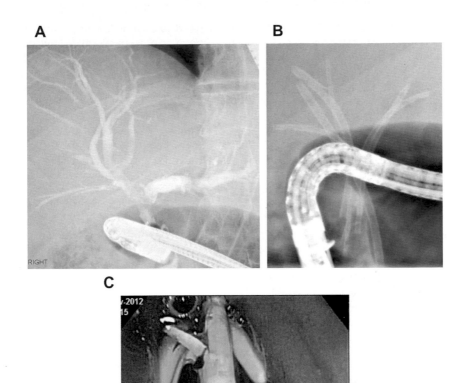

Fig. 1. Stricture caused by external beam radiation therapy. (*A*) Initial ERCP shows narrowing in the bifurcation extending into the intrahepatics. (*B*) After balloon dilation of stricture and initial placement of 2 stents, subsequent ERCP with upsizing and placement of multiple large-bore plastic stents are seen radiographically and (*C*) endoscopically.

with postsurgical strictures, chronic pancreatitis, and postorthotopic liver transplant (post-OLT) biliary strictures, with reported clinical success rates of 60%, 80%, and 50% respectively.[18–26] Uncovered SEMS have a median patency of approximately 20 months, and reinterventions are frequently required to manage stent occlusion from high rates of reactive tissue hyperplasia. In addition, stent embedment into the bile duct wall makes them nonremovable.[26] These factors limit the use of uncovered SEMS for long-term treatment of BBS and, as a result, uncovered SEMS are rarely, if ever, used for BBS.[27]

Fully covered SEMS (FCSEMS) are designed to prolong the duration of patency by preventing occlusion from reactive tissue hyperplasia and preventing tumor ingrowth. Removal is facilitated by preventing embedding of the metal wires into the bile duct. Treatment with FCSEMS is successful at the rate of about 80% to 90%.[17,28–33]

However, studies of FCSEMS so far have been limited by short follow-up, which limits confirmation of a durable response to stenting. High rates of stent migration have been reported with FCSEMS, ranging from 5% to 33% depending on the type of FCSEMS used,[31,32] and this has caused clinical concern because of the theoretically higher risk of biliary reobstruction, bowel obstruction, or perforation compared with plastic stents. A study by Park and colleagues[32] compared the use of 2 types of FCSEMS: flared-end stents versus anchoring flap stents. The study included 43 patients with biliary strictures of varying causes. No cases of migration occurred with the anchoring flap type of FCSEMS (22 patients) but the rate of migration for flared-end FCSEMS was 33% in 21 patients. All stents were easily removed at the end of the study.

Partially covered SEMS (PCSEMS) are uncovered at both the proximal and distal ends of the stent, which theoretically decreases the rate of stent migration, but increases the risk of tissue embedment, which may lead to difficultly in removing the stents. Kahaleh and colleagues[34] reported their findings on the use of PCSEMS in a study of 79 patients with biliary strictures secondary to multiple causes. The stent dwell time was 4 months on average, with a median follow-up of 1 year. Stricture resolution at follow-up was noted in 75% of patients, with a low rate of complications that included post-ERCP pancreatitis (4%), and stent migration (14%). All attempted PCSEMS removals were successful.

In a small study of 20 patients with biliary strictures caused by chronic pancreatitis, PCSEMS were highly effective in treating the stenosed ducts. Stricture resolution was achieved in 90% of patients after 6 months, with a 20% rate of stricture recurrence after a median time of 22 months. The following adverse events were each observed in 1 patient: stent migration, abdominal pain requiring stent removal after 1 month, postbiliary sphincterotomy bleeding requiring endoclip placement, and obstruction of the main pancreatic duct by the covered portion of the PCSEMS causing pancreatitis; subsequent infected pseudocyst formation required drainage.[35]

Short-term use of PCSEMS was evaluated in post-OLT anastomotic strictures. In a series of 22 patients who had PCSEMS placed for 2 months, the initial success rate of stricture dilation and expansion was 86%; however; the investigators noted a high recurrence rate, which approached 50%. Two patients were noted to have had complete stent migration, and 1 patient had a partial stent migration. Most concerning, difficulty was encountered during PCSEMS stent removal in 6 patients, requiring more than 1 procedure for removal.[36]

DISEASE-SPECIFIC MANAGEMENT OF BBS
Postoperative Strictures

Patients who undergo OLT are at highest risk of developing BBS with a rate of about 20% to 30%.[37,38] CCY follows distantly as the procedure with the second highest risk for BBS formation, at a rate of approximately 0.5%.[39–41]

Post-CCY biliary strictures

Multiple factors contribute to stricture formation following laparoscopic or open CCY, with confusion of the cystic duct with the CBD as the most common cause of intraoperative injury. Additional causes of CCY-associated biliary stricture include excessive traction on the gallbladder neck, biliary ischemia, unintentional electrocautery injury, and extension of thermal injury applied to a correctly recognized CBD.[42] The clinical and biochemical manifestations may be evident early in the postoperative period, and may be associated with jaundice and cholangitis, or with peritonitis caused by a bile leak. Delayed presentation is commonly related to ischemic injury or reanastomosis of the CBD, with the time to presentation dependent on the individual rate of fibrosis.

Endoscopic treatment of post-CCY biliary strictures has been shown to be successful, especially when 2 or more plastic stents are exchanged intermittently and remain in place for at least a 12-month period.[5,43–47] In addition, Bismuth I and II (distal) strictures are associated with better outcomes, compared with proximal hilar lesions (Bismuth III) (80% vs 25%, respectively).[6] A success rate of 74% to 90% at the end of the 12 months of treatment was reported, with a recurrence rate of 20% to 30% within 2 years of stent removal.[6,46] Long-term follow-up data (mean of 13.7 years) of 35 patients with postsurgical strictures showed good outcomes with endoscopic stenting: 4 patients (11.4%) had stricture recurrence, and 3 patients (8.6%) had acute cholangitis caused by common bile stones, all of which were treated endoscopically.[48] No further complications occurred in these patients after an additional mean follow-up of 7 years.

Post–liver transplant strictures

Several biliary complications may develop following OLT, including the formation of strictures, bile leaks, and biliary filling defects (such as casts, stones, and sludge).[49–51] BBS are the most common complication of OLT and may present at a variable period of time after OLT, ranging from days to more than 2 years.[52,53] So-called early strictures (<30 days after OLT) may be the result of CBD diameter mismatch between the donor and recipient, or they may be caused by surgical technique and are often located at the anastomosis. Hepaticojejunostomy is more likely to result in early stricture formation than duct-to-duct anastomosis, with end-to-end anastomosis being preferable. Late strictures (>30 days after OLT) may be associated with ischemic damage and require more aggressive and longer duration of endoscopic therapy, and result in a higher rate of retransplantation or surgical revision.[54–56]

Post-OLT strictures are further divided into anastomotic strictures (AS) and nonanastomotic strictures (NAS). AS are caused by focal stenosis at the junction of the recipient's CBD with the donor's common hepatic duct, and make up about 80% of post-OLT strictures. NAS after OLT respond less favorably to endoscopic therapy than AS, with up to 25% to 50% of patients with NAS ultimately expiring or undergoing retransplantation.[37] NAS have been strongly associated with ischemic injury to the biliary tree from causes such as hepatic artery thrombosis or stenosis and prolonged donor organ ischemic time.[57] Patients who undergo OLT with the transplanted liver being donated after cardiac death are at the highest risk of NAS, with a 37% reported NAS rate at 3 years of follow-up, versus a rate of 12% among patients in the same study who received a donation after brain death in which the donor was maintained on life-support before organ harvest.[58–61]

AS The appearance of a single, short stricture in the middle portion of the CBD in a patient after liver transplant suggests an AS, which accounts for up to 80% of biliary strictures following OLT.[62] Patients who develop a stricture within the first 1 to 2 months after OLT have the best response to endoscopic dilation and stent placement, with stricture resolution achievable after 3 months in most cases.[61] Patients with late presentation of AS often require 12 to 24 months of endoscopic stenting, with stent exchange every 3 months, to ensure a durable response to therapy. Long-term resolution of AS has been reported in 70% to 100% of patients who undergo balloon dilation and stenting and is superior to balloon dilation alone.[8,63–67] Furthermore, placement of increasing numbers of side-by-side plastic stents seems to be the most effective approach.[68] Recent results using fully covered metal stents have been encouraging (**Fig. 2**).

NAS Strictures that are more numerous, diffuse, and proximal to the anastomosis usually represent NAS, which often involving the hilum and intrahepatic biliary

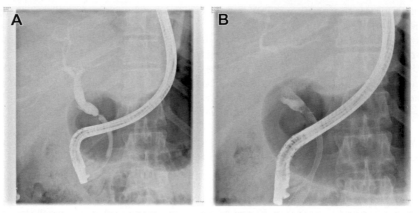

Fig. 2. FCSEMS for treatment of bile duct stricture. (A) Cholangiogram shows severe chole-dochal AS after liver transplant. (B) After placement of FCSEMS. Note: the stent was removed 4 months later following resolution of the stricture.

ducts.[9,69,70] From 10% to 25% of all strictures following OLT have been attributed to NAS.[54,71] Patients with NAS may have donor-recipient ABO blood-type incompatibility, or have had prolonged pretransplant ischemic time (cold or warm). Evaluation for hepatic artery thrombosis or stenosis by Doppler ultrasound and/or angiography by computed tomography or magnetic resonance imaging should be considered, because flow-limiting hepatic artery disease is a known cause of NAS and may require endovascular stenting, thrombolysis, or surgery.[72] A mean time of 10 months from OLT to diagnosis of NAS has been reported, although presentation is variable depending on the underlying cause.[73] NAS are less responsive to endoscopic therapy with a long-term response of 50% to 75%; however, biliary sludge extraction and stenting is advised and has been shown to reduce the need for repeat liver transplantation.[73–75] Furthermore, dilation and stenting for NAS can be considered as a bridge to retransplantation.[76] Patients require more endoscopic interventions over a prolonged time course, with 185 days median time to resolution of stenosis, compared with 67 days for AS.[9,77,78] However, patients with NAS are currently considered to have a poor prognosis and continued lifelong surveillance for stricture recurrence is often necessary.

Biliary-enteric strictures
Biliary-enteric strictures may occur after OLT with Roux-en-Y hepaticojejunostomy, partial liver resection, and pancreaticoduodenectomy (Whipple procedure). Because of alterations in intestinal luminal anatomy, endoscopic therapy for these strictures was once thought to be impossible. However, the use of colonoscopes and, more recently, the advent of balloon enteroscopes and wide-spread training of advanced therapeutic endoscopists have allowed such strictures to be accessed and treated with balloon dilation and stent placement (**Fig. 3**). Saleem and colleagues[79] noted a technical success rate of 70% for 56 patients with Roux-en-Y anatomy undergoing diagnostic single-balloon ERCP. Furthermore, Lee and colleagues[80] noted that balloon dilation alone was successful for 21 of 32 patients (66%) with bilioenteric strictures that occurred following surgical biliary reconstruction for post-CCY complications. The limitations of balloon ERCP for BBS therapy are long case times, significant endoscopic operator expertise and consistent case loads, limited availability of balloon enteroscopes (mostly limited to tertiary and quaternary referral

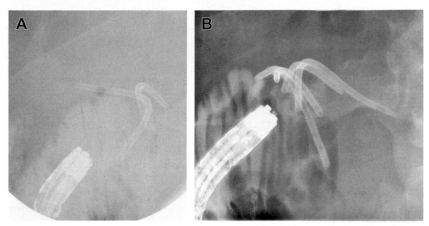

Fig. 3. Hepaticojejunal AS treated endoscopically. (*A*) Adult colonoscope in position at hepaticojejunostomy. Two 10-Fr plastic stents are placed. (*B*) Immediately after balloon dilation and placement of additional stents. Subsequent resolution of the stricture was achieved.

centers), and smaller channel sizes and therefore fewer endoscopic accessories. However, the potential for avoiding percutaneous drains and the need for surgical revisions are powerful factors to consider in favor of further training and development of balloon ERCP.

Chronic Pancreatitis-associated Biliary Strictures

Distal BBS are found in approximately 25% of patients with chronic pancreatitis.[81–84] Patients with signs of biliary obstruction should undergo decompression therapy to prevent cholangitis, secondary biliary cirrhosis, and choledocholithiasis.[85] Endoscopic therapy is a lower-morbidity alternative to surgical intervention, especially in patients who are poor surgical candidates.[86,87] Placement of multiple plastic stents (**Table 3**) has become the endoscopic therapy standard of care, because this achieves improved outcomes compared with placement of a single plastic stent.[6,35,84,88] However, BBS secondary to chronic pancreatitis (especially in patients with chronic calcifying pancreatitis) are more resistant to remodeling via stenting because of the resiliency of pancreatic fibrosis.[88,89] Approximately 80% of patients with chronic pancreatitis treated endoscopically may eventually develop relapse of strictures, with stent occlusion

Table 3
Results of studies of patients with chronic pancreatitis treated with multiple plastic stents

Author, Year (Reference)	Patients (n)	Stent Duration (mo)	Follow-up Period (mo)	Overall Success (%)
Draganov et al,[6] 2002	9	6	48[a]	44
Catalano et al,[84] 2004	12	14	47	92
Pozsar et al,[88] 2004	29[b]	21	12	60
Behm et al,[35] 2009	20	5	22	80
Regimbeau et al,[87] 2012	21	11[c]	44	76

[a] Includes 20 patients with other causes of BBS.
[b] All patients carried a diagnosis of chronic calcifying pancreatitis, which is considered difficult to treat endoscopically.
[c] Includes 12 patients who underwent covered metal stenting.

and migration commonly reported.[85,89–94] Endoscopic treatment may be less durable than surgery, but dilation and stenting can serve as a bridge to surgery.[87,95,96] Furthermore, endoscopic treatment may avoid surgical drainage procedures, such as the Puestow procedure (pancreaticojejunostomy), which has been shown to increase the beta-islet cell yield of patients with chronic pancreatitis who undergo total pancreatectomy with intrahepatic auto islet transplantation.[97,98]

PSC

Fibrotic strictures and saccular dilatations of the intrahepatic and extrahepatic bile ducts resemble beads on a string and radiographically suggest PSC.[99–101] Approximately 40% of patients with PSC develop so-called dominant strictures, which can cause biliary obstruction that require endoscopic therapy via balloon dilation alone to improve the forward flow of bile.[102–104] Stent placement has been shown to be detrimental in some patients with BBS caused by PSC, because complications including stent occlusion and cholangitis are observed more frequently than in patients undergoing balloon dilation alone.[105–107] The goals of endoscopic intervention are to balloon dilate the strictures to 18 to 24 Fr (6-mm–8-mm diameter), and to reduce the serum alkaline phosphatase level to 1.5 times the upper limit of normal.[108] Proper endoscopic therapy may lead to better outcomes than predicted by the Mayo model of PSC.[109–112] Short-term insertion of stents, for as short as approximately 10 days, may be safe and can be considered for PSC strictures if dilation alone is unsuccessful (**Fig. 4**); however, strictures should be routinely brushed for cytology because patients with PSC have a 20% to 30% risk of developing cholangiocarcinoma.[112–114] Because of the higher rate of cholangitis seen after biliary procedures in patients with PSC, routine periprocedural antibiotic prophylaxis is recommended; rates of post-ERCP pancreatitis, bleeding, and perforation seem to be similar to those in patients without PSC after ERCP.[72,115] In patients with secondary sclerosing cholangitis, treatment should be based on the underlying cause.[114]

Autoimmune Cholangiopathy

Autoimmune pancreatitis (AIP) is associated with the development of autoimmune cholangiopathy (AIC) in approximately 20% of patients, and is characterized by a lymphoplasmacytic infiltrate with immunoglobulin G4–positive cells.[114,116,117] Patients with AIC may develop biliary obstruction from fibrosis and inflammation at the head of the pancreas, which is typically treated with immunosuppressive doses of corticosteroids such as prednisone.[118] AIC may occur as an isolated biliary disease with or without AIP.[119,120] AIC is not limited to BBS development near the pancreatic head, and may cause biliary strictures at any point in the biliary tree or pancreatic ducts. Intrahepatic AIC strictures may appear similar to benign strictures caused by PSC but are generally more segmental and longer, and they frequently affect the distal CBD.[116] Stent placement can be performed to temporarily relieve biliary obstruction while patients undergo diagnosis, which is confirmed by a response and regression of strictures after starting treatment with corticosteroids.[121]

ENDOVASCULAR THERAPY–ASSOCIATED BBS

Percutaneous therapies for hepatocellular carcinoma, such as transarterial chemoembolization, radiofrequency ablation, and percutaneous ethanol injection have been recognized as causes of BBS. The mechanism of biliary injury following transarterial chemoembolization and percutaneous ethanol injection are likely to be collateral ischemia, whereas radiofrequency ablation may induce BBS development after

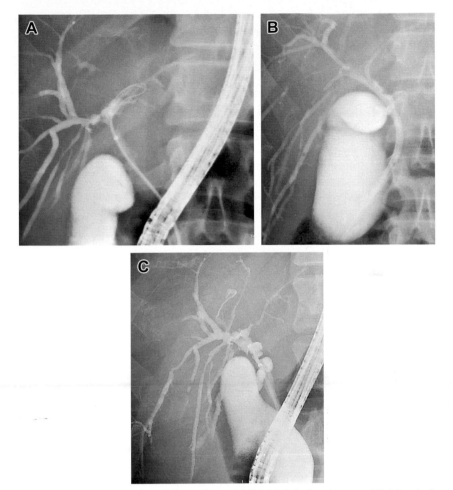

Fig. 4. PSC with complex benign hilar stricture. (*A*) Initial cholangiogram. (*B*) After balloon dilation and placement of multiple plastic stents. (*C*) After removal of stents, stricture resolution is seen.

extension of thermal injury to the target hepatocellular carcinoma tumor.[122–127] Cooling of the main bile ducts during radiofrequency ablation, by infusion of a chilled saline solution via endoscopic nasobiliary drainage tube or by choledochotomy, has been shown to prevent biliary stenosis in 2 small series of patients.[128,129]

SUMMARY

This article discusses the diverse causes of BBS, including strictures caused by postoperative adverse events, PSC, chronic pancreatitis, and ischemia. Endoscopic evaluation and treatment are the gold standards of therapy, with specific management based on correctly identifying the underlying cause, characteristics, and location of the stricture(s). The relative merits of ERCP with dilation, using plastic and self-expandable metal stents, are discussed. The most common therapy for BBS involves ERCP with balloon dilation and placement of multiple plastic stents in a side-by-side fashion followed by the periodic exchange of these stents for approximately 1 year to allow for expansion and remodeling of the stricture(s). The use of self-expandable removable metal stents for the treatment of BBS is under investigation; clinical trials are underway to determine the best management approach.

REFERENCES

1. Tee HP, James MW, Kaffes AJ. Placement of removable metal biliary stent in post-orthotopic liver. World J Gastroenterol 2010;16:3597–600.
2. Bismuth H. Postoperative strictures of the bile duct. In: Blumgart LH, editor. The biliary tract. Edinburgh (Scotland): Churchill Livingstone; 1982. p. 209–18.
3. Strasberg SM, Hertl M, Soper NJ. An analysis of the problem of biliary injury during laparoscopic cholecystectomy. J Am Coll Surg 1995;180:101–25.
4. DaVee T, Garcia JA, Baron TH. Precut sphincterotomy for selective biliary duct cannulation during endoscopic retrograde cholangiopancreatography. Ann Gastroenterol 2012;25(4):291–302.
5. Costamagna G, Pandolfi M, Mutignani M, et al. Long-term results of endoscopic management of postoperative bile duct strictures. Gastrointest Endosc 2001;54: 162–8.
6. Draganov P, Hoffman B, Marsh W, et al. Long-term outcome in patients with benign biliary strictures treated endoscopically with multiple stents. Gastrointest Endosc 2002;55:680–6.
7. Matlock J, Freeman ML. Endoscopic therapy of benign biliary strictures. Rev Gastroenterol Disord 2005;5:206–14.
8. Zoepf T, Maldonado-Lopez EJ, Hilgard P, et al. Balloon dilatation vs. balloon dilatation plus bile duct endoprostheses for treatment of anastomotic biliary strictures after liver transplantation. Liver Transpl 2006;12:88–94.
9. Thuluvath PJ, Pfau PR, Kimmey MB, et al. Biliary complications after liver transplantation: the role of endoscopy. Endoscopy 2005;37:857–63.
10. Lawrence C, Romagnuolo J, Payne KM, et al. Low symptomatic premature stent occlusion of multiple plastic stents for benign biliary strictures: comparing standard and prolonged stent change intervals. Gastrointest Endosc 2010;72: 558–63.
11. Dumonceau JM, Heresbach D, Devière J, et al. Biliary stents: models and methods for endoscopic stenting. Endoscopy 2011;43:617–26.
12. Somogyi L, Chuttani R, Croffie J, et al. Guidewires for use in GI endoscopy. Gastrointest Endosc 2007;65:571–6.
13. Costamagna G, Familiari P, Tringali A, et al. Multidisciplinary approach to benign biliary strictures. Curr Treat Options Gastroenterol 2007;10:90–101.
14. Baron TH, Morgan DE. Dilation of a difficult benign pancreatic duct stricture using the Soehendra stent extractor. Gastrointest Endosc 1997;46:178–80.
15. Ziebert JJ, DiSario JA. Dilation of refractory pancreatic duct strictures: the turn of the screw. Gastrointest Endosc 1999;49:632–5.
16. Baron TH, Poterucha JJ. Use of a small-caliber angioplasty balloon for the management of an impassable choledochocholedochal anastomotic biliary stricture. Liver Transpl 2008;14:1683–4.
17. Digestive Disease Week, American Society for Gastrointestinal Endoscopy meeting abstracts. May 2005, Chicago, Illinois, USA. Gastrointest Endosc 2005;61:AB77–309.
18. Foerster EC, Hoepffner N, Domschke W. Bridging of benign choledochal stenoses by endoscopic retrograde implantation of mesh stents. Endoscopy 1991;23:133–5.

19. O'Brien SM, Hatfield AR, Craig PI, et al. A 5-year follow-up of self-expanding metal stents in the endoscopic management of patients with benign bile duct strictures. Eur J Gastroenterol Hepatol 1998;10:141–5.
20. Roumilhac D, Poyet G, Sergent G, et al. Long-term results of percutaneous management for anastomotic biliary stricture. Liver Transpl 2003;9:394–400.
21. Deviere J, Cremer M, Baize M, et al. Management of common bile duct stricture caused by chronic pancreatitis with metal mesh self expandable stents. Gut 1994;35:122–6.
22. van Berkel AM, Cahen DL, van Westerloo DJ, et al. Self-expanding metal stents in benign biliary strictures due to chronic pancreatitis. Endoscopy 2004;36: 381–4.
23. Yamaguchi T, Ishihara T, Seza K, et al. Long-term outcome of endoscopic metallic stenting for benign biliary stenosis. World J Gastroenterol 2006;12: 426–30.
24. Eickhoff A, Jakobs R, Leonhardt A, et al. Self-expandable metal mesh stents for common bile duct stenosis in chronic pancreatitis: retrospective evaluation of long-term follow-up and clinical outcome pilot study. Z Gastroenterol 2003;41: 649–54.
25. Kahl S, Zimmermann S, Glasbrenner B, et al. Treatment of benign biliary strictures in chronic pancreatitis by self-expandable metal stents. Dig Dis 2002; 20:199–203.
26. Kahaleh M, Tokar J, Le T, et al. Removal of self-expandable metallic Wallstents. Gastrointest Endosc 2004;60:640–4.
27. van Boeckel PG, Vleggaar FP, Siersema PD. Plastic or metal stents for benign extrahepatic biliary strictures: a systematic review. BMC Gastroenterol 2009;9:96.
28. Kuo MD, Lopresti DC, Gover DD, et al. Intentional retrieval of Viabil stent-grafts from the biliary system. J Vasc Interv Radiol 2006;17:389–97.
29. Cahen DL, van Berkel AM, Oskam D, et al. Long-term results of endoscopic drainage of common bile duct strictures in chronic pancreatitis. Eur J Gastroenterol Hepatol 2005;17:103–8.
30. Traina M, Tarantino I, Barresi L, et al. Efficacy and safety of fully covered self-expandable metallic stents in biliary complications after liver transplantation: a preliminary study. Liver Transpl 2009;15:1493–8.
31. Mahajan A, Ho H, Sauer B, et al. Temporary placement of fully covered self-expandable metal stents in benign biliary strictures: midterm evaluation (with video). Gastrointest Endosc 2009;70:303–9.
32. Park do H, Lee SS, Lee TH, et al. Anchoring flap versus flared end, fully covered self-expandable metal stents to prevent migration in patients with benign biliary strictures: a multicenter, prospective, comparative pilot study (with videos). Gastrointest Endosc 2011;73:64–70.
33. Hu B, Gao DJ, Yu FH, et al. Endoscopic stenting for post-transplant biliary stricture: usefulness of a novel. J Hepatobiliary Pancreat Sci 2011;18:640–5.
34. Kahaleh M, Behm B, Clarke BW, et al. Temporary placement of covered self-expandable metal stents in benign biliary. Gastrointest Endosc 2008;67:446–54.
35. Behm B, Brock A, Clarke BW, et al. Partially covered self-expandable metallic stents for benign biliary strictures due to chronic pancreatitis. Endoscopy 2009;41:547–51.
36. Chaput U, Scatton O, Bichard P, et al. Temporary placement of partially covered self-expandable metal stents for. Gastrointest Endosc 2010;72:1167–74.
37. Pascher A, Neuhaus P. Bile duct complications after liver transplantation. Transpl Int 2005;18:627–42.

38. Verdonk RC, Buis CI, Porte RJ, et al. Biliary complications after liver transplantation: a review. Scand J Gastroenterol Suppl 2006;(234):89–101.
39. Balderramo D, Navasa M, Cardenas A. Current management of biliary complications after liver transplantation: emphasis. Gastroenterol Hepatol 2011;34:107–15.
40. MacFadyen BV Jr, Vecchio R, Ricardo AE, et al. Bile duct injury after laparoscopic cholecystectomy. The United States. Surg Endosc 1998;12:315–21.
41. Windsor JA, Pong J. Laparoscopic biliary injury: more than a learning curve problem. Aust N Z J Surg 1998;68:186–9.
42. Davidoff AM, Pappas TN, Murray EA, et al. Mechanisms of major biliary injury during laparoscopic cholecystectomy. Ann Surg 1992;215:196–202.
43. Huibregtse K, Katon RM, Tytgat GN. Endoscopic treatment of postoperative biliary strictures. Endoscopy 1986;18:133–7.
44. Geenen DJ, Geenen JE, Hogan WJ, et al. Endoscopic therapy for benign bile duct strictures. Gastrointest Endosc 1989;35:367–71.
45. Davids PH, Rauws EA, Coene PP, et al. Endoscopic stenting for post-operative biliary strictures. Gastrointest Endosc 1992;38:12–8.
46. Kassab C, Prat F, Liguory C, et al. Endoscopic management of post-laparoscopic cholecystectomy biliary strictures. Gastroenterol Clin Biol 2006;30:124–9.
47. Pozsar J, Sahin P, Laszlo F, et al. Endoscopic treatment of sphincterotomy-associated distal common bile duct. Gastrointest Endosc 2005;62:85–91.
48. Costamagna G, Tringali A, Mutignani M, et al. Endotherapy of postoperative biliary strictures with multiple stents: results. Gastrointest Endosc 2010;72:551–7.
49. Thuluvath PJ, Atassi T, Lee J. An endoscopic approach to biliary complications following orthotopic liver. Liver Int 2003;23:156–62.
50. Wojcicki M, Milkiewicz P, Silva M. Biliary tract complications after liver transplantation: a review. Dig Surg 2008;25:245–57.
51. Welling TH, Heidt DG, Englesbe MJ, et al. Biliary complications following liver transplantation in the model for end-stage. Liver Transpl 2008;14:73–80.
52. Bergman JJ, van den Brink GR, Rauws EA, et al. Treatment of bile duct lesions after laparoscopic cholecystectomy. Gut 1996;38:141–7.
53. Davidson BR, Rai R, Nandy A, et al. Results of choledochojejunostomy in the treatment of biliary complications after. Liver Transpl 2000;6:201–6.
54. Koneru B, Sterling MJ, Bahramipour PF. Bile duct strictures after liver transplantation: a changing landscape of the. Liver Transpl 2006;12:702–4.
55. Sanchez-Urdazpal L, Gores GJ, Ward EM, et al. Diagnostic features and clinical outcome of ischemic-type biliary complications. Hepatology 1993;17:605–9.
56. Pasha SF, Harrison ME, Das A, et al. Endoscopic treatment of anastomotic biliary strictures after deceased donor liver. Gastrointest Endosc 2007;66:44–51.
57. Dacha S, Barad A, Martin J, et al. Association of hepatic artery stenosis and biliary strictures in liver transplant. Liver Transpl 2011;17:849–54.
58. Foley DP, Fernandez LA, Leverson G, et al. Donation after cardiac death: the University of Wisconsin experience with liver. Ann Surg 2005;242:724–31.
59. de Vera ME, Lopez-Solis R, Dvorchik I, et al. Liver transplantation using donation after cardiac death donors: long-term. Am J Transplant 2009;9:773–81.
60. Pine JK, Aldouri A, Young AL, et al. Liver transplantation following donation after cardiac death: an analysis using. Liver Transpl 2009;15:1072–82.
61. Verdonk RC, Buis CI, Porte RJ, et al. Anastomotic biliary strictures after liver transplantation: causes and. Liver Transpl 2006;12:726–35.

62. Thethy S, Thomson B, Pleass H, et al. Management of biliary tract complications after orthotopic liver transplantation. Clin Transplant 2004;18:647–53.
63. Schwartz DA, Petersen BT, Poterucha JJ, et al. Endoscopic therapy of anastomotic bile duct strictures occurring after liver. Gastrointest Endosc 2000;51: 169–74.
64. Graziadei IW, Schwaighofer H, Koch R, et al. Long-term outcome of endoscopic treatment of biliary strictures after liver. Liver Transpl 2006;12:718–25.
65. Morelli J, Mulcahy HE, Willner IR, et al. Long-term outcomes for patients with post-liver transplant anastomotic biliary. Gastrointest Endosc 2003;58:374–9.
66. Holt AP, Thorburn D, Mirza D, et al. A prospective study of standardized nonsurgical therapy in the management of. Transplantation 2007;84:857–63.
67. Alazmi WM, Fogel EL, Watkins JL, et al. Recurrence rate of anastomotic biliary strictures in patients who have had. Endoscopy 2006;38:571–4.
68. Kulaksiz H, Weiss KH, Gotthardt D, et al. Is stenting necessary after balloon dilation of post-transplantation biliary. Endoscopy 2008;40:746–51.
69. Buis CI, Hoekstra H, Verdonk RC, et al. Causes and consequences of ischemic-type biliary lesions after liver. J Hepatobiliary Pancreat Surg 2006;13:517–24.
70. Sawyer RG, Punch JD. Incidence and management of biliary complications after 291 liver transplants. Transplantation 1998;66:1201–7.
71. Pfau PR, Kochman ML, Lewis JD, et al. Endoscopic management of postoperative biliary complications in orthotopic liver. Gastrointest Endosc 2000;52:55–63.
72. Abdelaziz O, Hosny K, Amin A, et al. Endovascular management of early hepatic artery thrombosis after living donor liver transplantation. Transpl Int 2012;25:847–56.
73. Tabibian JH, Asham EH, Goldstein L, et al. Endoscopic treatment with multiple stents for post-liver-transplantation. Gastrointest Endosc 2009;69:1236–43.
74. Rerknimitr R, Sherman S, Fogel EL, et al. Biliary tract complications after orthotopic liver transplantation with. Gastrointest Endosc 2002;55:224–31.
75. Rizk RS, McVicar JP, Emond MJ, et al. Endoscopic management of biliary strictures in liver transplant recipients. Gastrointest Endosc 1998;47:128–35.
76. Tung BY, Kimmey MB. Biliary complications of orthotopic liver transplantation. Dig Dis 1999;17:133–44.
77. Guichelaar MM, Benson JT, Malinchoc M, et al. Risk factors for and clinical course of non-anastomotic biliary strictures after. Am J Transplant 2003;3: 885–90.
78. Jagannath S, Kalloo AN. Biliary complications after liver transplantation. Curr Treat Options Gastroenterol 2002;5:101–12.
79. Saleem A, Baron TH, Gostout CJ, et al. Endoscopic retrograde cholangiopancreatography using a single-balloon enteroscope. Endoscopy 2010;42:656–60.
80. Lee AY, Gregorius J, Kerlan RK, et al. Percutaneous transhepatic balloon dilation of biliary-enteric anastomotic strictures after surgical repair of iatrogenic bile duct injuries. PLoS One 2012;7:e46478.
81. Wilson C, Auld CD, Schlinkert R, et al. Hepatobiliary complications in chronic pancreatitis. Gut 1989;30:520–7.
82. Stahl TJ, Allen MO, Ansel HJ, et al. Partial biliary obstruction caused by chronic pancreatitis. An appraisal of indications for surgical biliary drainage. Ann Surg 1988;207:26–32.
83. Aranha GV, Prinz RA, Freeark RJ, et al. The spectrum of biliary tract obstruction from chronic pancreatitis. Arch Surg 1984;119:595–600.
84. Catalano MF, Linder JD, George S, et al. Treatment of symptomatic distal common bile duct stenosis secondary to chronic. Gastrointest Endosc 2004;60:945–52.

85. Deviere J, Devaere S, Baize M, et al. Endoscopic biliary drainage in chronic pancreatitis. Gastrointest Endosc 1990;36:96–100.
86. Smits ME, Rauws EA, van Gulik TM, et al. Long-term results of endoscopic stenting and surgical drainage for biliary. Br J Surg 1996;83:764–8.
87. Regimbeau JM, Fuks D, Bartoli E, et al. A comparative study of surgery and endoscopy for the treatment of bile duct stricture in patients with chronic pancreatitis. Surg Endosc 2012;26:2902–8.
88. Pozsar J, Sahin P, Laszlo F, et al. Medium-term results of endoscopic treatment of common bile duct strictures in. J Clin Gastroenterol 2004;38:118–23.
89. Kahl S, Zimmermann S, Genz I, et al. Risk factors for failure of endoscopic stenting of biliary strictures in chronic. Am J Gastroenterol 2003;98:2448–53.
90. Barthet M, Bernard JP, Duval JL, et al. Biliary stenting in benign biliary stenosis complicating chronic calcifying. Endoscopy 1994;26:569–72.
91. Kiehne K, Folsch UR, Nitsche R. High complication rate of bile duct stents in patients with chronic alcoholic. Endoscopy 2000;32:377–80.
92. Vitale GC, Reed DN Jr, Nguyen CT, et al. Endoscopic treatment of distal bile duct stricture from chronic pancreatitis. Surg Endosc 2000;14:227–31.
93. Farnbacher MJ, Rabenstein T, Ell C, et al. Is endoscopic drainage of common bile duct stenoses in chronic pancreatitis. Am J Gastroenterol 2000;95:1466–71.
94. Eickhoff A, Jakobs R, Leonhardt A, et al. Endoscopic stenting for common bile duct stenoses in chronic pancreatitis. Eur J Gastroenterol Hepatol 2001;13:1161–7.
95. Buxbaum J. The role of endoscopic retrograde cholangiopancreatography in patients with pancreatic disease. Gastroenterol Clin North Am 2012;41:23–45.
96. Ito K, Fujita N, Noda Y, et al. Endoscopic treatment for biliary stricture secondary to chronic pancreatitis. Dig Endosc 2012;24(Suppl 1):17–21.
97. Sutherland DE, Radosevich DM, Bellin MD, et al. Total pancreatectomy and islet autotransplantation for chronic pancreatitis. J Am Coll Surg 2012;214:409–24 [discussion: 424–6].
98. Bellin MD, Sutherland DER, Robertson RP. Pancreatectomy and autologous islet transplantation for painful chronic pancreatitis: indications and outcomes. Hosp Pract (Minneap) 2012;40:80–7.
99. Pitt HA, Thompson HH, Tompkins RK, et al. Primary sclerosing cholangitis: results of an aggressive surgical approach. Ann Surg 1982;196:259–68.
100. Wiesner RH, LaRusso NF. Clinicopathologic features of the syndrome of primary sclerosing cholangitis. Gastroenterology 1980;79:200–6.
101. Chandok N, Hirschfield GM. Management of primary sclerosing cholangitis: conventions and controversies. Can J Gastroenterol 2012;26:261–8.
102. Tischendorf JJ, Hecker H, Kruger M, et al. Characterization, outcome, and prognosis in 273 patients with primary sclerosing. Am J Gastroenterol 2007;102:107–14.
103. Stiehl A, Rudolph G, Kloters-Plachky P, et al. Development of dominant bile duct stenoses in patients with primary sclerosing. J Hepatol 2002;36:151–6.
104. Bjornsson E, Olsson R. Dominant strictures in patients with primary sclerosing cholangitis-revisited. Am J Gastroenterol 2004;99:2281. United States.
105. Kaya M, Petersen BT, Angulo P, et al. Balloon dilation compared to stenting of dominant strictures in primary. Am J Gastroenterol 2001;96:1059–66.
106. Linder S, Soderlund C. Endoscopic therapy in primary sclerosing cholangitis: outcome of treatment and. Hepatogastroenterology 2001;48:387–92.
107. van Milligen de Wit AW, van Bracht J, Rauws EA, et al. Endoscopic stent therapy for dominant extrahepatic bile duct strictures in. Gastrointest Endosc 1996;44:293–9.
108. Al Mamari S, Djordjevic J, Halliday JS, et al. Improvement of serum alkaline phosphatase to <1.5 upper limit of normal predicts better outcome and reduced risk of

cholangiocarcinoma in primary sclerosing cholangitis. J Hepatol February 2013; 58(2):329–34.
109. Stiehl A, Rudolph G, Sauer P, et al. Efficacy of ursodeoxycholic acid treatment and endoscopic dilation of major duct. J Hepatol 1997;26:560–6.
110. Baluyut AR, Sherman S, Lehman GA, et al. Impact of endoscopic therapy on the survival of patients with primary sclerosing. Gastrointest Endosc 2001;53:308–12.
111. Gluck M, Cantone NR, Brandabur JJ, et al. A twenty-year experience with endoscopic therapy for symptomatic primary. J Clin Gastroenterol 2008;42:1032–9.
112. Chapman MH, Webster GJ, Bannoo S, et al. Cholangiocarcinoma and dominant strictures in patients with primary sclerosing cholangitis: a 25-year single-centre experience. Eur J Gastroenterol Hepatol 2012;24:1051–8.
113. Ponsioen CY, Lam K, van Milligen de Wit AW, et al. Four years experience with short term stenting in primary sclerosing cholangitis. Am J Gastroenterol 1999; 94:2403–7.
114. Novotný I, Dítě P, Trna J, et al. Immunoglobulin G4-related cholangitis: a variant of IgG4-related systemic disease. Dig Dis 2012;30:216–9.
115. Bangarulingam SY, Gossard AA, Petersen BT, et al. Complications of endoscopic retrograde cholangiopancreatography in primary. Am J Gastroenterol 2009;104:855–60.
116. Zen Y, Nakanuma Y. IgG4 cholangiopathy. Int J Hepatol 2012;2012:472376.
117. Chari ST, Smyrk TC, Levy MJ, et al. Diagnosis of autoimmune pancreatitis: the Mayo Clinic experience. Clin Gastroenterol Hepatol 2006;4:1010–6 [quiz: 934].
118. Chari ST. Current concepts in the treatment of autoimmune pancreatitis. JOP 2007;8:1–3. Italy.
119. Zen Y, Harada K, Sasaki M, et al. IgG4-related sclerosing cholangitis with and without hepatic inflammatory. Am J Surg Pathol 2004;28:1193–203.
120. Bjornsson E, Chari ST, Smyrk TC, et al. Immunoglobulin G4 associated cholangitis: description of an emerging clinical. Hepatology 2007;45:1547–54.
121. Small AJ, Loftus CG, Smyrk TC, et al. A case of IgG4-associated cholangitis and autoimmune pancreatitis responsive to. Nat Clin Pract Gastroenterol Hepatol 2008;5:707–12.
122. Kim HK, Chung YH, Song BC, et al. Ischemic bile duct injury as a serious complication after transarterial. J Clin Gastroenterol 2001;32:423–7.
123. Karmali S, Dixon E. Biliary stricture resulting from radiofrequency ablation. Am J Surg 2004;188:76–7.
124. Machi J, Uchida S, Sumida K, et al. Ultrasound-guided radiofrequency thermal ablation of liver tumors: percutaneous. J Gastrointest Surg 2001;5:477–89.
125. Rhim H, Yoon KH, Lee JM, et al. Major complications after radio-frequency thermal ablation of hepatic tumors. Radiographics 2003;23:123–34 [discussion: 134–6].
126. Chan MK, Kwok PC, Chan SC, et al. Percutaneous ethanol injection as a possible curative treatment for malignant. Cardiovasc Intervent Radiol 1999;22:326–8.
127. Tsai HM, Lin XZ, Chen CY. Computed tomography demonstration of immediate and delayed complications of. J Comput Assist Tomogr 2003;27:590–6.
128. Elias D, Sideris L, Pocard M, et al. Intraductal cooling of the main bile ducts during radiofrequency ablation. J Am Coll Surg 2004;198:717–21.
129. Ogawa T, Kawamoto H, Kobayashi Y, et al. Prevention of biliary complication in radiofrequency ablation for hepatocellular. Eur J Radiol 2010;73:385–90.

Endoscopic Management of Malignant Bile Duct Strictures

Kevin Webb, MD, Michael Saunders, MD*

KEYWORDS

- Stent • Stricture • Biliary • Malignant • Cholangiocarcinoma
- Photodynamic therapy • ERCP • Radiofrequency ablation

KEY POINTS

- Endoscopic stenting is the decompressive procedure of choice for unresectable malignant bile duct obstruction.
- The choice of stent (plastic versus metal, covered versus uncovered) is influenced by stricture location, expected patient survival, potential need for removability, and cost.
- For malignant hilar obstruction, a goal of stent placement resulting in more than 50% of liver volume drained should be achieved whenever possible, which frequently requires bilateral stent placement.
- Photodynamic therapy and radiofrequency ablation are promising endoscopic therapies for the treatment of malignant bile duct strictures.

INTRODUCTION

Many disease processes, arising from primary or metastatic disease in intrahepatic, extrahepatic, or hilar locations, can lead to malignant biliary strictures (**Table 1**). Until the 1980s, biliary-enteric surgical bypass was the treatment of choice for people with malignant pancreaticobiliary disease. However, in the last 20 years, endoscopic decompression, primarily through stent placement, has emerged as a therapeutic option offering lower overall cost, shorter hospitalization, and lower morbidity when compared with surgical intervention.[1] The goal of intervention is to relieve biliary obstruction that develops in 70% to 90% of patients with unresectable disease.[1] Obstruction can ultimately lead to jaundice, pruritus, secondary biliary cirrhosis, cholangitis, coagulopathy, and weight loss through malabsorption. Biliary decompression palliates these symptoms and improves quality of life but has not been shown to affect survival.[2,3]

BILIARY STENTING

With the push for less invasive and more cost-efficient measures in medicine, a variety of stents are now available for use in malignant pancreaticobiliary disease. The choice

Division of Gastroenterology, University of Washington Medical Center, 1959 NE Pacific Street, Box 356424, Seattle, WA 98195, USA
* Corresponding author.
E-mail address: michaels@medicine.washington.edu

Gastrointest Endoscopy Clin N Am 23 (2013) 313–331
http://dx.doi.org/10.1016/j.giec.2012.12.009
1052-5157/13/$ – see front matter Published by Elsevier Inc.

giendo.theclinics.com

Table 1
Causes of malignant bile duct strictures

Location	Lesion
Intrahepatic bile ducts	• Cholangiocarcinoma • Hepatocellular carcinoma • Metastatic disease
Extrahepatic bile duct	• Cholangiocarcinoma • Pancreatic cancer • Ampullary malignancy • Gallbladder cancer • Metastatic disease
Hilar region	• Cholangiocarcinoma • Bulky porta hepatis lymphadenopathy

seems relatively simple: plastic or metal? What seems simple from the surface can be layered with details, ultimately making one product more favorable than another for your patients. A preprocedural checklist should include lesion resectability, goals of care, life expectancy, location of the lesion, length of the lesion, covered versus uncovered, cost, and ultimately the physician's comfort with the product (**Box 1**). Once this is all considered, the procedure can finally begin.

Plastic Stents

Plastic stents have been used since the 1980s and are made from materials including Teflon, polyurethane, and polyethylene. Diameters range from 7.0F to 11.5F and lengths extend from 5 to 18 cm. Options include straight stents with flaps at each end, a single-pigtail stent, or double-pigtailed stent for anchoring purposes (**Fig. 1**). Insertion is via a push catheter over a guidewire. Plastic stents are very effective and are inexpensive when compared with their metallic counterparts; however, the short duration of stent patency, approximately 3 months, is a drawback. Stent occlusion can develop in the setting of sludge, tumor overgrowth, tissue debris, or bacterial colonization,[4] requiring repeat endoscopic retrograde cholangiopancreatographies (ERCP) every 3 months, or more frequently for stent occlusion, through the remainder of the patients' life.

Metal Stents

Self-expanding metal stents (SEMS) are configured into a cylinder by interwoven wires and are deployed from a preconstrained position within a delivery catheter, in

Box 1
Preprocedural checklist

• Lesion resectability and goals of care

• Life expectancy given stage of disease and comorbidities

• Location and length of the lesion

• Plastic versus self-expanding metal stents

• Covered versus uncovered

• Cost comparisons

• Physician comfort level with the procedure

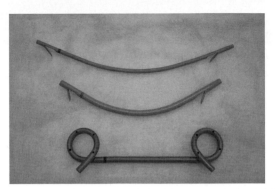

Fig. 1. Plastic stents: examples of straight and double-pigtailed plastic biliary stents. (*Courtesy of* Boston Scientific, Natick, MA; with permission.)

a through-the-scope manner (**Fig. 2**). These stents offer a larger diameter (6–8–10 mm sizes), which leads to an extended duration of stent patency (approximately 6 to 12 months). SEMS are more expensive than plastic and may not be removable because of tumor and tissue ingrowth. They can be made from 3 separate materials: stainless steel, nitinol (nickel and titanium combination), or Platinol (platinum core with nitinol encasement). Nitinol has been traditionally used, but there is a lack of evidence that any one material is superior to the others.[5,6]

Stents are uncovered, partially covered, or fully covered. The covering consists of a silicone, polycaprolactone, polyether polyurethane, polyurethane, or expanded polytetrafluoroethylene fluorinated ethylene propylene lining. After deployment, the stent expands into both the tumor and normal biliary epithelium through radial pressure in the following 24 to 48 hours.

Covered Versus Uncovered and Future Developments

There have been multiple studies comparing the patency of covered versus uncovered stents used in distal pancreaticobiliary malignancy (**Table 2**). The potential benefit of covered SEMS is removability, along with a theoretical longer patency rate. Studies have displayed reduced tumor ingrowth, but patency rates remained on par with uncovered SEMS because of tumor overgrowth, debris, sludge, and food impaction.[7–9] Potential disadvantages of fully covered stents include higher rates of stent migration, inability to use them at the hilum, and higher cost.

Uncovered SEMS are recommended in patients with intact gallbladders or hilar lesions to prevent cystic duct or major hepatic duct occlusion from the covered lining.

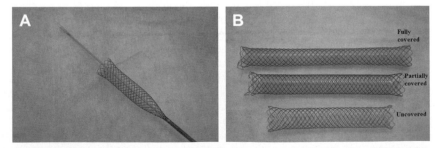

Fig. 2. Metal stents: (*A*) SEMS with delivery device and partial deployment. (*B*) Examples of a covered, partially covered, and uncovered biliary SEMS. (*Courtesy of* Boston Scientific Wallflex©, Natick, MA; with permission.)

Table 2
Distal malignant stricture: covered versus uncovered SEMS patency

Author	Covered SEMS Patency	Uncovered SEMS Patency	Significance
Yoon et al,[12] 2006	Mean of 398 d	Mean of 319 d	$P = .578$
Park et al,[13] 2006	Mean of 148.9 d	Mean of 143.5 d	$P = .531$
Telford et al,[27] 2010	Median of 357 d[a]	Median of 711 d	$P = .530$
Kullman et al,[28] 2010	154 d (Day when 25% of stents occluded)	199 d (Day when 25% of stents occluded)	$P = .348$
Saleem et al,[29] 2011	Weighted mean difference of + 60.56 d	Weighted mean difference of −60.56 d	$P = .001$

[a] Partially covered stents used.

Multiple studies have also demonstrated low rates of migration of uncovered SEMS in malignant biliary obstruction[10–14]; however, the disadvantages include tumor ingrowth and limited removability. The future of stent development is in the direction of drug-eluding stents incorporating chemotherapeutic agents, radioactive stents, and biodegradable stents.

Indications and Efficacy Introduction

Endoscopic biliary stenting is the therapeutic modality of choice to decompress the biliary system in pancreaticobiliary malignancies. Two variables should be considered before the procedure: the indication for decompression and the efficacy of the intervention. After these are considered and a plan is made, the intervention can be relatively straightforward.

Preoperative Decompression

The need for preoperative biliary decompression, however, is controversial. Placing a short, distal metal or plastic stent does not affect the surgeon's ability to perform a future pancreatoduodenectomy; however, the benefit of preoperative biliary drainage with regard to postoperative outcomes has been questioned.[15,16] Proceeding directly to surgery limits the number of interventions, potentially reducing costs and procedure-related complications. A recent multicenter randomized controlled trial included 202 patients with resectable pancreatic cancer. The patients were either taken to surgery within 1 week of diagnosis or had preoperative biliary drainage for 4 to 6 weeks followed by surgery. Significantly more serious complications were found in the biliary drainage group compared with those in the surgery alone group (74% vs 39%), although mortality rates were not significantly different.[17] This study was criticized for a 25% ERCP failure rate in addition to the use of plastic stents. However, previous retrospective studies have failed to show significantly different length of stay, infectious complications, readmission rates, and 30- and 90-day mortality rates between preoperative biliary decompression and surgery alone.[18]

Preoperative biliary decompression may improve symptoms, prevent complications of cholestasis, especially if there is a delay in surgical resection, and allow time for neoadjuvant chemotherapy in patients with locally advanced malignancy. In a recent retrospective study, 55 patients with resectable or borderline resectable pancreatic cancer were followed after receiving SEMS and neoadjuvant chemotherapy. Stent placement relieved obstruction in all of the patients, and the median time for chemotherapy was 104 days. The presence of the short biliary stent did not interfere with surgery in the 27 patients who underwent pancreatoduodenectomy.[19] The extent of liver dysfunction has also been suggested to be a major contributing factor to postoperative morbidity and mortality in regard to jaundice, secondary biliary cirrhosis, weight loss, and hypoalbuminemia, which can develop rapidly with unrelieved obstruction.[20]

Unknown Resectability

Unknown resectability leads to a significant clinical dilemma. A recent decision analysis evaluated several approaches in patients with unknown resectability and concluded that short-length SEMS is the preferred initial cost-minimizing strategy in patients with a distal common bile duct (CBD) stricture caused by suspected malignancy who are undergoing ERCP before definitive cancer staging.[21] The authors prefer short (4 cm), covered SEMS, especially if a histologic diagnosis has not been confirmed. For those patients with more proximal biliary strictures, plastic stents should generally be placed if a definitive diagnosis or staging has not been obtained or completed.

Distal: Plastic Versus Metal

Stenting in the case of unresectable malignancy for palliation is straightforward and is typically the initial endoscopic treatment, which only varies in terms of the lesion's location. Placing plastic stents is both effective and cost-effective and maintains the ability to remove or exchange the stent. However, the patency of plastic stents is typically 3 months because they eventually develop occlusion from sludge, bacterial colonization, or bacterial biofilm and require replacement.[4] Metal stents now help alleviate these issues with a prolonged duration of patency (median of 9 months) because of their increased diameter,[14,22] but metal stents come with higher costs and may not be removable. A large meta-analysis evaluated the outcomes of surgical bypass, endoscopically placed metal stents, and endoscopically placed plastic stents in patients with obstruction distal to the hilum. This study included almost 2500 patients from 24 separate studies. The results showed that SEMS produced similar outcomes to plastic stents in regard to decompression success but with improved patency rates, and the study concluded that SEMS are the treatment of choice in patients with unresectable distal malignant biliary obstruction.[1]

Numerous other randomized controlled trials have also compared plastic stents with SEMS and confirm longer patency, decreased hospitalization, decreased endoscopic procedures, and reduced overall cost in the SEMS group (**Table 3**).[22–26] SEMS should be standard of care in patients with unresectable distal pancreaticobiliary malignancy with life expectancy of more than 3–6 months.

Distal: Covered Versus Uncovered

Several trials compared stent patency rates of covered and uncovered SEMS in distal malignant biliary disease; a significant difference has not been shown (see **Table 2**).[12,13,27,28] The findings of a subsequent meta-analysis, however, contradicted these studies, showing that covered SEMS have prolonged stent patency (weighted

Table 3
Distal malignant strictures: plastic versus SEMS

Author	Plastic Stents	SEMS	Significance
Knyrim et al,[24] 1993	43% Stent failure rate	22% Stent failure rate	$P = .0035$
Prat et al,[25] 1998	3.2 mo (Median time for dysfunction)	4.8 mo (Median time for dysfunction)	Not reported
Kaassis et al,[22] 2003	5 mo (Median first obstruction)	Median not reached	$P = .007$

mean difference + 60.56 days) and prolonged survival (weighted mean difference + 68.76 days) compared with the uncovered SEMS. There was a trend toward increased stent migration, tumor overgrowth, and sludge formation with covered SEMS.[29] The choice of covered versus uncovered SEMS should be made on an individual basis in patients with distal malignant biliary obstruction depending on whether a tissue diagnosis has been obtained. If a tissue diagnosis has confirmed malignancy, then an uncovered stent is chosen. If no histologic diagnosis has been determined, a fully covered stent is appropriate to permit future removal if, as in certain cases, such as autoimmune pancreatitis and lymphoma, the obstruction may be resolved medically.

Hilar: Plastic Versus Metal Stents

Lesions in the hilum can be more technically challenging but should be stented, if technically feasible.[30] Hilar obstruction can be treated with plastic stents or uncovered SEMS as to not occlude drainage from the contralateral biliary system. In both retrospective and randomized controlled trials, SEMS outperformed plastic endoprosthesis with higher rates of successful drainage, prolonged survival, prolonged patency, and lower rates of adverse outcomes, including cholangitis, stent migration, perforation, or the need for unplanned ERCP/percutaneous transhepatic cholangiography (**Table 4**).[31–33]

Unilateral Versus Bilateral Drainage

The adequacy of unilateral or bilateral drainage continues to be debated in the setting of hilar lesions with therapy directed at palliation of obstructive symptoms. To relieve jaundice, approximately 25% to 30% of the liver needs to be drained[34]; however, unilateral drainage may incompletely relieve jaundice and increase the risk for cholangitis. Previous studies have shown variable outcomes in regard to successful decompression, stent patency, and complication rates.[35–37] In a recent 2-center retrospective study, cross-sectional imaging was used in 107 patients with hilar tumors to estimate liver volume drained by ERCP stenting. Patients were divided into groups according to the liver volume successfully drained: less than 30%, 30% to 50%, and greater than 50%. The investigators found that the main factor associated with effective drainage (defined as a decrease in serum bilirubin by 50% at day 30) was stents draining a volume greater than 50%, which frequently required bilateral stents. This group also displayed a longer median survival (119 vs 59 days, $P = .005$).[38] Conversely, intubating an atrophic sector (<30%) was not helpful and increased the risk of cholangitis. The

Table 4
Hilar malignant strictures: plastic versus SEMS

Author	Plastic Stent	SEMS	
Perdue et al,[31] 2008	32% Complications at day 30[a] 39% Stent-related adverse outcome rate	9% Complications at day 30[a] 12% Stent-related adverse outcome rate	$P = .027$ $P = .017$
Wagner et al,[32] 1993	50% Long-term stent failure rate Reinterventions for stent-related complications 2.4 ± 2.6 per pt	18.2% Long-term stent failure rate Reinterventions for stent-related complications 0.4 ± 0.5 per pt	NS NR
Sangchan et al,[33] 2012	46.3% Successful drainage Median survival 49 d	70.4% Successful drainage Median survival 126 d	$P = .011$ $P = .02$

Abbreviations: NR, Not reported, NS, not significant; pt, patient.
[a] Including occlusion, migration, perforation, and/or new cholangitis.

authors, therefore, consider high-quality cross-sectional imaging to be critical before endoscopic decompression of malignant hilar obstruction. Attempts should be made to maximize biliary drainage. If only unilateral drainage is possible, the dominant biliary system should be sought, based on preceding imaging studies. Draining more than 50% of the liver volume should be targeted, which may be achieved with unilateral or bilateral stenting (**Fig. 3**). The authors minimize contrast injection during the procedure, using only the minimum needed for effective stent placement. Care is taken to avoid injecting, intubating, or stenting atrophic (<30% of volume) segments. Stricture dilation using graded dilators (4F–7F, 5F–10F) and/or balloon dilation is performed to allow the large stents (SEMS or 10F plastic) and bilateral drainage if possible. When attempting bilateral drainage, the authors prefer placing a wire in each segment before deployment. If this is not successful, wire placement through the interstices of the stent followed by dilation can be attempted (**Fig. 4**). Finally, when attempting SEMS placement across hilar strictures, the type of SEMS chosen may be important because some are quite stiff and may be difficult to advance across tight and angulated strictures. The authors' preference is the 8-mm diameter uncovered Wallflex stent (Boston Scientific, Natick, Massachusetts), either unilaterally or bilaterally, across hilar strictures.

Complications

Complications related to ERCP and attempted biliary decompression can be significant, mainly because of the complex biliary anatomy related to the malignancy and the associated poor performance status of such patients. Complications can arise from the procedure itself, such as cardiopulmonary events, perforation, bleeding, and pancreatitis, or the complications can be stent specific, such as occlusion, migration, or infection (cholangitis, cholecystitis) (**Box 2**). The most common stenting complications remain occlusion and migration, occurring at higher rates in patients with malignant obstruction.

Stent occlusion

Stents occlude from debris, tissue ingrowth, or overgrowth. Plastic stents are particularly prone to occlusion secondary to debris. Electron microscopy studies have

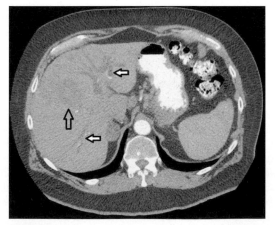

Fig. 3. Bilateral stenting to achieve more than 50% liver drainage in hilar malignancy. A patient with malignant hilar obstruction and jaundice. Computed tomography scan shows an intrahepatic mass in the right lobe of the liver (*clear arrow*) as well as dilated intrahepatic ducts bilaterally, left greater than right (*white arrows*). However, the left lobe is small and to drain at least 50% of the liver, bilateral stents would likely be needed.

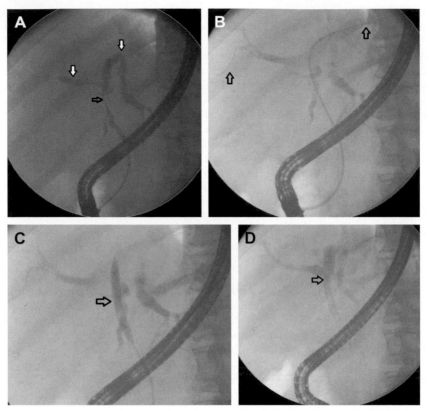

Fig. 4. Bilateral stenting to achieve more than 50% liver drainage in hilar malignancy. Same patient as **Fig. 3** with ERCP showing (*A*) a hilar stricture (*clear arrow*) and dilated intrahepatic ducts bilaterally (*white arrows*). (*B*) Successful guidewire access to both systems (*clear arrows*). (*C*) Balloon dilation of the stricture (*clear arrow*). (*D*) Despite dilation, after initial placement of the SEMS in the Left Hepatic Duct, right-sided placement was not feasible because of resistance at the level of the stricture. Successful bilateral SEMS placement was achieved by guidewire placement through the interstices (*clear arrow*) followed by dilation and eventual SEMS placement into the right system.

shown that the clogging material adheres to the inner surface of the stent through numerous tiny threads.[39] As previously mentioned, plastic stents tend to have patency of approximately 3 months[4] and require frequent replacement; SEMS have patency rates of approximately 9 months[14,22] and may be difficult to remove, especially for uncovered stents. A second stent can be successfully placed within the lumen of the occluded stent, which has been shown to be safe and effective.[40,41] SEMS are prone to tissue ingrowth requiring frequent procedures (**Fig. 5**). If removing an uncovered SEMS is desired, an effective method demonstrated by a small case series is to place a fully covered SEMS through the existing uncovered SEMS and then allow for necrosis of the tissue ingrowth during a short interval of 2 to 4 weeks before removing both stents.[42]

Stent migration
Stent migration rates for uncovered SEMS are low, around 1% to 2%, likely because of tumor and tissue embedding within the stent interstices.[10,12] Covered SEMS have

---

Box 2
Procedural complications

Endoscopy related

- Cardiopulmonary events
- Bleeding
- Perforation
- Pancreatitis

Stent related

- Occlusion
  - Tissue overgrowth, ingrowth, debris
- Migration
- Infection
  - Cholangitis, cholecystitis

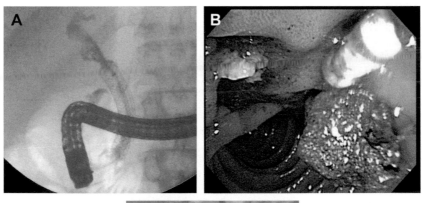

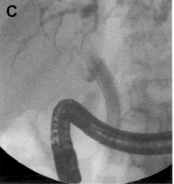

Fig. 5. (*A*) An occluded uncovered SEMS 10 months after placement for biliary obstruction caused by pancreatic cancer. (*B*) Stones and debris removed from within the stent and biliary tree with balloon sweep. (*C*) Placement of a second uncovered SEMS within the existing stent.

a comparably higher rate of migration, ranging from 6% to 8%.[7,8,11,12,43] Biliary sphincterotomy has long been thought to increase the rate of stent migration; but studies have only shown a trend toward higher migration rates with covered stents after sphincterotomy, and the question of superiority for stent migration remains unanswered.[44–46] If migration occurs after expansion, endoscopic argon plasma coagulation trimming has been reported as a safe and reproducible means of correcting stent migration or malposition.[47,48]

Infections

Ascending cholangitis remains the most common infectious complication from ERCP, stemming from incomplete drainage of an infected, obstructed biliary system. In a summary of almost 17 000 patients from prospective studies, the incidence rate was 1.4%.[49] Other large studies have shown similar rates (1.0%–2.2%).[50–52] Failure to completely drain an obstructed biliary system remains the most important predictor of post-ERCP biliary sepsis. Other risk factors for cholangitis include the procedure being performed at a small endoscopy center, combined percutaneous-endoscopic guided drainage, and malignant stricture stenting.[53,54] Cholecystitis has been associated with cystic duct occlusion from covered SEMS causing a functional gallbladder obstruction. Rates have been reported as high as 10%.[55,56] Caution should be used when deploying covered SEMS in patients with intact gallbladders.

PHOTODYNAMIC THERAPY

Since the 1970s, the incidence of cholangiocarcinoma has increased steadily in Western societies and now accounts for 2% of all gastrointestinal malignancies.[57,58] Unfortunately, less than 20% of patients are considered to have resectable tumors at the time of diagnosis.[59] Survival is typically measured in months after diagnosis, with most conventional therapies aimed at facilitating biliary decompression for symptomatic improvement. Alleviating jaundice through biliary stenting has not been associated with prolonging survival.[22,60,61] The efficacy of stenting is limited by stent patency; tissue remodeling does not occur through stenting alone. External beam radiotherapy and/or chemotherapy have also not been proven to prolong survival or adequately relieve jaundice,[62–65] leading toward a push for novel local therapies directed at not only palliating symptoms but also improving patient survival.

Photodynamic therapy (PDT) is an evolving and relatively new therapy in the management of inoperable cholangiocarcinoma that offers the possibility of remodeling the tumor mass.[66] This method is a local ablative method that combines a systemic photosensitizing agent followed by nonthermal light activation at a specific wavelength (**Fig. 6**). The photosensitizing agent, given intravenously, accumulates in malignant cells, and subsequent transpapillary or transcutaneous directed light activates the photosensitizing agent. This activation causes destruction of the neoplastic tissue through a photochemical process mediated by oxygen free radicals, mainly the singlet oxygen, which leads to the disturbance of microvasculature and the degradation of cell membranes and lysosomes.[67,68]

Description

There are 4 photosensitizing agents currently available for cholangiocarcinoma, with the hematoporphyrin derivatives (eg, Photosan-3, Photofrin II) being the most commonly used. Two to 4 days after systemic administration of the photosensitizing agent at a dose of 2 mg/kg, light activation is performed using a quartz fiber mounted with a cylindrical diffuser tip of 2 to 7 cm in length, coupled to a diode laser emitting

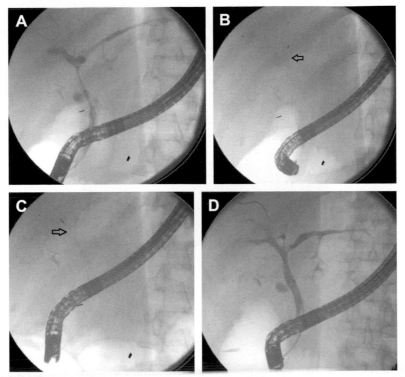

Fig. 6. Primary sclerosing cholangitis complicated by cholangiocarcinoma treated with PDT and chemoradiotherapy. (*A*) Pretreatment, (*B*) PDT fiber (*arrow*) in left intrahepatic duct, (*C*) PDT fiber (*arrow*) in right intrahepatic duct, and (*D*) 3 months after treatment.

a wavelength of 630 nm (**Fig. 7**). The energy density applied varies between 180 and 240 J/cm². The depth of ablative effect is limited by the absorption characteristics of the photosensitizer used and the resulting penetration depth of the appropriate wavelength. The depth of tumor necrosis with the hematoporphyrin derivatives is limited to 4 to 6 mm. The photosensitivity effects of the drug last for 4 to 6 weeks in decreasing intensity. These agents are also retained by the skin, leading toward potential phototoxicity as a potential side effect of PDT.[69]

Evidence for PDT

Many studies have looked at the use of PDT for cholangiocarcinoma, all with promising results. The first successful report was by McCaughan[70] in 1991, when he treated a single patient with unresectable cholangiocarcinoma with 7 sessions of PDT over a 4-year period.[70] This report was followed in the late 1990s with a prospective single-arm study by Ortner and colleagues[71] of 9 patients treated with combination Photofrin and biliary stenting. The results of the study showed prolonged survival (median 439 days), improved quality of life, and increased performance status. Several single-arm studies followed supporting the use of PDT in cholangiocarcinoma. The first randomized controlled trial was in 2003 comparing PDT plus stenting with stenting alone. The improvement in survival in the randomized PDT group was so impressive (median survival of 493 days with PDT plus stenting compared with 98 days in the stent alone group), the study was halted after the first 39 patients because it was thought to be unethical to continue randomization.[72] This study was criticized because

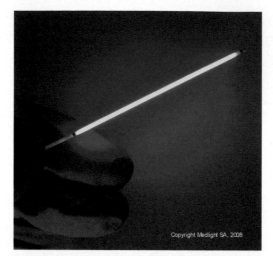

Fig. 7. PDT probe. A cylindrical light diffuser used for biliary PDT. (*Courtesy of* Medlight© SA, Switzerland; with permission.)

enrollment was limited to patients in whom biliary decompression was unsuccessful through stenting alone.[73]

Several studies followed in the 1990–2000s, all showing a significant reduction in serum bilirubin and increased survival with PDT compared with historical data (**Table 5**).[71,74–79] In one study, the presence of a visible mass on imaging and increased time between the diagnosis and PDT predicted a poorer survival rate after PDT in a multivariate analysis, suggesting that early intervention may provide better results.[76] Although many studies have been published in this area, most studies are small given the rarity of cholangiocarcinoma. A 2010 systematic review looked at all relevant studies (20 studies included) and concluded that PDT offered considerable benefit on survival and quality of life with few adverse effects and should be offered to patients with nonresectable cholangiocarcinoma.[80] The most common adverse event was cholangitis (27.5%) followed by phototoxicity (10.2%). It is difficult to tell how many cases of cholangitis are attributable to PDT because cholangitis is a complication of stenting alone. Given the high rate of cholangitis, patients should be given periprocedural antibiotics and stented. All studies were performed at expert tertiary medical centers and, thus, the results may not be generalized. The questions that remain include whether PDT in combination with chemoradiation therapy is beneficial

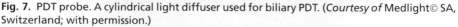

Table 5
Therapeutic effect of PDT for malignant biliary strictures

Author	Serum Bilirubin Before/After Treatment	Median Survival in PDT + Stent Groups
Ortner et al,[71] 1998	318/103	439 d
Berr et al,[75] 2000	11.2/1.1	330 d
Ortner et al,[72] 2003	9.4/2.3	16.4 mo
Zoepf et al,[79] 2005	2.75/1.3	21 mo
Prasad et al,[76] 2007	6.1/3.5	214 d
Kahaleh et al,[78] 2008	8.3/3.5	16.2 mo

in regard to survival and whether this modality can be used as a bridge for definitive therapy, such as surgical resection or transplantation.

RADIOFREQUENCY ABLATION

Radiofrequency ablation (RFA), delivered either percutaneously or interoperatively, has been used for decades as a heat delivery system for the destruction of primary and secondary hepatic tumors via localized necrosis.[81–83] Preliminary animal studies have paved the way for a promising novel endoscopic therapy for patients with malignant bile duct obstruction.[84,85]

Description

RFA uses radio waves for heat production, which leads to injury to abnormal cells. The Habib EndoHPB (EMcision UK, London, United Kingdom) is a novel device that has recently been approved to assist in localized destruction of tissue during endoscopic procedures. This catheter is a bipolar 8F catheter, 180 cm useable length, with 2 stainless steel electrodes 8 mm apart, 5 mm from the distal tip (**Fig. 8**). The catheter is compatible with endoscopes that have a working channel of 3.2 mm or greater and is introduced over a 0.035-in guidewire into the biliary system. This probe is activated at 10 W of energy for 90 seconds at a time, which produces local coagulation necrosis over a 2.5 cm length. Depending on the length of the stricture, sequential applications can be applied. The device is then removed with subsequent stent insertion.

Evidence for RFA

One recent study looked at the efficacy of endoscopically applied RFA in malignant bile duct obstruction. Steel and colleagues[86] performed RFA in 22 patients (16

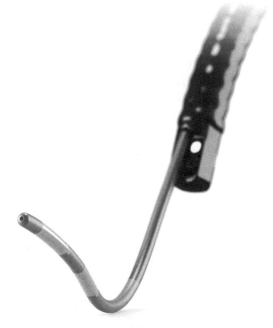

Fig. 8. RFA probe. The Habib EndoHPB bipolar RFA catheter. (*Courtesy of* François Poulin, EMcision International, Montreal, QC; with permission.)

pancreatic cancer, 6 cholangiocarcinoma) with unresectable malignant bile duct obstruction in an open-label pilot study at a single tertiary care unit between 2009 and 2010. RFA was successfully delivered in 21 of the 22 patients enrolled, with all 21 patients demonstrating stent patency at day 30. At day 90, 3 patients had stent occlusions and one patient died of disease progression (the stent was patent). Complications included biochemical pancreatitis and rigors, and 2 patients required percutaneous cholecystostomies. The known complications of RFA including hemorrhage and abscess formation at the site of the RFA[82,83] were not experienced in this study. This study concluded that RFA in the biliary system is safe and effective; however, randomized studies with longer follow-up are needed. Monga and colleagues[87] subsequently published a successful case report showing pictures and video before and after RFA treatment of a 1.5-cm mid-CBD stricture diagnosed as cholangiocarcinoma. Further studies are needed to evaluate RFA over a longer period, evaluating stricture resolution and survival, stent patency, complications, and cost-effectiveness.

SUMMARY

Endoscopic-guided therapy, primarily with stent placement, directed at palliation of malignant biliary obstruction, has evolved greatly over the last 3 decades, becoming the procedure of choice for biliary decompression. The endoscopic goal is for adequate biliary drainage to palliate obstructive symptoms but also to limit the number of interventions in the patients' remaining life. A preprocedural plan should be made through a multidisciplinary approach and should address key questions specific to each patient, including potential for resection, life expectancy, goals of care, location of the lesion, and costs. Cross-sectional imaging is critical before proceeding with attempted biliary decompression, especially for hilar strictures. Endoscopically directed biliary therapies, such as PDT and RFA, hold promise to improve patient outcomes for those with locally advanced or unresectable disease.

REFERENCES

1. Moss AC, Morris E, Leyden J, et al. Malignant distal biliary obstruction: a systematic review and meta-analysis of endoscopic and surgical bypass results. Cancer Treat Rev 2007;33:213–21.
2. Geer RJ, Brennan MF. Prognostic indicators for survival after resection of pancreatic adenocarcinoma. Am J Surg 1993;165:68–72.
3. Levy MJ, Baron TH, Gostout CJ, et al. Palliation of malignant extrahepatic biliary obstruction with plastic versus expandable metal stents: an evidence based approach. Clin Gastroenterol Hepatol 2004;2:273–85.
4. Donelli G, Guaglianone E, Di Rosa R, et al. Plastic biliary stent occlusion: factors involved and possible preventive approaches. Clin Med Res 2007;5:53–60.
5. Chun HJ, Kim ES, Hyun JJ, et al. Gastrointestinal and biliary stents. J Gastroenterol Hepatol 2010;25(2):234.
6. Chen YK, Jakribettuu V, Springer EW, et al. Safety and efficacy of argon plasma coagulation trimming of malpositioned and migrated biliary metal stents: a controlled study in the porcine model. Am J Gastroenterol 2006;101(9):2025.
7. Ornellas LC, Stefanidis G, Chuttani R, et al. Covered Wallstents for palliation of malignant biliary obstruction: primary stent placement versus reintervention. Gastrointest Endosc 2009;70(4):676.
8. Kahaleh M, Tokar J, Conaway MR, et al. Efficacy and complications of covered Wallstents in malignant distal biliary obstruction. Gastrointest Endosc 2005;61(4):528.

9. Kahaleh M, Brock A, Conaway MR, et al. Covered self-expandable metal stents in pancreatic malignancy regardless of resectability: a new concept validated by a decision analysis. Endoscopy 2007;39(4):319.

10. Loew BJ, Howell DA, Sanders MK, et al. Comparative performance of uncoated, self-expanding metal biliary stents of different designs in 2 diameters: final results of an international multicenter, randomized, controlled trial. Gastrointest Endosc 2009;70(3):445.

11. Yang KY, Ryu JK, Seo JK, et al. A comparison of the Niti-D biliary uncovered stent and the uncovered Wallstent in malignant biliary obstruction. Gastrointest Endosc 2009;70(1):45.

12. Yoon WJ, Lee JK, Lee KH, et al. A comparison of covered and uncovered Wall-stents for the management of distal malignant biliary obstruction. Gastrointest Endosc 2006;63(7):996.

13. Park do H, Kim MH, Choi JS, et al. Covered versus uncovered wallstent for malignant extrahepatic biliary obstruction: a cohort comparative analysis. Clin Gastroenterol Hepatol 2006;4(6):790.

14. Yoon WJ, Ryu JK, Yang KY, et al. A comparison of metal and plastic stents for the relief of jaundice in unresectable malignant biliary obstruction in Korea: an emphasis on cost effectiveness in a country with a low ERCP cost. Gastrointest Endosc 2009;70:284–9.

15. Laurent A, Tayar C, Cherqui D. Cholangiocarcinoma: preoperative biliary drainage (Con). HPB (Oxford) 2008;10:126.

16. Nimura Y. Preoperative biliary drainage before resection for cholangiocarcinoma (Pro). HPB (Oxford) 2008;10:130.

17. Van der Gaag NA, Rauws EA, van Eijck CH, et al. Preoperative biliary drainage for cancer of the head of the pancreas. N Engl J Med 2010;362:129.

18. Coates JM, Beal SH, Russo JE, et al. Negligible effect of selective preoperative biliary drainage on perioperative resuscitation, morbidity, and mortality in patients undergoing pancreaticoduodenectomy. Arch Surg 2009;144:841.

19. Aadam AA, Evans DB, Khan A, et al. Efficacy and safety of self-expandable metal stents for biliary decompression in patients receiving neoadjuvant therapy for pancreatic cancer: a prospective study. Gastrointest Endosc 2012;76:67.

20. Su CH, Tsay SH, Wu CC, et al. Factors influencing postoperative morbidity, mortality, and survival after resection for hilar cholangiocarcinoma. Ann Surg 1996;223:384.

21. Chen VK, Arguedas MR, Baron TH. Expandable metal biliary stents before pancreaticoduodenectomy for pancreatic cancer: a Monte-Carlo decision analysis. Clin Gastroenterol Hepatol 2005;3:1229.

22. Kaassis M, Boyer J, Dumas R, et al. Plastic or metal stents for malignant stricture of the common bile duct? Results of a randomized prospective study. Gastrointest Endosc 2003;57(2):178–82.

23. Carr-Locke DL, Ball TJ, Connors PJ, et al. Randomized, controlled trial of metal stents for malignant obstruction of the common bile duct. Gastrointest Endosc 1993;39:310A.

24. Knyrim K, Wagner HJ, Pausch J, et al. A prospective, randomized, controlled trial of metal stents for malignant obstruction of the common bile duct. Endoscopy 1993;25:207–12.

25. Prat F, Chapat O, Ducot B, et al. Randomize trial of endoscopic drainage methods for inoperable malignant strictures of the common bile duct. Gastrointest Endosc 1998;47:1–7.

26. Moses PL, Alan BN, Gordon SR, et al. A randomized multicenter trial comparing plastic to covered metal stents for palliation of lower malignant biliary obstruction. Gastrointest Endosc 2006;63:AB289.

27. Telford JJ, Carr-Locke DL, Baron TH, et al. A randomized trial comparing uncovered and partially covered self-expandable metal stents in the palliation of distal malignant biliary obstruction. Gastrointest Endosc 2010;72:907.

28. Kullman E, Frozanpor F, Söderlund C, et al. Covered versus uncovered self-expandable nitinol stents in the palliative treatment of malignant distal biliary obstruction: results from a randomized, multicenter study. Gastrointest Endosc 2010;72:915.

29. Saleem A, Leggett CL, Murad MH, et al. Meta-analysis of randomized trials comparing the patency of covered and uncovered self-expandable metal stents for palliation of distal malignant bile duct obstruction. Gastrointest Endosc 2011; 74:321.

30. Larghi A, Tringali A, Lecca PG, et al. Management of hilar biliary strictures. Am J Gastroenterol 2008;103:458.

31. Perdue DG, Freeman ML, DiSario JA, et al. Plastic versus self-expanding metallic stents for malignant hilar biliary obstruction: a prospective multicenter observational cohort study. J Clin Gastroenterol 2008;42:1040.

32. Wagner HJ, Knyrim K, Vakil N, et al. Plastic endoprostheses versus metal stents in the palliative treatment of malignant hilar biliary obstruction. A prospective and randomized trial. Endoscopy 1993;25:213.

33. Sangchan A, Kongkasame W, Pugkhem A, et al. Efficacy of metal and plastic stents in unresectable complex hilar cholangiocarcinoma: a randomized controlled trial. Gastrointest Endosc 2012;76:93.

34. Dowsett JF, Vaira D, Hatfield AR, et al. Endoscopic biliary therapy using the combined percutaneous and endoscopic technique. Gastroenterology 1989; 96:1180.

35. Deviere J, Baize M, de Toeuf J, et al. Long-term follow-up of patients with hilar malignant stricture treated by endoscopic internal biliary drainage. Gastrointest Endosc 1988;34:95.

36. De Palma GD, Galloro G, Siciliano S, et al. Unilateral versus bilateral endoscopic hepatic duct drainage in patients with malignant hilar biliary obstruction: results of a prospective, randomized, and controlled study. Gastrointest Endosc 2001; 53:547.

37. Naitoh I, Ohara H, Nakazawa T, et al. Unilateral versus bilateral endoscopic metal stenting for malignant hilar biliary obstruction. J Gastroenterol Hepatol 2009;24:552.

38. Vienne A, Hobeika E, Gouya H, et al. Prediction of drainage effectiveness during endoscopic stenting of malignant hilar strictures: the role of liver volume assessment. Gastrointest Endosc 2010;72(4):736–8.

39. Weickert U, Zimmerling S, Eickhoff A, et al. Comparative scanning electron microscopic study of biliary and pancreatic stents. Z Gastroenterol 2009;47(4):347.

40. Togawa O, Kawabe T, Isayama H, et al. Management of occluded uncovered metallic stents in patients with malignant distal biliary obstructions using covered metallic stents. J Clin Gastroenterol 2008;42(5):546.

41. Rogart JN, Boghos A, Rossi F, et al. Analysis of endoscopic management of occluded metal biliary stents at a single tertiary care center. Gastrointest Endosc 2008;68(4):676.

42. Hirdes MM, Siersema PD, Houben MH, et al. Stent-in-stent technique for removal of embedded esophageal self-expanding metal stents. Am J Gastroenterol 2011; 106(2):286–93.

43. Soderlund C, Linder S. Covered metal versus plastic stents for malignant common bile duct stenosis: a prospective, randomized, controlled trial. Gastrointest Endosc 2006;63(7):986.

44. Artifon EL, Sakai P, Ishioka S, et al. Endoscopic sphincterotomy before deployment of covered metal stent is associated with greater complication rate: a prospective randomized control trial. J Clin Gastroenterol 2008;42(7):815.

45. Banerjee N, Hilden K, Baron TH, et al. Endoscopic biliary sphincterotomy is not required for transpapillary SEMS placement for biliary obstruction. Dig Dis Sci 2011;56(2):591.

46. Davids PH, Groen AK, Rauws EA, et al. Randomised trial of self-expanding metal stents versus polyethylene stents for distal malignant biliary obstruction. Lancet 1992;340(8834–8835):1488.

47. Vanbiervliet G, Piche T, Caroli-Bosc FX, et al. Endoscopic argon plasma trimming of biliary and gastrointestinal metallic stents. Endoscopy 2005;37(5):434.

48. Christiaens P, Decock S, Buchel O, et al. Endoscopic trimming of metallic stents with the use of argon plasma. Gastrointest Endosc 2008;67(2):369.

49. Andriulli A, Loperfido S, Napolitano G, et al. Incidence rates of post-ERCP complications: a systematic survey of prospective studies. Am J Gastroenterol 2007;102(8):1781.

50. Anderson DJ, Shimpi RA, McDonald JR, et al. Infectious complications following endoscopic retrograde cholangiopancreatography: an automated surveillance system for detecting postprocedure bacteremia. Am J Infect Control 2008; 36(8):592.

51. Williams EJ, Taylor S, Fairclough P, et al. Risk factors for complication following ERCP: results of a large-scale, prospective multicenter study. Endoscopy 2007; 39(9):793.

52. Wang P, Li ZS, Liu F, et al. Risk factors for ERCP-related complications: a prospective multicenter study. Am J Gastroenterol 2009;104(1):31.

53. Loperfido S, Angelini G, Benedetti G, et al. Major early complications from diagnostic and therapeutic ERCP: a prospective multicenter study. Gastrointest Endosc 1998;48(1):1.

54. Freeman ML, Nelson DB, Sherman S, et al. Complications of endoscopic biliary sphincterotomy. N Engl J Med 1996;335(13):909.

55. Suk KT, Kim HS, Kim JW, et al. Risk factors for cholecystitis after metal stent placement in malignant biliary obstruction. Gastrointest Endosc 2006;64(4):522.

56. Fumex F, Coumaros D, Napoleon B, et al. Société Française d'Endoscopie Digestive. Similar performance but higher cholecystitis rate with covered biliary stents: results from a prospective multicenter evaluation. Endoscopy 2006; 38(8):787.

57. Welzel TM, et al. Impact of classification of hilar cholangiocarcinomas (Klatskin tumors) on the incidence of intra- and extrahepatic cholangiocarcinoma in the United States. J Natl Cancer Inst 2006;98:873–5.

58. Shaib Y, El-Serag HB. The epidemiology of cholangiocarcinoma. Semin Liver Dis 2004;24:115–25.

59. Jarnagin WR, et al. Staging, resectability, and outcome in 225 patients with hilar cholangiocarcinoma. Ann Surg 2001;234(4):507–17.

60. Chang WH, Kortan P, Haber GB. Outcome in patients with bifurcation tumors who undergo unilateral versus bilateral hepatic drainage. Gastrointest Endosc 1998; 47(5):354–62.

61. Prat F, et al. Predictive factors for survival of patients with inoperable malignant distal biliary strictures: a practical management guideline. Gut 1998;42(1):76–80.

62. Shinchi H, et al. Length and quality of survival following external beam radiotherapy combined with expandable metallic stent for unresectable hilar cholangiocarcinoma. J Surg Oncol 2000;75(2):89–94.

63. Bowling TE, et al. A retrospective comparison of endoscopic stenting alone with stenting and radiotherapy in non-resectable cholangiocarcinoma. Gut 1996; 39(6):852–5.
64. Rao S, et al. Phase III study of 5FU, etoposide and leucovorin (FELV) compared to epirubicin, cisplatin and 5FU (ECF) in previously untreated patients with advanced biliary cancer. Br J Cancer 2005;92(9):1650–4.
65. Glivelius B, et al. Chemotherapy improves survival and quality of life in advanced pancreatic and biliary cancer. Ann Oncol 1996;7(6):593–600.
66. Berr F, et al. Neoadjuvant photodynamic therapy before curative resection of proximal bile duct carcinoma. J Hepatol 2000;32:352–7.
67. Abels C. Targeting of the vascular system of solid tumours by photodynamic therapy (PDT). Photochem Photobiol Sci 2004;3(8):765–71.
68. Dougherty TJ, et al. Photodynamic therapy. J Natl Cancer Inst 1998;90(12): 889–905.
69. Zoepf T. Photodynamic therapy of cholangiocarcinoma. HPB (Oxford) 2008;10: 161–3.
70. McCaughan JS Jr, et al. Photodynamic therapy to treat tumors of the extrahepatic biliary ducts. A case report. Arch Surg 1991;126:111–3.
71. Ortner MA, et al. Photodynamic therapy of nonresectable cholangiocarcinoma. Gastroenterology 1998;114:536–42.
72. Ortner MA, et al. Successful photodynamic therapy for nonresectable cholangiocarcinoma: a randomized prospective study. Gastroenterology 2003; 125(5):1355.
73. Gores GJ. A spotlight on cholangiocarcinoma. Gastroenterology 2003;125: 1536–8.
74. Rumalla A, Baron TH, Wang KK, et al. Endoscopic application of photodynamic therapy for cholangiocarcinoma. Gastrointest Endosc 2001;53:500–4.
75. Berr F, Weidmann M, Tannapfel A, et al. Photodynamic therapy for advanced bile duct cancer: evidence for improved palliation and extended survival. Hepatology 2000;31:291–8.
76. Prasad GA, Wang KK, Baron TH, et al. Factors predicting survival in patients with cholangiocarcinoma treated with photodynamic therapy. Clin Gastroenterol Hepatol 2007;5:743–8.
77. Dumoulin FL, Gerhardt T, Fuchs S, et al. Phase II study of photodynamic therapy and metal stent as palliative treatment for nonresectable hilar cholangiocarcinoma. Gastrointest Endosc 2003;57:860–7.
78. Kahaleh M, et al. Unresectable cholangiocarcinoma: comparison of survival in biliary stenting alone versus stenting with photodynamic therapy. Clin Gastroenterol Hepatol 2008;6(3):290–7.
79. Zoepf T, Jakobs R, Arnold JC, et al. Palliation of nonresectable bile duct caner: improved survival after photodynamic therapy. Am J Gastroenterol 2005;100: 2426–30.
80. Gao F, Yu B, et al. Systematic review: photodynamic therapy for unresectable cholangiocarcinoma. J Hepatobiliary Pancreat Sci 2010;17:125–31.
81. Cho YK, Kim JK, Kim MY, et al. Systemic review of randomized trials for hepatocellular carcinoma treated with percutaneous ablation therapies. Hepatology 2009;49:453–9.
82. Mulier S, Ruers T, Jamart J, et al. Radiofrequency ablation versus resection for resectable colorectal liver metastases: time for a randomized trial? An update. Dig Surg 2008;25:445–60.

83. Sutherland LM, Williams JA, Padbury RT, et al. Radiofrequency ablation of liver tumors: a systematic review. Arch Surg 2006;141:181–90.
84. Khorsandi S. In vivo experiments for the development of a novel bipolar radiofrequency probe (EndoHPB) for the palliation of malignant biliary obstruction. EASL Monothematic Conference, June 12-14, 2008. Liver cancer: from molecular pathogenesis to new therapies (P97).
85. Khorsandi SE, Zacharoulis D, Vavra P, et al. The modern use of radiofrequency energy in surgery, endoscopy, and interventional radiology. Eur Surg 2008;40: 204–10.
86. Steel AW, Postgate AJ, Khorsandi S, et al. Endoscopically applied radiofrequency ablation appears to be safe in the treatment of malignant biliary obstruction. Gastrointest Endosc 2011;73(1):149–53.
87. Monga A, Gupta R, Ramchamdani M, et al. Endoscopic radiofrequency ablation of cholangiocarcinoma: a new palliative treatment modality. Gastrointest Endosc 2011;74(4):935–7.

Biliary Manifestations of Systemic Diseases

Zaree Babakhanian, MD, John A. Donovan, MD*

KEYWORDS

- Systemic disease • Biliary manifestations • Bile duct imaging
- Endoscopic approaches

KEY POINTS

- Systemic illnesses can cause bile duct injuries and biliary tract disease.
- Biliary tract disease accompanying systemic illnesses is most often characterized by cholestasis, with or without clinical jaundice and mild liver enzyme abnormalities.
- Bile duct changes caused by immunoglobulin 4 cholangiopathy must be distinguished from pancreatic cancer and cholangiocarcinoma.
- Critical illness, regardless of cause, can cause bile duct injury mimicking sclerosing cholangitis.
- Acquired immune deficiency syndrome cholangiopathy is a bile duct disease of diminishing importance in the era of highly active antiretroviral therapy therapy.

INTRODUCTION

Biliary manifestations of systemic disease are common. Cholestasis causing clinical jaundice, hyperbilirubinemia, and nonspecific liver enzyme abnormalities are common sequels to systemic inflammatory and infectious conditions. Less often, but importantly, systemic illnesses cause more direct injury to the biliary tract (**Box 1**). Endoscopic evaluations of these biliary tract involvements that complicate systemic illnesses are sometimes indicated and of proven therapeutic benefit.

IGG4-ASSOCIATED CHOLANGITIS

IgG4-related systemic disease (ISD) is a recently recognized, multisystem, fibroinflammatory condition characterized by IgG4-rich lymphoplasmacytic infiltration of affected organs and increased serum IgG4. Of the disease variants, autoimmune pancreatitis is

No disclosures.
Division of Gastrointestinal and Liver Diseases, Keck School of Medicine, University of Southern California, 2011 Zonal Avenue, HMR 101, Los Angeles, CA 90033, USA
* Corresponding author.
E-mail address: jdonovan@usc.edu

Gastrointest Endoscopy Clin N Am 23 (2013) 333–346
http://dx.doi.org/10.1016/j.giec.2012.12.001
1052-5157/13/$ – see front matter © 2013 Elsevier Inc. All rights reserved.

giendo.theclinics.com

Box 1
Systemic diseases with biliary manifestations

Immunoglobulin G4 (IgG4) cholangiopathy

Sclerosing cholangitis in critically Ill patients (SC-CIP)

Acquired immune deficiency syndrome (AIDS) cholangiopathy

Cystic fibrosis

Sarcoidosis

Sickle cell disease

Graft-versus-host disease (GVHD)

Mycobacterium tuberculosis

Lymphoma

Histiocytosis X

---

the best studied. In 2001, increased serum IgG4 was described in patients with auto-immune pancreatitis (AIP).[1] IgG4-related systemic disease has since been associated with effects in multiple organs.[2–4] IgG4-associated cholangitis (IAC) is the biliary manifestation of ISD. Cases of biliary strictures that were previously reported in autoimmune pancreatitis and steroid-responsive biliary strictures were probably IAC related.[5]

IgG4-associated cholangitis can resemble primary sclerosing cholangitis (PSC), cholangiocarcinoma, or pancreatic cancer and needs to be distinguished from these conditions so that unnecessary surgery can be avoided and appropriate medical therapy can be initiated.[6] Patients with IAC are usually men in their sixth decade presenting with obstructive jaundice, weight loss, and mild abdominal discomfort.[7] Coexisting inflammatory bowel disease should suggest the diagnosis of PSC rather than IAC.[6,7] Alkaline phosphatase levels are usually 4 to 5 times the upper limit of normal (ULN) and are accompanied by increased total bilirubin and mild aspartate aminotransferase (AST) and alanine aminotransferase (ALT) increases.[7] Carbohydrate antigen (CA) 19-9 levels of more than 100 IU/mL usually indicate cases of cholangiocarcinoma rather than IAC.[7]

Increased serum IgG4 is present at diagnosis in most (75%), but not all, patients with IAC.[7,8] In contrast, less specific IgG4 increases can occur in patients with biliary strictures from other causes including PSC[9,10] and cholangiocarcinoma.[8] Increased IgG4 values (>140 mg/dL) are 64% to 78% sensitive and 88% specific in discriminating IAC from cholangiocarcinoma. Increasing the IgG4 cutoff value to more than 280 mg/dL decreases sensitivity to 34% to 50% and increases the specificity for the diagnosis of IAC to 97%.[8]

The nonspecific cholangiogram findings in IgG4-associated cholangitis are shown by the results of cholangiography in a series of 53 patients described by Ghazale[7]:

- Intrapancreatic biliary strictures resembling those seen pancreatic cancer (51%)
- Proximal extrahepatic biliary strictures resembling cholangiocarcinoma (9%)
- Intrahepatic biliary strictures resembling those seen in PSC (8%)
- Multifocal strictures with combinations of the first 3 findings (32%)

Findings from endoscopic transpapillary intraductal ultrasound that better distinguish IAC from cholangiocarcinoma include smooth outer and inner margins of imaged strictures and homogeneous internal echoes.[11] The measured bile duct thickness in areas of normal-appearing (uninvolved) bile ducts seen by cholangiography can be of additional clinical importance. A duct wall thickness of 0.8 mm was 95% sensitive and 90.9% specific in differentiating IAC from cholangiocarcinoma, and a wall thickness of 1 mm was 85% sensitive and 100% specific for IAC.[11]

The diagnosis of IgG4 cholangiopathy cannot be established by endoscopic retrograde cholangiopancreatography (ERCP) alone. The occasional finding of IgG4-positive cells in cases of PSC and cholangiocarcinoma limits this finding's ability to establish or confirm a diagnosis of IAC.[7,11,12] In IAC cases, ERCP serves an adjunctive and complimentary role to other diagnostic methods. Ampulla of Vater and transpapillary bile duct biopsies in patients with IAC often do not show classic histologic findings. The presence of IgG4 immunostained cells (>10 stained cells/high-power field) and absence of malignant cells support a suspected diagnosis of IAC.[7] Biopsies from both the ampulla and bile duct increase the probability of finding IgG4-positive cells. Kawakami and colleagues[12] showed that 21 of 29 (72%) patients had more than 10 IgG4-positive cells in at least 1 biopsy specimen.

An algorithm has been suggested for diagnosing and managing IAC using the HISORt (histology, imaging, serology, other organ involvement, response to steroid therapy) criteria (**Table 1**).[7] Patients with unexplained biliary strictures are considered to have IAC when core biopsies or surgical specimens from biliary or pancreatic tissues show features of IAC or AIP.[7,13] Unexplained biliary strictures with classic imaging findings of AIP plus increased IgG4 results also confirm a diagnosis of IAC.[7] The diagnosis of IAC is probable in patients with unexplained biliary strictures when 2 or more of the following conditions are present: (1) increased serum IgG4, (2) pancreatic imaging suggesting AIP,[13] (3) the presence of other organ involvement with IgG4-related disease, or (4) bile duct biopsy showing more than 10 IgG4-positive

Table 1 HISORt criteria of IAC	
Feature	**Characteristic**
Histology of the bile duct	Lymphoplasmacytic infiltrate with >10 IgG4-positive cells/hpf within and around the bile ducts with associated obliterative phlebitis and storiform fibrosis. See text regarding bile duct biopsy specimens
Imaging of the bile duct	One or more strictures involving intrahepatic, proximal extrahepatic, or intrapancreatic bile ducts Fleeting/migrating biliary strictures
Serology	Increased IgG4
Other organ involvement	Pancreas: imaging or histology consistent with AIP or suggesting AIP Retroperitoneal fibrosis Renal involvement Salivary/lacrimal gland enlargement IgG4 immunostaining of involved organs shows ≥10 IgG4-positive cells/hpf The presence of IBD suggests PSC rather than IAC
Response to steroid therapy	Improvement of liver tests and biliary strictures

Abbreviations: hpf, high-power field; IBD, inflammatory bowel disease.

cells/high-power field.[7] In this group of patients, the diagnosis of IAC is confirmed by response to steroid therapy.

Clinical response, indicated by lessening of bile duct strictures, is expected in patients with IAC treated with steroids (**Fig. 1**).[5] Nonresponse in patients with suspected IAC indicates the possibility of a different diagnosis that most often includes pancreatic or biliary malignancy.[7] Biliary stent placement before steroid therapy can lead to more rapid resolution of symptoms and allow ERCP with possible stent removal after 6 to 8 weeks of steroid treatment.[7] Relapse of disease can occur with steroid withdrawal and is more common in patients with proximal strictures.[7,14] Maintenance therapies with azathioprine and mycophenolate mofetil have been described.[7] Overall, the prognosis for treated patients with IAC seems to be good, although long-term studies proving efficacy are lacking.

SCLEROSING CHOLANGITIS IN CRITICALLY ILL PATIENTS

Sclerosing cholangitis in critically ill patients (SC-CIP) is a secondary sclerosing cholangitis seen in severely ill patients without biliary obstruction, PSC, or other preexisting biliary diseases. A wide array of underlying disease processes in the critically ill are associated with this condition, including severe pneumonia, bacterial sepsis, polytrauma, and burn injuries.[15,16] Affected patients, regardless of the type of critical illness, commonly require prolonged intensive care unit confinements, mechanical ventilation, and vasopressor support. There are no specific patient demographics with regard to age or sex associated with SC-CIP; in one report, patients with SC-CIP ranged in age from 16 to 73 years.[16]

The pathogenesis of biliary duct damage in SC-CIP is thought to be secondary to ischemic injury.[15,17,18] The intrahepatic bile ducts receive blood exclusively from the peribiliary vascular plexus and are highly sensitive to ischemic injury. Arterial hypoperfusion related to severity of illness may cause ischemic injury of the bile duct epithelium, which in turn may lead to biliary cast formation (**Fig. 2**) and SC-CIP.[17] Gelbamann and colleagues[15] performed chemical analyses on biliary casts from patients with SC-CIP, and protein, presumably from necrotic biliary epithelium, was the main component.

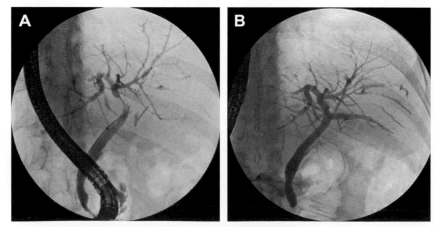

Fig. 1. IgG4-associated sclerosing cholangitis with intrahepatic strictures mimicking PSC (A) before treatment, and (B) after 12 weeks of steroid therapy. (*From* Ghazale A, Chari ST, Zhang L, et al. Immunoglobulin G4-associated cholangitis: clinical profile and response to therapy. Gastroenterology 2008;134:710; with permission from Elsevier.)

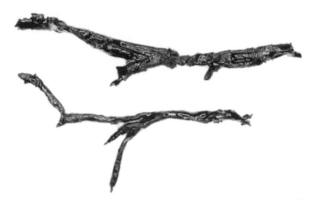

Fig. 2. Extracted biliary casts that resemble the intrahepatic ductal system. (*From* Ruemmele P, Hofstaedter F, Gelbmann CM. Secondary sclerosing cholangitis. Nat Rev Gastroenterol Hepatol 2009;6:287–95; with permission from Macmillan Publishers Ltd.)

Cholestasis of SC-CIP is generally noticed within the first 1 to 2 weeks after the initial physiologic insult and injury.[15,19] Early in development, SC-CIP can be difficult to differentiate from sepsis-associated cholestasis. SC-CIP is a progressive disorder, whereas sepsis-associated cholestasis typically resolves with recovery from the underlying condition.[20] Marked increase of serum alkaline phosphatase is the most prominent laboratory abnormality in this condition, with levels commonly more than 1000 U/L and usually associated with clinical and laboratory evidence of jaundice. Mild increases 2 to 3 times the ULN of AST and ALT are typical.[15,16,19]

In patients with SC-CIP, ultrasound with Doppler should be performed to evaluate patency of the hepatic artery and to exclude hepatic or portal vein thrombosis. Ultrasound examinations are otherwise not helpful in diagnosing SC-CIP. Bile duct obstruction causing dilatation in SC-CIP is unusual. Magnetic resonance cholangiopancreatography (MRCP) showed intrahepatic strictures in a small series of SC-CIP cases.[21]

ERCP plays a key role in diagnosing SC-CIP. Dynamic cholangiogram findings can worsen with disease progression (**Box 2**).[15,16]

ERCP also has a therapeutic role for patients with SC-CIP, allowing dilation and stenting of strictures. Multiple sessions of ERCP are sometimes required.[16] Extracting biliary casts (**Fig. 3**) and debris by balloon catheter or Dormia basket results in clinical

---

Box 2
Cholangiogram findings and disease progression

- Intrahepatic bile duct cast formation leading to intraductal filling defects early in disease course

- Multiple irregular intrahepatic biliary strictures of variable degree occurring several weeks after onset of cholestasis

- Advancing rarefaction of small bile ducts and progressive sclerosis several months after onset of cholestasis

- Dominant strictures of the right or left hepatic ducts

- Common bile duct (CBD) is generally unremarkable except in cases of filling defects from biliary casts migration

- Biliary casts resembling intrahepatic ductal system

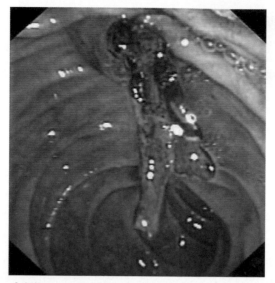

Fig. 3. Extraction of biliary casts through the papilla of Vater. (*From* Ruemmele P, Hofstaedter F, Gelbmann CM. Secondary sclerosing cholangitis. Nat Rev Gastroenterol Hepatol 2009;6:287–95; with permission from Macmillan Publishers Ltd.)

and biochemical improvements with decreasing bilirubin and alkaline phosphatase.[15,19] Nasobiliary drainage and saline lavage do not remove biliary casts from smaller intrahepatic ducts inaccessible to endoscopic intervention.[15]

Failure of endoscopic therapies to improve SC-CIP predicts poor outcomes. In long-term follow-up of 29 patients with SC-CIP, 19 patients died, 3 patients required orthotropic liver transplantation, 4 patients were registered for transplantation, and 3 patients showed signs of severe cholestasis.[18] Ursodeoxycholic acid (UDCA) used in combination with endoscopic treatments may transiently improve the clinical course but does not seem to affect progression.[16] Prescription of UDCA in 16 of the 29 patients followed longitudinally was thought to be of limited efficacy.[18]

AIDS CHOLANGIOPATHY

Biliary manifestations in patients with AIDS were first described before the advent of highly active antiretroviral therapy (HAART). The associated type of secondary sclerosing cholangitis was initially classified as AIDS-related sclerosing cholangitis and later as AIDS cholangiopathy. In a report of 3 patients with AIDS and biochemical evidence of cholestatic liver disease, all 3 patients had stenosis of the distal CBD and irregularity of the intrahepatic bile ducts.[22] A larger series later described variable ERCP findings in 26 patients with AIDS and suspected biliary tract disease.[23]

In contemporary patients, the diagnosis of AIDS cholangiopathy should be considered in untreated human immunodeficiency virus (HIV) disease and unexplained cholestasis. HIV-infected patients with AIDS cholangiopathy usually have low cluster of differentiation 4 (CD4) counts and evidence of opportunistic infection. CD4 counts are typically less than 200×10^6/L and most patients have a CD4 count less than 50×10^6/L.[24] Multiple opportunistic infections, most commonly by *Cryptosporidium* and cytomegalovirus species, are implicated as causes of AIDS-associated cholangiopathy.[22,23,25]

Patients with AIDS cholangiopathy present with complaints of right upper quadrant and epigastric pain. Fever is present in approximately one-half of patients. Liver profiles reflect cholestasis but clinical jaundice is rare. The most striking laboratory abnormality is a marked increase of serum alkaline phosphatase to 6 or 7 times the ULN. Serum transaminases are typically increased only 2 to 3 times the ULN.[23,26,27]

Noninvasive imaging by ultrasound is the initial study of choice in evaluating patients with AIDS and suspected bile duct injury. Ultrasound findings include minimal to marked dilatation of the intrahepatic and extrahepatic bile ducts, and thickening of the CBD wall. A normal transabdominal ultrasound should not, however, preclude further imaging and diagnostic considerations in patients with suspected bile duct disease, because ultrasound examination fails to show biliary abnormalities in 11% to 28% of cases.[23,25,27] MRCP and endoscopic ultrasound (EUS) were not available during the early descriptions of AIDS cholangiopathy so reports of MRCP and EUS findings in these patients are lacking.

Since the early reports of the disease, ERCP has been the predominate mode of bile duct study used to confirm a diagnosis of AIDS cholangiopathy. Cholangiogram results can be categorized into 4 major findings, described in **Box 3**.[23] Papillary stenosis with intrahepatic ductal irregularities resembling sclerosing cholangitis is the most common finding, occurring in approximately 50% to 70% of cases (**Fig. 4**).[23,26,27]

ERCP can facilitate the diagnosis of opportunistic infections in patients with AIDS cholangiopathy. Intra-ampullary biopsies after sphincterotomy or biopsies of the major papilla when sphincterotomy is not performed can be of diagnostic importance.[23,25,28] *Cryptosporidium* and cytomegalovirus species are the most commonly recovered organisms from obtained biopsy specimens.[23,25,28] Aspirated bile can also be examined and cultured.[25] The presence of opportunistic organisms in biopsied tissue or collected bile predicts poor outcomes.[24] Despite this observation, the clinical significance of microorganisms in biliary samples is difficult to assess, because species-specific treatments do not improve AIDS cholangiopathy.[27]

ERCP has an important therapeutic role in the treatment of patients with AIDS cholangiopathy. Multiple studies show that endoscopic sphincterotomy improves abdominal pain caused by papillary stenosis.[23,25-28] Despite the symptomatic relief, there is no expected survival benefit after sphincterotomy. In a large study of 94 patients over 20 years, the adjusted hazard ratio resulting from endoscopic sphincterotomy was not statistically significant (adjusted hazard ratio 0.67, 95% confidence interval 0.40–1.11).[24]

AIDS cholangiopathy is an increasingly rare diagnosis in the era of HAART and medically controlled HIV disease. In a series of AIDS cholangiopathy cases between 1983 and 2001, 68 patients were diagnosed before, and only 23 cases after, 1993.

Box 3
Four major findings of cholangiogram results

- Distal CBD stricture with proximal dilatation of CBD (papillary stenosis) and intrahepatic ductal irregularities resembling sclerosing cholangitis
- Distal CBD stricture with proximal dilatation of CBD (papillary stenosis) and normal intrahepatic ducts
- Normal extrahepatic ducts with irregularities of the intrahepatic ducts resembling sclerosing cholangitis
- Long extrahepatic bile duct strictures with or without intrahepatic abnormalities

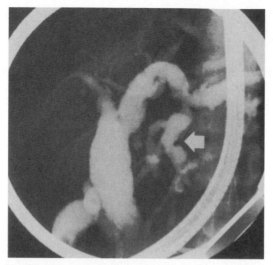

Fig. 4. Diffuse intrahepatic sclerosing cholangitis and papillary stenosis. Markedly abnormal intrahepatic ducts with dilatation and focal stricturing (*arrow*). (*From* Cello JP. Acquired immunodeficiency syndrome cholangiopathy: spectrum of disease. Am J Med 1989;86:542; with permission from Elsevier.)

The prognosis of patients with AIDS cholangiopathy depends on the underlying HIV-related condition.[24] Patients with limited access to treatment, or who are medically noncompliant, remain at risk for worsening AIDS and complications including AIDS cholangiopathy.

CYSTIC FIBROSIS

Cystic fibrosis (CF) is an autosomal recessive multiorgan disease caused by mutations in the gene that encodes for the cystic fibrosis transmembrane conductance regulator (CFTR). Mucosal obstruction of exocrine glands is the main contributor to morbidity in affected patients.[29] The lungs and the pancreas are the most commonly involved organs. Improved care and survival of patients with CF have exposed other targeted tissues to disease that includes hepatobiliary disorders.[30]

In the liver, CFTR is expressed in biliary epithelial cells and participates in bile excretion.[31] CFTR dysfunction causes mucous plugging of bile ductules in some patients with CF. Progressive inflammation can evolve to focal biliary fibrosis, cirrhosis, and further complications.[32]

The biliary manifestations of CF include sclerosing cholangitis like involvement of the intrahepatic bile ducts, CBD strictures, choledocholithiasis, and rare intrahepatic biliary stones. Patient presentations and laboratory evaluations are often nonspecific and may fail to identify those with biliary involvement. In one study, only 3 of 20 patients with CF-related liver disease complained of abdominal pain; 2 of the 3 had choledocholithiasis.[33] The most striking liver test abnormality, when present, is an increased alkaline phosphatase increased 2 to 4 times the ULN.[33,34]

Ultrasound is an insensitive tool for detecting duct abnormalities in this population. In 2 studies of patients with CF-associated biliary disease, ultrasound imaging failed to show abnormalities of the intrahepatic and/or extrahepatic ducts.[33,34] Despite these limitations, ultrasound is recommended as an initial screening examination when CF-related disease is suspected.[35] Magnetic resonance cholangiography is more specific and is the preferred imaging modality to evaluate CF patients with biliary tract disease. A prospective study of magnetic resonance cholangiogram features in these patients included biliary abnormalities resembling sclerosing cholangitis in patients without clinical, laboratory, or ultrasound data suggesting biliary tract disease.[36] Intrahepatic biliary abnormalities were seen in 18 of 26 patients undergoing MRCP. Nine of these 18 patients did not have clinical evidence of liver or biliary disease.[35] In another series, 13 of 20 patients had abnormalities of the intrahepatic or extrahepatic biliary ducts seen on MRCP.[37]

Cholangiography findings in adults with CF are shown in **Box 4**.[33–35,37,38]

Optimal treatments for CF-related biliary disease are not well reported and evidence supporting endoscopic therapy for intra/extrahepatic biliary abnormalities in CF is lacking. Therapeutic ERCP intervention, on a case-to-case basis, should be dictated by the likelihood of success in the correction of a specific bile duct abnormality (ie, choledocholithiasis, dominant stricture) causing illness. Early detection of biliary tract manifestations of CF and the use of UDCA have been advocated, but there are no data showing improved outcomes relative to the progression of bile duct disease, development of secondary biliary cirrhosis, the need for liver transplantation, or death.[39]

SARCOIDOSIS

Sarcoidosis is a multiorgan disease characterized by noncaseating granulomas in affected organs. Although infrequent, hepatic sarcoidosis is considered by some experts to be more underreported than rare.[40] The broad spectrum of liver disease caused by sarcoidosis ranges from asymptomatic hepatic granulomas to diffuse hepatic involvement leading to chronic liver disease and cirrhosis with a need for liver transplantation.[41–43] Biliary involvement in sarcoidosis has been most often described in case reports.[42,44,45] Sarcoidosis-related biliary tract injuries vary from small intralobular bile duct changes mimicking primary biliary cirrhosis to larger intrahepatic and extrahepatic bile duct changes similar to those characteristic of PSC.

Whether hepatic sarcoidosis causes biliary disease resembling PSC or whether sarcoidosis can coexist independently with PSC is not clear. The presence of inflammatory bowel disease and serum antineutrophil cytoplasmic antibody in a patient with sarcoidosis is more suggestive of a rare coexistence with PSC. Case reports argue that individual patients are affected by either secondary sclerosing cholangitis caused by sarcoidosis or by independent PSC in the liver of the patient with systemic sarcoidosis.[45,46] The importance of this distinction lies in the treatment and overall prognosis of patients with sarcoidosis who may have bile duct injury responsive to steroid treatment.

Box 4
Cholangiography findings in adults

- Beading and strictures of the intrahepatic ducts
- Minor variations in caliber caused by strictures of right and/or left intrahepatic ducts
- CBD strictures[a]
- Choledocholithiasis of extrahepatic and intrahepatic ducts (rare)

[a] CBD strictures have been reported with high frequency by some investigators[38] but have not been consistently shown as prevalent by others.[33,34]

Patients with sarcoidosis involving the biliary tree may present with abdominal pain, weight loss, and, occasionally, jaundice.[41,44] A cholestatic biochemical profile characterized by increased serum alkaline phosphatase is most typical. Although these symptoms and laboratory findings are nonspecific, they should prompt further investigation for bile duct involvement in a patient with diagnosed sarcoidosis or with signs and symptoms of systemic illness suggesting the diagnosis.[47] Liver biopsies showing noncaseating granulomas in the context of systemic illness with biliary tract disease should also raise the possibility of sarcoidosis-related biliary disease.[40]

ERCP findings are generally similar to those found in PSC. Various ERCP findings from case reports are described in **Box 5**.[42–45,48]

Steroid therapy for sarcoidosis with biliary tract involvement can improve ERCP[42] and biochemical findings in some cases.[45] The role of endoscopy in the management of biliary sarcoidosis is not clear, although dominant strictures can be dilated and stented. Individual patient and clinical conditions should dictate ERCP and endoscopic interventions.

SICKLE CELL DISEASE

Sickle cell disease (SCD) is an inherited cause of chronic hemolytic anemia with multiple end-organ effects.[49] Right upper quadrant pain and jaundice in a patient with SCD suggests a wide differential diagnosis that includes acute sickle cell hepatic crisis, sickle cell intrahepatic cholestasis, and choledocholithiasis.[50] Gallstones are a frequent complication of SCD and, by one prospective report, are present in one-half of patients with homozygous SCD by the age of 22 years.[51] Chronic hemolysis and the released bilirubin stored in the gallbladder enable the precipitation of pigmented gallstones that are characteristically black.[49]

Patients with SCD who have cholestatic jaundice and a normal biliary ultrasound should be further evaluated by MRCP or EUS before ERCP. One report found that 42 of 79 (53%) patients with SCD who also had cholestatic jaundice and normal ultrasound results had normal ERCP findings.[52] Among all patients undergoing ERCP, approximately 25% had dilatation of the bile ducts without an obstructive cause. The investigators surmised that this nonobstructive cholangiopathy might be caused by sickling in end arteries of the biliary arterial tree leading to hypoxic bile duct injury and dilatation.[52] SCD causing an ischemic cholangiopathy characterized by multiple stenoses of the intrahepatic ducts has also been proposed but more rare.[53]

Choledocholithiasis was reported in approximately 39% of patients with SCD and cholestatic jaundice evaluated by ERCP.[52] Preoperative ERCP before cholecystectomy has been advocated for those patients with indications of CBD stones including

---

Box 5
ERCP findings form case reports

- Dominant stricture of distal right hepatic duct without proximal intrahepatic duct dilatation. Less prominent segmental strictures and dilatations in other intrahepatic bile ducts. Normal CBD.

- Multiple strictures and dilatations of intrahepatic ducts.

- Multiple segmental strictures in the intrahepatic bile ducts. High-grade CBD stricture.

- Left hepatic duct stenosis with proximal dilatation. Beaded intrahepatic ducts.

- Common hepatic duct narrowing and dilatation of intrahepatic bile ducts.

choledocholithiasis on imaging, cholelithiasis with a dilated CBD, biochemical evidence of obstructive jaundice, or a history of pancreatitis.[54]

GVHD

GVHD is a potentially devastating event following allogeneic bone marrow, hematopoietic stem cell and, less frequently, solid organ transplantation. The incidence of GVHD is greater after donation from an unrelated donor. Donor-derived T-cell activation and an immune-related attack of targeted organs in the immunosuppressed recipient is the mechanism of injury.[55] Systemic manifestations include skin, liver, and gastrointestinal disorders. Hepatic involvement of variable severity is related to multiple factors, including sepsis, medication-induced injury, and sinusoidal occlusive disease after preconditioning before hematopoietic engraftment. Intrahepatic cholestasis and jaundice are the most common clinical findings, although an acute hepatitis like presentation may also occur.[56]

Direct injury of the biliary tract by GVHD is most often mediated by an immunologic injury of small and medium-sized bile ducts leading to vanishing bile duct syndromes and progressive cholestasis. Ketelsen and colleagues[57] studied computed tomography imaging of the gallbladder and CBD in 27 patients with hepatic or gastrointestinal GVHD after allogeneic hematopoietic stem cell transplantation. Findings included increased enhancements of the gallbladder and CBD and increased enhancement and dilatation of the duodenum. Measured increases in CBD diameters were more common in these patients than in stem cell recipients without GVHD (67% vs 12%; $P<.0001$). The investigators implicated GVHD-related inflammation of the major papilla and sphincter of Oddi dysfunction as reasons for the differences.[57]

There are limited data regarding the usefulness of ERCP in evaluating patients with GVHD and bile duct changes after transplantation. Kim and colleagues[58] reported ERCP findings in a group of 40 hematopoietic stem cell recipients. Three recipients with hepatic GVHD were in a subset of patients with normal-appearing CBD. When present, strictures were most often malignant and predicted mortality.[58]

OTHER CONDITIONS

Bile duct injuries have been reported, in small or single case series, in a variety of other conditions with systemic involvements. Important among these are rare descriptions of *mycobacterium tuberculosis*,[59] malignant lymphomas,[60] and histiocytosis X[61] causing focal bile duct strictures and obstruction.

SUMMARY

Multiple target organs may be injured as a result of systemic illness. When involved, injuries to the biliary tract are most often manifested by cholestasis and abnormal liver tests with or without clinical jaundice. Noninvasive imaging may help in diagnosis. More often, ERCP is needed for a more sensitive evaluation, better diagnosis, and effective treatment.

REFERENCES

1. Hamano H, Kawa S, Horiuchi A, et al. High serum IgG4 concentrations in patients with sclerosing pancreatitis. N Engl J Med 2001;344:732–8.
2. Hamaguchi Y, Fujimoto M, Matsushita Y, et al. IgG4-related skin disease, a mimic of angiolymphoid hyperplasia with eosinophilia. Dermatology 2011;223:301–5.

3. Kakudo K, Li Y, Taniguchi E, et al. IgG4-related disease of the thyroid glands. Endocr J 2012;59:273–81.
4. Cornell LD. IgG4-related kidney disease. Curr Opin Nephrol Hypertens 2012;21: 279–88.
5. Bjornsson E, Chari ST, Smyrk TC, et al. Immunoglobulin G4 associated cholangitis: description of an emerging clinical entity based on review of the literature. Hepatology 2007;45:1547–54.
6. Nakazawa T, Naitoh I, Hayashi K, et al. Diagnostic criteria for IgG4-related sclerosing cholangitis based on cholangiographic classification. J Gastroenterol 2012;47:79–87.
7. Ghazale A, Chari ST, Zhang L, et al. Immunoglobulin G4-associated cholangitis: clinical profile and response to therapy. Gastroenterology 2008;134:706–15.
8. Oseini AM, Chaiteerakij R, Shire AM, et al. Utility of serum immunoglobulin G4 in distinguishing immunoglobulin G4-associated cholangitis from cholangiocarcinoma. Hepatology 2011;54:940–8.
9. Mendes FD, Jorgensen R, Keach J, et al. Elevated serum IgG4 concentration in patients with primary sclerosing cholangitis. Am J Gastroenterol 2006;101: 2070–5.
10. Alswat K, Al-Harthy N, Mazrani W, et al. The spectrum of sclerosing cholangitis and the relevance of IgG4 elevations in routine practice. Am J Gastroenterol 2012;107:56–63.
11. Naitoh I, Nakazawa T, Ohara H, et al. Endoscopic transpapillary intraductal ultrasonography and biopsy in the diagnosis of IgG4-related sclerosing cholangitis. J Gastroenterol 2009;44:1147–55.
12. Kawakami H, Zen Y, Kuwatani M, et al. IgG4-related sclerosing cholangitis and autoimmune pancreatitis: histological assessment of biopsies from Vater's ampulla and the bile duct. J Gastroenterol Hepatol 2010;25:1648–55.
13. Chari ST, Smyrk TC, Levy MJ, et al. Diagnosis of autoimmune pancreatitis: the Mayo Clinic experience. Clin Gastroenterol Hepatol 2006;4:1010–6.
14. Alderlieste YA, van den Elzen BD, Rauws EA, et al. Immunoglobulin G4-associated cholangitis: one variant of immunoglobulin G4-related systemic disease. Digestion 2009;79:220–8.
15. Gelbmann CM, Rummele P, Wimmer M, et al. Ischemic-like cholangiopathy with secondary sclerosing cholangitis in critically ill patients. Am J Gastroenterol 2007; 102:1221–9.
16. Engler S, Elsing C, Flechtenmacher C, et al. Progressive sclerosing cholangitis after septic shock: a new variant of vanishing bile duct disorders. Gut 2003;52: 688–93.
17. Ruemmele P, Hofstaedter F, Gelbmann CM. Secondary sclerosing cholangitis. Nat Rev Gastroenterol Hepatol 2009;6:287–95.
18. Kulaksiz H, Heuberger D, Engler S, et al. Poor outcome in progressive sclerosing cholangitis after septic shock. Endoscopy 2008;40:214–8.
19. Jaeger C, Mayer G, Henrich R, et al. Secondary sclerosing cholangitis after long-term treatment in an intensive care unit: clinical presentation, endoscopic findings, treatment, and follow-up. Endoscopy 2006;38:730–4.
20. Chand N, Sanyal AJ. Sepsis-induced cholestasis. Hepatology 2007;45:230–41.
21. Scheppach W, Druge G, Wittenberg G, et al. Sclerosing cholangitis and liver cirrhosis after extrabiliary infections: report on three cases. Crit Care Med 2001;29:438–41.
22. Margulis SJ, Honig CL, Soave R, et al. Biliary tract obstruction in the acquired immunodeficiency syndrome. Ann Intern Med 1986;105:207–10.

23. Cello JP. Acquired immunodeficiency syndrome cholangiopathy: spectrum of disease. Am J Med 1989;86:539–46.
24. Ko WF, Cello JP, Rogers SJ, et al. Prognostic factors for the survival of patients with AIDS cholangiopathy. Am J Gastroenterol 2003;98:2176–81.
25. Ducreux M, Buffet C, Lamy P, et al. Diagnosis and prognosis of AIDS-related cholangitis. AIDS 1995;9:875–80.
26. Benhamou Y, Caumes E, Gerosa Y, et al. AIDS-related cholangiopathy. Critical analysis of a prospective series of 26 patients. Dig Dis Sci 1993;38:1113–8.
27. Bouche H, Housset C, Dumont JL, et al. AIDS-related cholangitis: diagnostic features and course in 15 patients. J Hepatol 1993;17:34–9.
28. Schneiderman DJ, Cello JP, Laing FC. Papillary stenosis and sclerosing cholangitis in the acquired immunodeficiency syndrome. Ann Intern Med 1987;106:546–9.
29. Rowe SM, Miller S, Sorscher EJ. Cystic fibrosis. N Engl J Med 2005;352: 1992–2001.
30. Bhardwaj S, Canlas K, Khai C, et al. Hepatobiliary abnormalities and disease in cystic fibrosis. Epidemiology and outcomes through adulthood. J Clin Gastroenterol 2009;43:858–64.
31. Curry MP, Hegarty JE. The gallbladder and biliary tract in cystic fibrosis. Curr Gastroenterol Rep 2005;7:147–53.
32. Colombo C. Liver disease in cystic fibrosis. Curr Opin Pulm Med 2007;13:529–36.
33. O'Brien S, Keogan M, Casey M, et al. Biliary complications in cystic fibrosis. Gut 1992;33:387–91.
34. Nagel RA, Javaid A, Meire HB, et al. Liver disease and bile duct abnormalities in adults with cystic fibrosis. Lancet 1989;2:1422–5.
35. Feranchak AP. Hepatobiliary complications of cystic fibrosis. Curr Gastroenterol Rep 2004;6:221–9.
36. Durieu I, Pellet O, Simonot L, et al. Sclerosing cholangitis in adults with cystic fibrosis: a magnetic resonance cholangiographic prospective study. J Hepatol 1999;30:1052–6.
37. King LJ, Scurr ED, Murugan N, et al. Hepatobiliary and pancreatic manifestations of cystic fibrosis: MR imaging appearances. Radiographics 2000;20:767–77.
38. Gaskin KJ, Waters DL, Howman-Giles R, et al. Liver disease and common-bile-duct stenosis in cystic fibrosis. N Engl J Med 1988;318:340–6.
39. Debray D, Kelly D, Houwen R, et al. Best practice guidance for the diagnosis and management of cystic fibrosis-associated liver disease. J Cyst Fibros 2011;10: S29–36.
40. Devaney K, Goodman ZD, Epstein MS, et al. Hepatic sarcoidosis. Clinicopathologic features in 100 patients. Am J Surg Pathol 1993;17(12):1272–80.
41. Ebert EC, Kierson M, Hagspiel KD. Gastrointestinal and hepatic manifestations of sarcoidosis. Am J Gastroenterol 2008;103:3184–92.
42. Alam I, Levenson SD, Ferrell LD, et al. Diffuse intrahepatic biliary strictures in sarcoidosis resembling sclerosing cholangitis. Case report and review of the literature. Dig Dis Sci 1997;42:1295–301.
43. Tombazzi C, Waters B, Ismail MK, et al. Sarcoidosis mimicking primary sclerosing cholangitis requiring liver transplantation. Ann Hepatol 2008;7:83–6.
44. Rezeig MA, Fashir BM. Biliary tract obstruction due to sarcoidosis: a case report. Am J Gastroenterol 1997;92:527–8.
45. Maambo E, Brett AS, Vasudeva R, et al. Hepatobiliary sarcoidosis presenting as sclerosing cholangitis: long-term follow-up. Dig Dis Sci 2007;52:3363–5.
46. Lidar M, Langevitz P, Livneh A, et al. Sclerosing cholangitis associated with systemic sarcoidosis. J Clin Gastroenterol 2003;36:84–5.

47. Thomas KW, Hunninghake GW. Sarcoidosis. JAMA 2003;289:3300–3.
48. Romero-Gomez M, Suarez-Garcia E, Otero MA, et al. Sarcoidosis, sclerosing cholangitis, and chronic atrophic autoimmune gastritis: a case of infiltrating sclerosing cholangitis. J Clin Gastroenterol 1998;27:162–5.
49. McCavit TL. Sickle cell disease. Pediatr Rev 2012;33:195.
50. Banerjee S, Owen C, Chopra S. Sickle cell hepatopathy. Hepatology 2001;33: 1021–8.
51. Bond LR, Hatty SR, Horn ME, et al. Gall stones in sickle cell disease in the United Kingdom. Br Med J 1987;295:234–6.
52. Issa H, Al-Haddad A, Al-Salem A. Sickle cell cholangiopathy: an endoscopic retrograde cholangiopancreatography evaluation. World J Gastroenterol 2009; 15:5316–20.
53. Hillaire S, Gardin C, Attar A, et al. Cholangiopathy and intrahepatic stones in sickle cell disease: coincidence or ischemic cholangiopathy? Am J Gastroenterol 2000;95:300–1.
54. Issa H, Al-Salem AH. Role of ERCP in the era of laparoscopic cholecystectomy for the evaluation of choledocholithiasis in sickle cell anemia. World J Gastroenterol 2011;17:1844–7.
55. Blazer BR, Murphy WJ, Abdedi M. Advances in graft-versus-host disease biology and therapy. Nat Rev Immunol 2012;12:443–58.
56. Hogan W, Maris M, Storer B. Hepatic injury after nonmyeloablative conditioning followed by allogeneic hematopoietic cell transplantation: a study of 193 patients. Blood 2004;103(1):78–84.
57. Ketelsen D, Vogel W, Bethge W, et al. Enlargement of the common bile duct in patients with acute graft vs host disease: what does it mean? Am J Roentgenol 2009;193(3):w181.
58. Kim H, Alousi A, Lee J, et al. Role of ERCP in patients after hematopoietic stem cell transplantation. Gastrointest Endosc 2011;74:817.
59. Chong VH, Lim KS. Hepatobiliary tuberculosis. Singapore Med J 2010;51: 744–51.
60. Menias CO, Prasad S, Wang HL, et al. Mimics of cholangiocarcinoma: spectrum of disease. Radiographics 2008;28(4):1115–29.
61. Thompson HH, Pitt HA, Lewin KJ. Sclerosing cholangitis and histiocytosis X. Gut 1984;25:526–30.

Endoscopic Approach to the Patient with Benign or Malignant Ampullary Lesions

Hyung-Keun Kim, MD[a,b], Simon K. Lo, MD[b,c],*

KEYWORDS

- Endoscopic papillectomy • Ampullectomy • Pancreaticoduodenectomy
- Ampullary adenoma • Ampullary cancer

KEY POINTS

- Adenoma is the most common benign ampullary lesion and clinically most important because of its potential to undergo malignant transformation to ampullary cancer. Adenocarcinoma is the most common malignant ampullary lesion.
- Endoscopic examination using side-viewing duodenoscopy with tissue sampling is typically needed to establish the diagnosis. However, endoscopic biopsy may not detect intramural tumor and early focal adenocarcinoma.
- Endoscopic ultrasonography or transpapillary intraductal ultrasonography can provide more detailed and accurate information on the extent of ampullary tumors, including the dimensions, echogenicity, involvement of duodenal layers, and possibly regional lymph node status.
- Endoscopic papillectomy is regarded as a curative treatment of ampullary adenoma and may be a curative treatment of ampullary adenoma with high-grade intraepithelial neoplasia/in situ tumor. The current data also suggest that when an endoscopically resected specimen has a well-differentiated intramucosal cancer with clear margins and no angiolymphatic invasion, subsequent radical surgery may not be necessary.
- There is no standardized technique for endoscopic removal of ampullary tumors (eg, submucosal injection, endoscopic resection, electrocautery setting, pancreatic stenting, biliary stenting, pancreatic or biliary sphincterotomy), because of complexity of the procedure.
- Future randomized, long-term, follow-up studies are required to address many unresolved issues and to provide evidence for future consensus in this field.

The author has nothing to disclose.
[a] Division of Gastroenterology, Department of Internal Medicine, The Catholic University of Korea College of Medicine, Uijeongbu St. Mary's Hospital, 65-1, Guemo-dong, Uijeongbu 480-717, Republic of Korea; [b] Cedars-Sinai Medical Center, 8700 Beverly Boulevard, Room 7511, Los Angeles, CA 90048, USA; [c] David Geffen School of Medicine at UCLA, Los Angeles, CA 90095, USA
* Corresponding author. Cedars-Sinai Medical Center, 8700 Beverly Boulevard, Room 7511, Los Angeles, CA 90048.
E-mail address: simon.lo@cshs.org

INTRODUCTION

Tumors of the major duodenal papilla, also known as ampullary tumors, are rare, with an approximate 5% incidence of all gastrointestinal neoplasms.[1] It has a reported prevalence of 0.04% to 0.12% of the general population, based on autopsy series.[2,3] These tumors seem to be detected more frequently with increasing performance of upper endoscopic examination and endoscopic retrograde cholangiopancreatography (ERCP). Adenoma is the most common benign ampullary tumor.[1] Ampullary adenomas seem to follow the adenoma-to-carcinoma sequence in progression, similar to that of colorectal cancer.[4–6] Endoscopic biopsy of ampullary tumors carries an alarming 30% false-negative rate for detecting carcinoma-in-situ and invasive carcinoma.[7] Thus, there is a need for complete resection.

Historically, radical surgery with pancreaticoduodenectomy (Whipple procedure) was considered the standard treatment of ampullary tumors.[8,9] However, this operation has considerable morbidity (27%–52%) and mortality (3%–9%)[8–12] and is rarely performed for the treatment of known benign ampullary tumors. Rather, a limited surgery with transduodenal local excision (ampullectomy) is more commonly performed. Although surgical ampullectomy is associated with fewer morbidities (19%–33%) and mortalities (0%–3%) than pancreaticoduodenectomy,[12–14] there is concern about the high recurrence rate of up to 35%.[12,15]

An attractive treatment modality for benign ampullary tumors is endoscopic therapy, which mainly consists of endoscopic resection and thermal ablation. First described in the 1980s,[16–20] numerous cases and cohort series of endoscopic papillectomy (EP), both retrospective and prospective, have been reported.[20–49] These series have provided ample evidence that endoscopic ampullectomy or snare resection can be used as first-line therapy for benign ampullary adenoma. However, there remain concerns about endoscopic ampullectomy, including its technical difficulties, complications, incomplete removal, and a high rate of recurrence. Recently, preoperative assessment with endoscopic ultrasonography (EUS) has enabled identification of early or focal ampullary cancer for endoscopic ampullectomy. However, the consensus on how and when to use endoscopic ampullectomy has not been fully established.

This article reviews the approach to the patient with benign or malignant ampullary lesion.

BENIGN AND MALIGNANT AMPULLARY LESIONS

Benign ampullary tumors are rare and include adenoma, lipoma, fibroma, lymphangioma, leiomyoma, hamartoma, hemangioma, and carcinoid and neurogenic tumor.[50–53] Of these benign tumors, adenoma is the most common[1] and clinically most important, because of its potential to undergo malignant transformation to ampullary cancer.[4–6] Adenoma is classified histopathologically, according to its microscopic architecture, as tubular, villous, or tubulovillous. Ampullary adenoma may occur sporadically or in the context of genetic syndromes, such as familial adenomatous polyposis (FAP). The major duodenal papilla is a common site of extracolonic adenoma in FAP.[54] The risk of ampullary adenomas and adenocarcinomas is increased 200-fold to 300-fold in such genetic polyposis syndromes.[55]

The primary malignant ampullary tumors are adenocarcinoma, lymphoma, neuroendocrine, and signet ring cell carcinoma.[51,53] Metastatic neoplasms include malignant melanoma, hypernephroma, and lymphoma.[51] Of these malignant lesions, adenocarcinoma is the most common. Malignancies of the distal common bile duct, head of pancreas, duodenum, and major duodenal papilla are collectively referred to as periampullary cancer.[56] Of these regional neoplastic lesions, ampullary adenocarcinoma has perhaps the highest rate of resectability and the best prognosis.[57,58] This may be, in part, because the anatomic location allows symptoms and presentation to occur earlier, and also in part because adenocarcinoma of the papilla tends histologically to be more differentiated.[59] **Fig. 1** shows the various benign or malignant ampullary lesions.

Neuroendocrine Tumors

Primary neuroendocrine tumors of the ampulla of Vater are rare and constitute a heterogeneous group of neoplasms both clinically and morphologically.[60] As with neuroendocrine tumors in other sites, 2 morphologic variants of neuroendocrine neoplasms in the ampulla have been recognized: benign neuroendocrine tumors, known as carcinoid tumors, and high-grade neuroendocrine carcinomas, which show malignant behavior and have recently been characterized as small cell carcinomas or large cell neuroendocrine carcinomas.[61–63] They are often recognized as

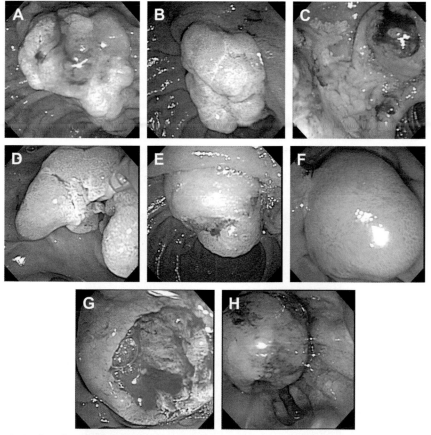

Fig. 1. Various benign or malignant ampullary lesions. (*A*) Adenoma in patient with FAP. (*B*) Large ampullary adenoma. (*C*) Ampullary adenoma with huge laterally spreading tumor. (*D*) Laterally spreading tumor over the papilla. (*E*) Ampullary cancer. (*F*) Bulging papilla with periampullary cancer. (*G*) Ampullary cancer with spontaneous hemorrhage. (*H*) Large ampullary neuroendocrine tumor.

a submucosal, round or oval mass, which may have overlying ulcerations (**Fig. 2**).[64] The natural histories of ampullary carcinoid and high-grade neuroendocrine carcinoma are not well established. However, according to the recent study using data from the National Cancer Institute's SEER (Surveillance Epidemiology and End Results) program from 1973 to 2006, there were 82 carcinoid tumors and 57 high-grade neuroendocrine carcinomas[65]; Of these 57, 42 were neuroendocrine carcinomas; 9 were small cell carcinomas; and 6 were large cell neuroendocrine carcinomas. The mean size of ampullary carcinoid tumors was 1.76 cm and high-grade neuroendocrine carcinoma was 3.05 cm. The frequency of lymph node metastasis was 28.5% for carcinoid tumors and 62% for high-grade neuroendocrine carcinomas. Although there have been several reports of endoscopic treatment of small carcinoid tumors arising from the duodenum,[66] the standard treatment of ampullary carcinoid tumor and high-grade neuroendocrine carcinoma is surgery. Endoscopic resection may be appropriate in selected patients, but the selection criteria have yet to be defined.

DIAGNOSIS AND LOCAL STAGING

Side-viewing duodenoscopy and ERCP are typically needed for a detailed evaluation of all ampullary tumors. They provide information not only on the size and lateral mucosal margins but also on the presence and extent of intraductal growth by cholangiogram and pancreatogram. Because there is a wide range in the endoscopic appearance of ampullary tumors, endoscopic assessment alone is not entirely reliable for diagnosis. Thus, tissue sampling is always required to establish the diagnosis. However, even endoscopic biopsy of the ampullary tumor has been criticized as inaccurate, with reported diagnostic accuracies ranging from 62% to 83% (**Fig. 3**).[67–69] Malignant transformation is frequently focal, and up to 50% of ampullary villous adenomas contain foci of adenocarcinoma at the time of diagnosis.[70] Aggressive but careful tissue sampling with large forceps biopsies, snare excision, or postsphincterotomy biopsies of the interior portions of the papilla is sometimes needed. Of these

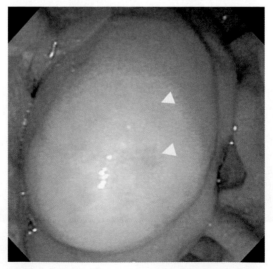

Fig. 2. Large submucosal, oval ampullary neuroendocrine tumor with several tiny erosions (*white arrowheads*).

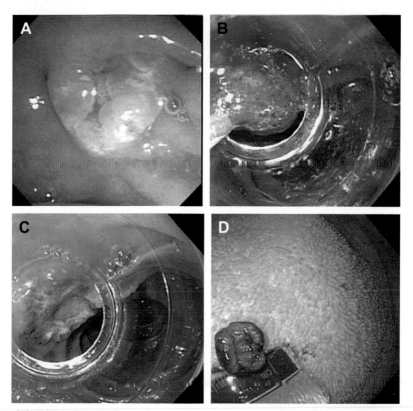

Fig. 3. (*A*) This patient with small ampullary lesion was referred for ampullary adenoma diagnosed by endoscopic forceps biopsy. (*B*) EP using mucosectomy cap was performed for the definite diagnosis. (*C*) Clean postpapillectomy site. (*D*) A pathologic sample about 1 cm in size was obtained; the pathologic diagnosis was foveolar metaplasia.

methods, endoscopic sphincterotomy may be most helpful for confirmation of an intramural tumor, especially in cases of unexplained common bile duct or pancreatic duct dilatation.[20,71] However, obtaining biopsy specimens after endoscopic sphincterotomy is associated with the complications of ERCP. Coagulated or necrotic tissue induced by sphincterotomy may be difficult to interpret histologically.[71] Some experts advocate for the use of sphincterotomy to overcome the shortcomings of taking small superficial biopsy and it also functions as a therapeutic tool.[72] However, other endoscopists prefer to avoid splitting the papilla to allow en bloc endoscopic removal later.

Various methods have been adopted to help assess the lateral and depth of involvement of ampullary tumors. Kim and colleagues[59] used methylene blue and indigo carmine to distinguish neoplastic from normal tissue. Uchiyama and colleagues[73] reported that magnifying endoscopy and narrow-band imaging could reasonably predict histology in 14 patients with an enlarged ampulla. Recently, Itoi and colleagues[74] prospectively compared narrow-band imaging and indigo carmine in the enhancement of the lateral margins before EP in 14 patients. These investigators found that the ability of narrow-band imaging to highlight tumor margin was statistically significantly better than that of indigo carmine. However, these studies have limitations, such as examination with a forward-viewing endoscope, small sample sizes, and nonrandomized designs. Nonetheless, using narrow-band imaging (**Fig. 4**) or

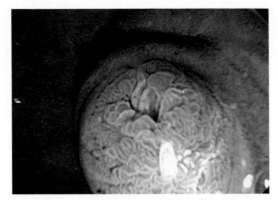

Fig. 4. Narrow-band imaging may enhance visual inspection of mucosal involvement and lateral tumor margin in the ampullary lesion.

conventional chromoendoscopy may enhance visual inspection of mucosal involvement of ampullary tumors.

EUS

EUS and transpapillary intraductal ultrasonography (IDUS) can provide more detailed and accurate information regarding the extent of ampullary tumors, including dimensions, echogenicity, involvement of duodenal layers, and possibly regional lymph node status (**Fig. 5**). EUS findings are helpful in differentiating benign adenomas from malignancies and may guide optimal treatment modality.[75] There have been many studies assessing the usefulness of EUS in T and N staging of ampullary lesions (**Table 1**).[76–86] In the published series, the overall T staging accuracy of EUS for ampullary tumors ranged from 56% to 91% and N staging accuracy from 50% to 81%. There are a few studies comparing EUS with other imaging modalities. Cannon and colleagues[80] reported their experience of staging 50 patients with EUS, computed tomography (CT), and magnetic resonance imaging (MRI). EUS was more accurate than CT and MRI for T staging (78% vs 24% in EUS vs CT; $P<.01$, 78% vs 46% in EUS vs MRI; $P = .07$). N staging had similar results (68% vs 59% vs 77%; $P>.05$). Chen and colleagues[83] compared EUS with CT and ultrasonography (US) in 21 patients with ampullary lesion. EUS was superior to CT and US in both T staging (EUS 75%, CT 5%, US 0%) and N staging (EUS 50%, CT 33%, US 0%). As seen in these studies, EUS is essential to assess T staging of ampullary lesion and less so for N staging. EUS is less accurate in the presence of a biliary stent (nonstenting: T, 83%–84%, N, 100%; stenting: T, 71%–72%, N, 75%),[80,83] particularly with its tendency to understage T2/T3 carcinomas.[80]

IDUS

Unlike EUS with frequencies of 7.5 to 10 MHz, the higher frequency (20–30 MHz) IDUS probe can be inserted through the working channel of the duodenoscope into the common bile duct.[79] Thus, high-resolution IDUS performed in a plane perpendicular to the duct may be more suitable than conventional EUS for staging benign and malignant ampullary lesions (**Table 2**).[79,82,85] Menzel and colleagues[82] reported that IDUS was significantly superior to EUS and CT in tumor visualization (100% vs 59.3% vs 29.6%, respectively). The overall accuracy in tumor diagnosis for IDUS (88.9%; 24 of 27) was significantly superior to EUS (56.3%; 9 of 16) ($P = .05$). Ito and

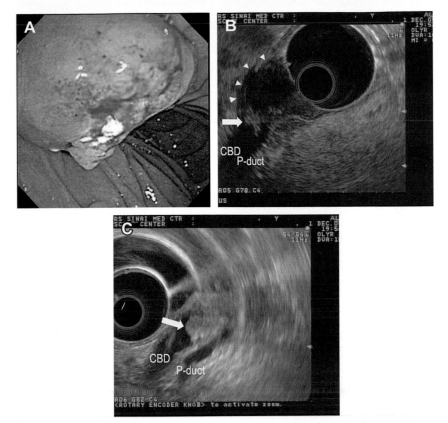

Fig. 5. (A) Large ampullary cancer with irregular mucosal surface, shallow erosions, and spontaneous bleeding. (B) EUS shows a mixed echogenic mass with irregular margin, suggesting invasion into proper muscle layer (*white arrowheads*) and intraductal extension (*white arrow*). (C) EUS shows hyperechogenic intraductal involvement (*white arrow*) in biliary tract.

colleagues[85] compared IDUS against EUS in 40 patients with an ampullary neoplasm before surgery (n = 30) or EP (n = 10). Tumor depiction by IDUS and EUS was achieved in 100% and 95% of the patients, respectively. The overall accuracy by IDUS and EUS in T staging was 78% and 63%, respectively (*P* = .14). In those 10 patients who underwent EP, the accuracy of IDUS and EUS in T staging was 100% and 80%, respectively. Thus, IDUS seems to be more valuable than conventional EUS in tumor assessment; however, it is more invasive and has little capacity to evaluate for lymph node involvement.

Current Recommendations of EUS/IDUS

A recent survey of ampullectomy practices was performed involving 46 expert biliary endoscopists from both tertiary-care centers and private practices in America and Canada. Before EP was performed, EUS was "always" used by 67% of respondents, used "sometimes" in 31%, and "never" in 2%.[87] Although EUS and IDUS are now widely available, there is no established consensus regarding whether all patients with ampullary lesions should undergo EUS before therapy. Several recommendations have been made regarding indication of EUS and they are largely related to size,

Table 1
Diagnostic accuracy of EUS of T staging and N staging in ampullary lesions

Reference	Patients	Modality	Overall T Accuracy (%)	T1 Accuracy (%) (n)	T2 Accuracy (%) (n)	T3 Accuracy (%) (n)	T4 Accuracy (%) (n)	N Accuracy (%) (n)
Yasuda et al,[76] 1988	12	EUS	83					
Mitake et al,[77] 1990	28	EUS	89		100	75		
Tio et al,[78] 1996	32	EUS	84	60 (3/5)	92 (12/13)	91 (11/12)	50 (1/2)	
Itoh et al,[79] 1997	32	EUS	91	d1 ≥100 (19/19)		d2 100 (1/1)	panc(+) 75 (9/12)	
Cannon et al,[80] 1999	50	EUS	78[a]	100 (16/16)	53 (8/15)	75 (12/16)	100 (3/3)	68
		CT	24					59
		MRI	46					77
Kubo et al,[81] 1999	35	EUS	74	67 (6/9)	71 (10/14)	83 (10/12)		63
Menzel et al,[82] 1999	16	EUS	56					
Chen et al,[83] 2001	21	EUS	75	67 (2/3)	88 (7/8)	67 (6/9)		50
		CT	5					33
		US	0					0
Skordilis et al,[84] 2002	17	EUS	82	78		84		71
Ito et al,[85] 2007	40	EUS	63	62 (13/21)	45 (5/11)	88 (7/8)		
Artifon et al,[86] 2009	27	EUS	74[b]	0 (0/2)	85 (11/13)	75 (9/12)		81[b]
		CT	52					56

Abbreviations: d0, tumor limited to Oddi muscle layer; d1, tumor invading the duodenal submucosal layer; d2, tumor invading the duodenal muscularis propria layer; panc(+), tumor invading the pancreas (pancreatic parenchyma).
[a] $P<.01$ in EUS versus CT, $P = .07$ in EUS versus MRI.
[b] P not significant.

Table 2
Diagnostic accuracy of IDUS of T staging and N staging in ampullary lesions

Reference	Patients	Modality	Overall T Accuracy (%) (n)	N Accuracy (%)	Sensitivity (%)	Specificity (%)
Itoh et al,[79] 1997	32	IDUS	88		67[a]	91[a]
		EUS	91		67[a]	96[a]
Menzel et al,[82] 1999	27	IDUS	89[b] (24/27)	93	100[c]	75[c]
		EUS	56 (9/16)		63[c]	50[c]
Ito et al,[85] 2007	40	IDUS	78[d] (100% in EP group)			
		EUS	63 (80% in EP group)			

[a] For lymph node metastases.
[b] P = .05 in comparison of overall T accuracy between IDUS versus EUS.
[c] For T staging.
[d] P = .14 in comparison of overall T accuracy between IDUS versus EUS.

endoscopic appearance, and histologic grade. One large retrospective study advocated performing EUS from a cost-efficacy standpoint on patients with (1) high-grade dysplasia or intramucosal cancer revealed on biopsy, (2) features of unresectability, or (3) lesions larger than 2 cm.[39] Baillie[88] suggested that lesions less than 1 cm in diameter or those that do not have suspicious signs of malignancy (ulceration, induration, bleeding) would not require EUS evaluation; however, EUS should be indicated in large ampullary adenomas (>3 cm). Thus, Lim and colleagues[89] have proposed criteria for evaluation by IDUS/EUS: (1) size greater than 3 cm, (2) malignant features observed on endoscopy, or (3) biopsy-proven high-grade dysplasia or carcinoma-in-situ/T1 in a patient unfit for surgery. However, even lesions of 2 cm in size may harbor carcinoma and thus EUS is reasonable to perform. If carcinoma is identified on biopsy, radical surgery is likely the treatment of choice and the diagnostic value of EUS is minimized.

INDICATIONS FOR EP

The American Society of Gastrointestinal Endoscopy (ASGE) published guidelines in 2006 that stated that endoscopic removal of ampullary adenocarcinoma cannot be endorsed for routine management, and high-grade dysplasia is not a contraindication to endoscopic removal.[90] However, because of the lack of long-term results based on large study populations, indication for EP has not yet been fully established.

According to the published studies, most criteria for EP include the following: (1) size less than 4 to 5 cm, (2) no endoscopic evidence of malignancy, (3) benign histology, and (4) no ductal invasion. Although there is a report that ampullary tumors up to 8 cm in diameter have been successfully resected piecemeal,[41] many investigators recommend that lesions 4 to 5 cm or larger should not be treated endoscopically.[21,25,26,31,45,47]

Endoscopically benign features of ampullary adenomas include pale lobulated appearance, soft consistency, regular margin, and the absence of ulceration, excessive friability, or spontaneous bleeding.[21,26,30,31] As the ASGE guideline stated, many investigators include high-grade dysplasia in earlier forceps biopsy specimens as an indication for EP but exclude adenocarcinoma for endoscopic excision.[30,45–47] Extension of adenoma into the distal common bile duct or the pancreatic duct is often regarded as a contraindication for EP.[26,28,30–32,34–36,39,43–45,47,48] In 1 retrospective study, ampullary adenoma that had extended to the biliary or the pancreatic duct could be removed endoscopically in only a few patients.[31] There is only 1 prospective study that compared the outcomes of EP for ampullary tumors with and without intraductal growth (31 vs 75 patients).[33] The success rate was significantly higher in the group without intraductal growth (46% vs 83%, $P<.001$). Surgery for incomplete removal or recurrence was needed more frequently for the patients with intraductal growth than for those without (37% vs 12%, $P<.001$). Therefore, the investigators suggested that endoscopic removal, in experienced hands, was still feasible when the tumor had limited intraductal involvement. Some experts further proposed that this limited intraductal growth should be defined as less than 1 cm in length.[72,91] In addition, some studies recommended using the ability to elevate tumor by submucosal injection as a criterion for EP.[26,32] Failure to achieve a cleavage plane with submucosal injection has been shown as the strongest predictor of malignancy, followed by EUS T stage.[32]

Early-Stage Ampullary Cancer

Traditionally, pancreaticoduodenectomy or pylorus-preserving pancreaticoduodenectomy has been considered to be the standard treatment of ampullary cancer, whereas EP is regarded as a curative treatment of ampullary adenoma. High-grade dysplasia is generally included in the benign adenoma group and is treated similarly, although more evidence to support this approach is needed.[72,90] The more delicate question is whether adenomas harbor T1 cancer, defined as tumor limited to the ampulla or the sphincter of Oddi, according to the TNM classification. It remains to be determined whether subsequent radical surgery is necessary despite complete endoscopic removal of early-stage ampullary cancer (**Fig. 6**).

There have been a few anecdotal publications on endoscopic removal of ampullary adenoma containing T1 cancer in patients unfit for surgery.[92,93] Recently, the increased application of EUS and IDUS has contributed to more accurate staging of early ampullary cancer and, in turn, expanded indications for EP that include early, localized intramucosal ampullary cancer (**Table 3**).[37,48,49] In a retrospective study in which focal cancer was defined as a lesion involving only mucosa with size less than

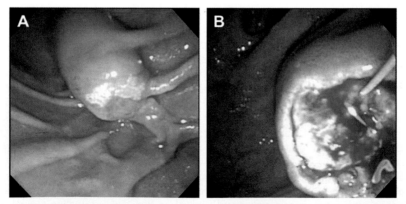

Fig. 6. (A) Duodenoscopic examination shows small ampullary adenoma with some whitish granular mucosal change. (B) After endoscopic ampullectomy, this small lesion was diagnosed as small adenoma with focal cancer. For the definite therapy, a Whipple operation was performed, but no residual cancer lesion was found in the surgical pathology.

Table 3
Clinical studies of EP on patients with HGIN/Tis or T1 cancer

Reference	Design	Patients	Indication	Malignant Foci (%)	Recurrence in Malignancy	HGD	Recurrence in HGD (%)	Endoscopic Success (%)	Follow-up (mo)
Yoon et al,[37] 2007	R	23	HGIN/Tis or focal T1 cancer in ampullary adenoma	10 (43): all negative margin 6/10: EP only 4/10: PD (no residual)	0/10 0/6	13 (57): all negative margin 10/13: EP only 3/13: PD (no residual)	0/13 0/10	16/16 (100)	HGIN/Tis: 27, T1: 32
Ito et al,[48] 2012	R	28 16 (MT) 12 (PT)	Adenoma or well-differentiated adenocarcinoma confined to the papilla of Vater (T1) without tumor spread into the bile/pancreatic duct	12 (43) 8 (50) 4 (33)			4/28 (14) 3 (19) 1 (8)	24/28 (86) 13/16 (81) 11/12 (92)	15 41[a]
Salmi et al,[49] 2012	P	61	T1N0 lesion without invasion of the orifice by EUS	13 (21) 4/13 (38): negative margin->EP only 5/13: PD (1 patient: no residual) 4/13: palliative treatment	0/4 0/1	11 (18)	0/11	37/45 (82)	36

Abbreviations: HGD, high grade dysplasia; HGIN/Tis, high-grade intraepithelial neoplasia/in situ tumor; MT, modified technique; P, prospective; PD, pancreatic duct; PT, previous technique; R, retrospective.
[a] $P = .016$ in comparison of follow-up duration between MT and PT groups.

one-fourth the diameter of main adenoma, 13 patients had high-grade intraepithelial neoplasia/in situ tumor (HGIN/Tis) and 10 patients had focal T1 cancer in ampullary adenoma that were resected by EP.[37] All patients had clear resection margins. Of these patients, 10 with HGIN/Tis and 6 with focal T1 cancer did not undergo additional surgery and had no signs of recurrence of cancer or disease-related deaths during the follow-up period (a mean of 27 months for HGIN/Tis and 32 months for focal T1 cancer). In a recent prospective study, 61 patients had an EUS revealing a T1N0 lesion without invasion of the orifice.[49] Of these 61 patients, 13 malignant lesions were treated endoscopically. Five of these 13 patients with negative margins were treated solely by EP with 3-year and 4-year follow-up showing no recurrence.

Apart from complete resection, lymphovascular invasion seems to be another decisive prognostic criterion in the treatment of T1 ampullary cancers.[72] A few studies have addressed the issue of lymphovascular invasion in early-stage ampullary cancer (**Table 4**). In a retrospective study of 201 patients who had undergone pancreatico-duodenectomy for ampullary cancer, 67 patients with a histologic diagnosis of pTis (n = 5) or pT1 (n = 62) cancer were analyzed.[94] Lymph node metastasis occurred in 6 (9.0%) and mucosal tumor infiltration along the common bile duct or pancreatic duct was observed in 15 (22.4%) of these patients with pTis or pT1 cancer. Recurrence was confirmed in 12 (18.2%) of these patients and resulted in disease-related deaths in all of them. Thus, the investigators recommended that pancreaticoduodenectomy be performed to achieve adequate radical resection, even in early ampullary cancer. In another retrospective study of 159 patients with a final diagnosis of ampullary cancer after curative surgical resection, microlymphovascular invasion was present in 56.7% (17/30) of T1 cancers but was absent in all HGIN/Tis specimens.[95] These investigators also recommended that surgical resection be performed for the T1 stage ampulla of Vater cancer because of the high rate of lymphovascular invasion. On the contrary, 2 recent studies show no lymphovascular or lymph node metastasis in patients with HGIN/Tis and focal T1 cancer.[37,95,96] One of these reports is a retrospective multicenter review of 216 patients with ampullary cancer. Those patients with early-stage ampullary cancer of less than 2 cm, with a well-differentiated histology and no angiolymphatic invasion (n = 13) had no lymph node metastasis and no recurrence during a median follow-up of 35.9 months.[96] Collectively, these 4 studies show the incidence of lymph node metastasis of about 10% in patients with T1 cancer. With regards to lymph node involvement in HGIN/Tis, there are too few patients (n = 22) to draw a conclusive statement. Nonetheless, there was no lymph node metastasis in these 22 patients with HGIN/Tis. Therefore, EP may be a curative treatment of ampullary adenoma with HGIN/Tis. The current data also suggest that when an endoscopically resected specimen has a well-differentiated intramucosal cancer with clear margins and no angiolymphatic invasion, subsequent radical surgery may not be necessary. However, large, prospective studies with long-term follow-up are needed to yield conclusive evidence for these settings.

TECHNIQUE FOR EP

There is no standardized technique for endoscopic removal of ampullary tumors because of complexity of the procedure, and **Table 5** shows its complexity in the published series. The term ampullectomy refers to removal of the entire ampulla of Vater and is a surgical term for procedures that require reimplantation of the distal common bile duct and pancreatic duct within the duodenal wall (**Fig. 7**). Technically, when endoscopic resections of lesions at the major papilla are performed, only tissue from the nonductal papilla can be removed endoscopically, and thus the term EP

Table 4
Lymph node metastasis, microlymphatic invasion, and follow-up results in early-stage ampullary cancer

Reference (Number of Patients)	LN Metastasis (%)	MLV Invasion (%)	Ductal Mucosa Involvement (%)	Recurrence (%)	Death (%)
Yoon et al[94] (n = 201)					
pTis, pT1	6/67 (9.0)		15/67 (22.4)	12/66 (18.2)[a]	
Tumor size ≤1 cm	5/43 (11.6)				
W/D	24/102 (23.5)				
pTis, pT1 + ≤ 1 cm	1/19 (5.3)				
pTis, pT1 + W/D	4/53 (7.5)				
≤1 cm + W/D	3/21 (14.3)				
Lee et al[95] (n = 159)					
pTis	0/6 (0)	0/6 (0)			
pT1	3/30 (10.0)	17/30 (56.7)[b]			
Yoon et al[37] (n = 83)[c]					
HGIN/Tis	0/11 (0)			0/10 (0) for 27 mo	0/10 (0) for 27 mo
Focal T1[d]	0/4 (0)		0/6 (0)	0/6 (0) for 32 mo	0/6 (0) for 32 mo
pT1	6/56 (10.7)		10/56 (17.9)		
Woo et al[96] (n = 216)					
pTis	0/5 (0)			0	
pT1	5/57 (8.8)			4 (7.0)	5 (8.8)
pTis, pT1	5/62 (8.1)				
pTis, pT1 + <2 cm	2/29 (6.9)				
pTis, pT1 + <2 cm + W/D	0/16 (0)			0 for 86 mo	0 for 86 mo
pTis, pT1 + <2 cm + W/D + no angiolymphatic invasion	0/13 (0)			0 for 36 mo	0 for 36 mo

Abbreviations: LN, lymph node; MLV, microlymphovascular; W/D, well-differentiated.
[a] Recurrence occurred in all pT1 patients.
[b] $P = .02$ in comparison of microlymphovascular invasion between pTis versus pT1.
[c] EP = 23, surgery = 60.
[d] Focal was defined as a lesion involving only mucosa with size less than one-fourth the diameter of main adenoma.

(**Figs. 8** and **9**) is more appropriate than the term endoscopic ampullectomy. Nonetheless, the 2 terms are often used interchangeably in the literature.[90,97]

Submucosal Injection

Several investigators have advocated the routine use of submucosal injection immediately before EP.[24,26,32,35,36] Fluids injected into the submucosa have included saline solution, epinephrine, methylene blue, and viscous material such as hydroxypropyl methylcellulose.[98,99] The reported volumes of injected fluid are not standardized and vary widely. Submucosal injection may prevent unnecessary resection attempts,

Table 5
Techniques of EP

Reference	Patients	Submucosal Injection	Routine PD Stent	Routine Biliary Stent	Routine PD Sphincterotomy	Routine Biliary Sphincterotomy	Electrical Current	Adjunctive Ablation
Ponchon et al,[20] 1989	11	No	No	No	No	Yes (pre-R)		Nd:YAG, argon laser
Binmoeller et al,[21] 1993	25		No, 4%				Pure cutting	
Greenspan et al,[22] 1997	8		Yes, 100%	Yes, 88%				YAG laser photocoagulation, 75%
Martin et al,[23] 1997	14	Saline, 57%	71%	29%		50% (pre-R), 1 at ampullectomy		APC, 7%
Park et al,[24] 2000	6	Saline	No	No	No	No	Blended	
Vogt et al,[25] 2000	18		No	No, 50%				APC, 17%
Desilets et al,[26] 2001	13	1:20,000 saline/Epi	Yes, 85% (pre-R, 5F)	23%	Yes (pre-R)	Yes (pre-R)	Pure coagulation	APC, 38%, bipolar electrocautery, 15% probe
Zadorova et al,[27] 2001	16		No			Yes		APC
Norton et al,[28] 2002	26		No, 36% (5-F)		No, 8%	Yes	Blended	Monopolar coagulation, 38%, APC, 8%
Catalano et al,[30] 2004	103	No	Yes 88% (5- to 7-F)	No, 33% (7- to 10-F)	As needed	4%	Blended	APC, 17%, Nd:YAG, 3%, multipolar, 14%
Cheng et al,[31] 2004	55	1:10,000 Epi, 27%	Yes, 75% (3, 4, 5-F, before or after)	No	As needed	As needed	Endocut	Multipolar, APC, snare tip coagulation
Kahaleh et al,[32] 2004	56	Saline or 1:100,000 Epi	No, 7% (7-F)	No	Yes (pre-R)	Yes (pre-R)		APC

Study	N					13% [a]	71% [a]	Pure cutting	Monopolar, APC
Bohnacker et al,[33] 2005	106	No	Yes (7-F)	No	No	13% [a]	71% [a]	Pure cutting	Monopolar, APC
Harewood et al,[34] 2005	19	No	Yes, 53% vs No (5-F)	No	No	No	Yes	Blended or Endocut (most cases)	
Eswaran et al,[35] 2006	51	1:20,000 Epi	Yes (pre-R, 3-F or 5-F)	No	No	Yes (pre-R)	Yes (pre-R)		APC
Katsinelos et al,[36] 2006	14	1:10,000 Epi/dextrose 50%	No, 29%	No, 64% (10-F)	No, 64% (10-F)	Yes (pre-R), 5-F	Yes (pre-R), 10-F	Blended	Heater probe
Yoon et al,[37] 2007	16							Blended	APC
Boix et al,[38] 2009	21	No	No, 0			Yes (pre-R)	Yes (pre-R)	Blended	APC
Irani et al,[39] 2009	102	Some cases [b]	Yes (3-F)	Yes (pre-R in 3/4 providers)	Yes (10-F, 7-F)	Yes (pre-R in 3/4 providers)	Yes (pre-R in 3/4 providers)	Blended	APC
Jung et al,[40] 2009	22	1:10,000 saline/Epi, some cases	14%	41%	41%	32%	41%	Endocut	
Hooper et al,[41] 2010	10 (LST-P) / 15 (C)	No / No	Yes, 90% (5-F)	No, 30%	No, 30%	No	No	Endocut Q	No APC / No APC
Hwang et al,[42] 2010	11		Yes (pre-R, 5-F)	No	No	No	No	Endocut	APC, 73%
Igarashi et al,[43] 2010	36	No	Yes (7-F)	Yes (7-F)	Yes (7-F)	No	No	Autocut [c]	
Yamao et al,[44] 2010	36	No	Yes 97%, (7-F)	Yes, 81%, (5-F)	Yes, 81%, (5-F)	No	No	Endocut	APC
Harano et al,[45] 2011	28	Saline, 43%	Yes, 82% (5-F)	Yes, 75% (7-F)	Yes, 75% (7-F)	No	No	Endocut	
Jeanniard-Malet et al,[46] 2011	42	No	No, 62% (5-F, 7-F)	No, 24	No, 24		24%	Pure current	

(continued on next page)

Table 5
(continued)

Reference	Patients	Submucosal Injection	Routine PD Stent	Routine Biliary Stent	Routine PD Sphincterotomy	Routine Biliary Sphincterotomy	Electrical Current	Adjunctive Ablation
Patel et al,[47] 2011	38	No	Some->Yes (3-F or 5-F)	No	Some	Some	Blended-> Endocut	APC
Ito et al,[48] 2012	16 (MT)	No	Yes	Yes (7-F)	Yes	Yes	Endocut	APC
	12 (PT)	No	Yes (5F)	No	No	No	Pure cutting	APC
Salmi et al,[49] 2012	61	31%[d]	Yes after 2006, 60% (5-F)				Pure cutting 75%, Endocut 25%	

Abbreviations: APC, argon plasma coagulation; C, conventional adenoma; D, diathermic snare; Epi, epinephrine solution; LST-P, giant laterally spreading tumors of the papilla; MT, modified technique; Nd:YAG, neodymium-yttrium aluminum garnet; PD, pancreatic duct; pre-R, preresection; PT, previous technique; S, standard polypectomy snare.

[a] If intraductal growth was identified, preresection sphincterotomy was performed.

[b] Only for lesions with lateral extensions and flat.

[c] High-frequency surgical equipment, PSD-60.

[d] If lateral duodenal sides were affected.

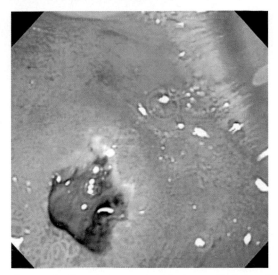

Fig. 7. Duodenoscopic examination shows postsurgical ampullectomy site. A small irregular black-brown adherent clot and reimplanted distal common bile duct is found in the duodenal wall.

because the inability to elevate the lesion is predictive of scarring or deep tissue involvement by invasive cancer.[26,32] Adding epinephrine to an injection solution may also decrease the risk of bleeding[26,32,35,36]; however, 1 retrospective study[31] showed that there was no difference in the bleeding rates between the EP performed without epinephrine mixed submucosal injection (5.9%, 3/51) and with it (5.3%, 1/19). However, these claims have not been validated with randomized controlled trials. In addition, submucosal injection can make it difficult to capture the lesion with a snare and may blur the margins of the tumor.[91] Thus, many investigators do not recommend submucosal injection as a routine step.[30,33,34,38,39,41,43,44,46–48] Most experts do not recommend fluid injection before proceeding with EP.[100–103]

Endoscopic Resection

Of the various commercially available snares, standard polypectomy snares have been used in most reports.[21,26,30,39,41,47] Some experts suggest that the thin wire maximizes current density for swift transection and minimizes stalling and dispersion of the energy, which may cause injury to the pancreatic orifice and late occurrence of sphincter stenosis.[102] However, there is no evidence that confirms the advantage of 1 type of snare over another.[90]

Snare position during papillectomy is also not standardized. The snare can be opened either from a cephalad to caudal (upside down) direction (see **Figs. 8C** and **9B**) or in the caudal-to-cephalad orientation. Most published reports have not specified the orientation of the snare during the procedure, but at least 3 studies[32,43,48] have advocated snaring the tumor in the upside down orientation. The argument in favor of the upside down approach is that the opened snare typically pushes the nonpapillary tissue back, and it is easy to visualize the tissue as it is being captured. Further, wire slippage from the tissue rarely occurs.

If a lesion can be completely ensnared, en bloc resection similar to the standard polypectomy can be performed (see **Figs. 8C** and **9B**). Whether en bloc or

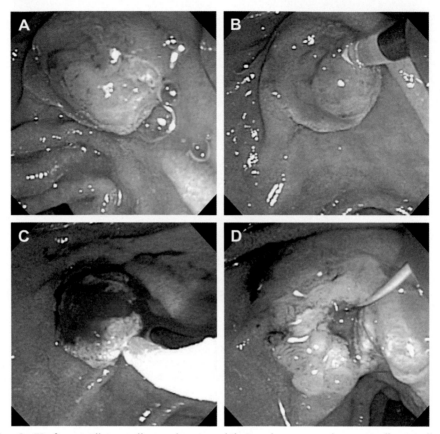

Fig. 8. EP for small ampullary adenoma. (*A*) Duodenoscopy shows small ampullary adenoma. (*B*) Cannulation was performed for cholangiography and pancreatography before the resection of ampullary adenoma. (*C*) Snaring ampullary lesion using standard polypectomy snare was performed from a cephalad to caudal (upside down) direction. (*D*) After resection of ampullary adenoma, a guidewire was positioned for inserting prophylactic pancreatic duct stent at the clean papillectomy base.

piecemeal resection is the best method for eradication of an ampullary tumor remains to be resolved, but, generally, en bloc resection is the preferred technique.[101–103] En bloc resection provides a complete tissue sample for precise pathologic evaluation and shortens the procedure time. Balloon-catheter-assisted EP has also been advocated to facilitate en bloc resection of flat papillary tumors.[91] Mucosectomy cap–assisted ampullectomy has also been used successfully in this setting (**Fig. 10**).[104] For larger lesions (>2 cm in diameter) or in cases in which an attempt at en bloc resection has left visible neoplastic tissue in place, piecemeal resection is commonly performed. Desilets and colleagues[26] recommend piecemeal resection because it is believed to decrease the risk of perforation. However, piecemeal resection could increase the chance of tumor seeding, increase the number of ERCP sessions required for eradication, and render precise histopathologic assessment of resection specimens impossible.[91] Nonetheless, en bloc and piecemeal resection have both been extensively used to address the lesions of various sizes and architecture.[20,21,25,27,30,31,33,35–40,44,45,48]

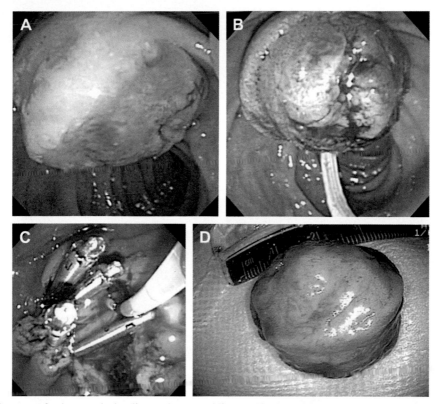

Fig. 9. EP for large tubulovillous adenoma. (*A*) Duodenoscopy shows large ampullary lesion containing nodular, uneven granular overlying mucosa and tiny hemorrhagic spots. (*B*) Snaring large ampullary lesion with en bloc was performed from a cephalad to caudal (upside down) direction. (*C*) After en bloc resection, 4 hemoclips were applied for bleeding control and cannulation was performed for the prophylactic pancreatic duct stenting. (*D*) Retrieved, large ampullary tumor sample was about 3 cm in size, and the diagnosis was tubulovillous adenoma with superficial cancer.

Electrocautery Settings

There is no consensus regarding the mode of electrical current used for EP. Some investigators advocate the use of pure cutting current to avoid edema and cautery injuries caused by the coagulation mode,[21,33,46,48] although 1 study[26] used the pure coagulation current. In most published reports, blended current is the most widely used.[24,28,30,34,36–39,47] The Endocut mode of the ERBE generator (ERBE USA Inc., Marietta, GA, USA) seems to be used increasingly because it allows effective cutting according to the properties of the tissue.[31,40–42,44,45,48]

Pancreatic Stenting

Postpapillectomy pancreatitis is one of the most feared complications. Several studies have suggested that prophylactic pancreatic stenting might reduce the risk of postpapillectomy pancreatitis (**Fig. 11, Table 6**).[27,30,31,45] The theoretic possibility that it can minimize the risk of papillary stenosis has not been fully confirmed. Some investigators advocate routinely placing pancreatic stents,[22,26,30,31,33,35,39,41,43–45,48] but others

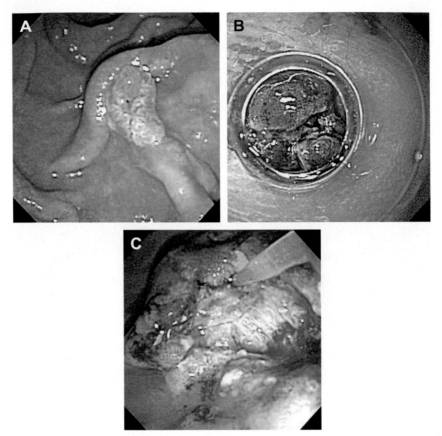

Fig. 10. (*A*) Duodenoscopy shows a small flat and whitish granular ampullary adenoma. (*B*) A mucosectomy cap, attached to the tip of an endoscope, was used to perform cap-assisted ampullectomy. (*C*) After resection, cannulation was performed for the prophylactic pancreatic duct stenting.

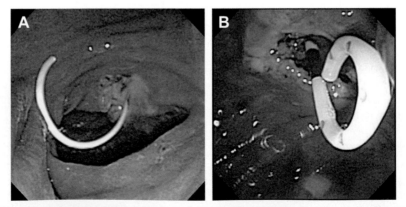

Fig. 11. (*A*) A 3-F stent without flaps was placed after endoscopic resection of ampullary lesion. (*B*) A 5-F stent was placed after endoscopic resection of ampullary lesion.

Table 6
Pancreatitis according to the presence or absence of prophylactic pancreatic duct stent, stenting, and sphincterotomy

Reference	Pancreatitis (%)			P Value	Routine PD Stent	Routine Biliary Stent	Routine PD Sphincterotomy	Routine Biliary Sphincterotomy
		PD Stent (%)	No Stent (%)					
Zadorova et al,[27] 2001	2 (13)	(0)	(20)	NR	No			Yes
Norton et al,[28] 2002	4 (15)	2/10 (20)	2/18 (11)	0.5	No, (5-F)		No, 8%	Yes
Catalano et al,[30] 2004	5 (5)	3/91 (3.3)	2/12 (17)	NR	Yes (5- to 7-F)	No, 33% (7- to 10-F)	As needed	4%
Cheng et al,[31] 2004	5 (9)	4/41 (9.6)	1/4 (25)	0.33	Yes, (3-F, 4-F, 5-F)	No	As needed	As needed
Bohnacker et al,[33] 2005	13 (6)	NR (11)	NR (14)	>0.05	Yes (7-F)	No	13%[a]	71%[a]
Harewood et al,[34] 2005	3 (16)	0/10 (0)	3/9 (33)	0.02[b]	Yes vs No (5-F)	No	No	Yes
Katsinelos et al,[36] 2006	1 (7)	0/4	1/10	NR	No	No, 64% (10-F)	Yes (preresection)	Yes (preresection)
Irani et al,[39] 2009	10 (10)	NR	NR	NR	Yes (3-F)	Yes (10-F, 7-F)	Yes (preresection in 3/4 providers)	Yes (preresection in 3/4 providers)
Hooper et al,[41] 2010	0	0/9 (5F)	0/1	NR	Yes (5-)	No; 30% (30)	No	No
Yamao et al,[44] 2010	3 (8)	2/35 (6)	1/1 (100)	NR	Yes (7-)	Yes, 81% (5-F)	No	No
Harano et al,[45] 2011	2 (7)	0/23 (0)	2/5 (40)	NR	Yes (5-F)	Yes 75% (7-F)	No	No
Jeanniard-Malet et al,[46] 2011	6 (14)	4/26 (15)	2/16 (13)	NR	No, (5-, 7-F)	No, 24%	Some	24%
Patel et al,[47] 2011	3 (8)	1/20 (5)	2/18 (11)	0.62	Some→Yes (3-F or 5-F)	No	Some	Some
Salmi et al,[49] 2012	6 (10)	1/36 (3)	5/25 (20)	<0.05[c]	Yes after 2006 (5-F)			
Total	63 (8.2)	17/305 (5.6)	21/119 (17.6)					

Abbreviations: NR, not reported; PD, pancreatic duct.

[a] If intraductal growth was identified, preresection sphincterotomy was performed.
[b] P = .02 in comparison of pancreatitis between PD stent and no PD stent groups.
[c] P<.05 in comparison of pancreatitis between PD stent and no PD stent groups.

argue for selected use only when delayed drainage of the pancreatic duct is noted after EP.[21,23,28,32,36,46,47]

Two studies have provided evidence in support of prophylactic pancreatic stenting. The only prospective, randomized, controlled trial[34] showed that prophylactic pancreatic stenting during EP significantly decreased postpapillectomy pancreatitis in the stent group (0% vs 33%, $P = .02$). Although this study had calculated the necessary number of patients to be enrolled as 25 in each arm, the study was stopped by the site's institutional review board based on the high observed rate of pancreatitis in the nonstent group after 19 patients (10 stented, 9 nonstented) had been randomized. All 3 patients who developed postpapillectomy pancreatitis were in the nonstent group (3/9, 33%). Therefore, this study concluded that "a protective effect is conferred by pancreatic stent placement in reducing postpapillectomy pancreatitis. Further large-scaled studies are required to confirm benefit." Recently, another prospective cohort study[49] reported on the outcomes of EP performed on 61 patients. Beginning in 2006, pancreatic stent placement was routinely performed on 36 patients; it was not attempted on the 25 patients treated before 2006. Postpapillectomy pancreatitis developed in 3% (1/36) of the patients for whom pancreatic stenting was planned, although there was a 20% failure rate for stent insertion. On the contrary, 20% (5/25) of the patients in whom there was no attempt at pancreatic stenting developed pancreatitis ($P<.05$). Based on their experience, these investigators advocated performing pancreatic stenting on all patients who underwent EP.

The optimal duration of pancreatic stenting has not been established. The literature has reports of stenting duration that range from 24 hours to 3 months.[21,28,30,34,40] To minimize stent-induced ductal changes, some investigators advocate short duration for 1 to 3 days.[28,34,42] Other investigators have recommended that the stents are left in place until the second session of endoscopic examination, which is frequently performed 1 to 2 months after EP. The remaining pancreatic stent may protect the pancreatic duct orifice during the follow-up examination, when additional endoscopic excision and thermal ablation may be needed.[26,30,33,39] Pancreatic stents of various diameters, lengths, and shapes have been reported for use in EP in the literature. Some investigators suggest that a 3-F stent without flaps be used to minimize stent-induced ductal injuries and promote spontaneous migration, because of its small caliber (see **Fig. 11**A).[105] However, a recent randomized controlled study shows no statistically significant difference in spontaneous passage by 2 weeks between the 5-F (n = 38) and 3-F (n = 40) (68.4% vs 75.0%, $P = .617$) stents. In addition, placement of 5-F stents is easier, faster, and requires usage of fewer wires than that for 3-F pancreatic stents.[106] In the published series, 5-F pancreatic stents have been used most commonly (see **Fig 11**B),[26,28,30,31,34,41,42,45–49] followed by 7-F,[30–33,43,44,46] and then 3-F stents.[31,35,39,47]

The timing of pancreatic stenting before or after EP is controversial.[88] Many investigators who routinely inserted a pancreatic stent during EP placed it after endoscopic resection of the ampullary tumor.[22,23,30,33,39,41,43–45,48] Even an experienced interventional endoscopist might be afraid of failing to identify the pancreatic orifice after removing the ampullary tumor. Thus, some investigators advocate placing a pancreatic stent before endoscopic resection.[26,35,42] Furthermore, preresection pancreatic stenting may protect the pancreatic duct orifice from electrosurgical thermal injury. However, having a stent protruding from the pancreatic orifice may hinder complete excision of the tumor. Some expert groups recommend reserving prepapillectomy pancreatic stenting for smaller lesions, because accessing the pancreatic orifice after resection of the large ampullary lesions is easy.[103] A recent survey of 46 biliary endoscopists showed that participants overwhelmingly favored always placing a prophylactic pancreatic stent, with 86% placing it after EP rather than before resection (23%).[87] Although appropriate prospective randomized controlled studies are desirable to confirm this protective effect, prophylactic pancreatic stenting seems to have become an established practice in EP.

Biliary Stenting

Prophylactic biliary stenting is generally not necessary. Similar to the goal of preventing postpapillectomy pancreatitis, placing a biliary stent after EP may prevent postpapillectomy cholangitis. In a few recent studies, some investigators have advocated routine placement of prophylactic biliary stent after EP,[43–45] and others even recommend the routine performance of both biliary sphincterotomy and biliary stenting to protect patients from the small risk of cholangitis.[39,48] Even although the evidence is lacking, prophylactic biliary stent placement may be considered if the bile duct orifice is not clearly visible and if there is difficulty in cannulation after resection of the tumor.[97]

Pancreatic or Biliary Sphincterotomy

Pancreatic or biliary sphincterotomy during EP may enhance pancreaticobiliary drainage after papillectomy, simplify attempts to access the biliary and pancreatic duct for stent placement, and assist in postprocedure surveillance.[90] There is no consensus as to whether these maneuvers should be performed at all, much less before or after the papillectomy.[20,23,26–28,32,34–36,38,39,48]

In the published series, some investigators routinely performed only biliary sphincterotomy before or after EP[20,23,27,28,34]; other groups performed biductal preresection sphincterotomy.[26,32,35,36,38,39] Biductal preresection sphincterotomy may potentially avoid the difficulty in identifying the pancreatic or biliary orifice once the papilla has been manipulated or snared. This practice may also provide postprocedure drainage, which in turn lowers the risk of pancreatitis, cholangitis, and even late strictures.[26,32,35] However, there are also some concerns over the safety and efficacy of biductal preresection sphincterotomy. Preresection sphincterotomy may add substantial risk of bleeding or perforation.[28] In addition, tissue cutting, mechanical manipulations, and thermal injury exerted during preresection sphincterotomy may alter the anatomy of the resected specimen and make precise histopathologic evaluation of the tumor difficult.[97,107] It is not always possible to perform sphincterotomy safely because of difficulty defining landmarks, especially in the larger lesions. There has been no study to address whether these complications are the direct results of sphincterotomy or tumor resection.

To further confuse the picture, there are endoscopists who routinely perform preresection pancreatic stenting after biductal preresection sphincterotomy[26,35] and others who perform postresection biductal stentings routinely.[39] It remains unclear if there is any benefit derived from stenting after preresection biductal sphincterotomy.

A recent Japanese study[48] advocated a modified technique of EP, which consists of resection with the Endocut mode (ERBE electrosurgical generator), followed by postresection biductal sphincterotomy and biductal stenting. This technique has been performed on 16 patients since April 2007. Before this time, EP was performed with a cutting current, followed by only pancreatic stenting in 12 patients. Using the modified technique was associated with significantly lower frequency of complications than using the previous technique (6% (1/16) versus 75% (9/12), $P = .00078$). However, prospective, randomized studies should be performed.

Additional Ablative Therapies

Snare resection of small remnant lesions at the EP session can occasionally be performed with the mucosectomy cap.[104] In most cases, ablative therapy is the only technically feasible means to destroy the retained tissue.[90,97] Ablative therapy is also useful for a recurrent adenomatous tissue not amenable to snare resection.[31,97,103] Modalities for thermal ablation include argon plasma coagulation (APC), monopolar/multipolar electrocoagulation,[26,28,30,31,33] and neodymium-yttrium aluminum garnet (Nd:YAG) laser photoablation.[20,22,30] Among these methods, APC is the most frequently used because of its widespread availability and easy targeting for superficial tissue destruction.[20,26–28,30–33,35,37–39,44,47,48] A recent survey of 46 biliary endoscopists confirmed APC as the favored adjunct modality (83%) for removing residual adenomatous tissue.[87] The lack of tissue for histopathologic evaluation because of lesion destruction is a major drawback of the thermal ablation method,[20,59] and thus any suspicious area should be biopsied before ablation.[90] Thermal ablation is used mostly as a complementary technique when EP is incomplete.[59,97]

There has been no randomized controlled trial that compared individual ablative modalities. One retrospective multicenter study[30] addressed the efficacy of adjunct thermal ablation after EP. Thermal ablation was used in 37 of the 103 patients using a variety of technologies (18 APC, 14 multipolar electrocoagulation, 3 Nd:YAG laser photoablation). The overall success rate of EP was similar among patients who had ablation (30/37, 81%) compared with those who did not (52/66, 78%). There was a trend for a higher rate of recurrence in patients not treated with thermal ablation (9/66, 14% vs 1/37, 3%), but the difference did not reach statistical significance $(P = .22)$.

PUBLISHED OUTCOMES
Clinical Success and Recurrence

The results of EP for ampullary tumors in the published studies are summarized in **Table 7**. In these reported series, success rates for EP range from 29% to 100%, with an overall success rate of about 79%.[20–33,35–42,44–49] The recurrence rates of ampullary adenoma after EP range from 0% to 33%, with an overall incidence of about 12%.[20–22,24–31,33,36–49] Predictors of successful endoscopic resection in 1 retrospective multicenter study included age older than 48 years, lesion size less than 24 mm, and male gender.[30] In another study, a small lesion size (<2 cm) and the absence of dilated ducts were associated with a successful outcome.[39] Risk factors for recurrence included larger size and high-grade dysplasia.[39,47,108] Some studies argued that size had not been definitely linked to increased likelihood of recurrence.[59,109] Often the recurrent tissue is small, histologically benign, without intraductal growth and is thus easily amenable to endoscopic eradication.[25,30,31,36,38,44,46,47]

The reported success rates of EP vary widely. There are several reasons: different study designs, no standardized inclusion criteria, no standardized techniques, and different sample sizes. Importantly, the definition of EP has not been agreed. Conventionally, success may be defined as complete excision of the lesion on visual inspection.[97] Some investigators consider success as the outcome regardless of the number of treatment sessions,[35] and other investigators define success as the absence of recurrence on long-term follow-up.[39,44] Yet other investigators include recurrence during long-term follow-up that is easily treated endoscopically in the category of success.[30,31,38] To compare the outcomes between studies, a consensus on the definition of success is needed. To clearly define a recurrence versus residual lesion, 1 study has suggested that at least 1 endoscopy with a biopsy specimen showing no residual tissue is required, along with a 3-month interval between the end of the treatment and the diagnosis of a recurrence.[39]

Complications

The complications of EP are generally divided into early (acute pancreatitis, bleeding, perforation, cholangitis) and late (papillary stenosis),[90,97] and the published results are summarized in **Table 8**. The overall morbidity rate in these series is 19% (range 5%–56%), with the breakdown of overall individual complication rates as follows: pancreatitis, 10% (range 0%–33%); bleeding, 4% (range 0%–30%); cholangitis, 0.6% (range 0%–13%); perforation, 0.4% (range 0%–7%); cholecystitis, 0.2% (range 0%–10%); and papillary stenosis, 1.4% (range 0%–10%).

Death was rare and has been reported in 2 patients, and thus the overall mortality was 0.09%. Both of these patients developed severe postpapillectomy pancreatitis, resulting in death, and did not have the pancreatic duct stent placed.[23,32] Biductal pre-resection sphincterotomy was performed in 1 of 2 patients.[32] Acute pancreatitis is a feared and the most common complication after EP, although most cases are mild. It is difficult to address exactly the issue of whether postpapillectomy pancreatitis results from resection, the choice of electrocautery setting, or other intraprocedural manipulations, including sphincterotomy, stenting, and additional ablation. Bleeding is the second common complication and is also affected by multiple technical issues during EP. Perforation is a rare complication of EP and may be caused by a sphincterotomy and not tumor resection.[28] One study[39] reported 2 perforations in 102 patients. These 2 perforations occurred in the patients with extensive lateral extension of the lesion and invasive cancer, leading the investigators to speculate underlying malignancy and lateral extension as a risk for bleeding and perforation. Papillary stenosis is a late complication of EP. In 1 retrospective multicenter study, papillary stenosis occurred more frequently in the patients without pancreatic duct stents (8.3%, 1/12) than with stents (2.2%, 2/91).[30] Determining if prophylactic pancreatic stenting can reduce the risk of papillary stenosis requires a large-scale long-term follow-up study to answer the question.

POSTPAPILLECTOMY SURVEILLANCE

Because of the risk of recurrence after EP, endoscopic surveillance is mandatory. However, there is no standard guideline as to the interval and duration of surveillance. In general, published reports describe initial surveillance examination at 3 to 6 months after the index procedure and then regular follow-up at 3-month to 6-month intervals.[20,25,27,30,36,41,47,49] Some investigators performed initial surveillance examination at 1 month,[24,26,31,35,40,45,48] and a few investigators even suggested initial examination at as early as 7 days.[43,44] In most reports, regular surveillance was recommended for a minimum 1 year and then yearly or at longer intervals.[20,25,27,36,41–43,47,48] **Fig. 12** shows the postampullectomy figure during the endoscopic surveillance.

An initial surveillance examination generally involves endoscopy with ERCP and multiple biopsies. A cholangiogram and a pancreatogram should be routinely obtained during surveillance to rule out the possibility of intraductal residual or recurrent lesions. Lesions found to contain areas of high-grade dysplasia may need to be ablated and followed closely.[90] Whether all subsequent surveillance procedures should incorporate ERCP remains to be determined. End points for surveillance of the sporadic ampullary adenomas have not been established. Patients with FAP should undergo surveillance at 3-year intervals.[30] ASGE guidelines recommend that a reasonable approach for sporadic ampullary polyps is to adopt a surveillance policy similar to

Table 7
Outcomes of EP

Reference	Design	Patients	FAP (%)	Endoscopic Success (%)	Recurrence Rate (%)	Malignant Foci (%)	Follow-up (mo)
Ponchon et al,[20] 1989	R	11		10/11 (91)	1/11 (9)	2 (18)	39
Binmoeller et al,[21] 1993	R	25	NR	23/25 (92)	6/23 (26)	0	37
Greenspan et al,[22] 1997	A	8		6/8 (75)	2/8 (25)	2 (25)	12
Martin et al,[23] 1997	A	14	6 (43)	6/12 (50)	NR	0	31
Park et al,[24] 2000	R	6		4/6 (67)	0/4 (0)	2 (33)	21
Vogt et al,[25] 2000	R	18		12/18 (67)	6/18 (33)	1 (6)	75
Desilets et al,[26] 2001	R	13	7 (54)	12/13 (92)	0/12 (0)	0	19
Zadorova et al,[27] 2001	R	16	1 (6)	13/16 (81)	3/16 (19)	0	
Norton et al,[28] 2002	R	26	15 (58)	12/26 (46)	2/21 (10)	1 (4)	9
Saurin et al,[29] 2003	R	24		16/24 (67)	1/16 (6)	0	66
Catalano et al,[30] 2004	R, M	103	30 (29)	83 (80)	10/103 (10)	6 (6)	36
Cheng et al,[31] 2004	R	55	14 (26)	28/38 (74)	9/27 (33)	7 (13)	30
Kahaleh et al,[32] 2004	P	56		30/35 (86)		21 (38)	
Bohnacker et al,[33] 2005	P	106 75; IDG(−) 31; IDG(+)a	5 (5)	73 (73) 60 (83) 13 (46)b	15 (15) 11 (15) 4 (15)	9 (8)	40 42 35
Eswaran et al,[35] 2006	R	29 (>3 cm) 22 (1–3 cm)	9 (31) 12 (55)	25/29 (86) 22/22 (100)		3 (10) 0 (0)	
Katsinelos et al,[36] 2006	R	14	4 (29)	11/14 (79)	2/11 (18)	3 (21)	28

Study	Design	No.		Complete resection	Recurrence	Complications	Follow-up
Yoon et al,[37] 2007	R	16		16/16 (100)	0/16	6 (38)	27 (HGIN/Tis), 32 (T1)
Boix et al,[38] 2009		21		6/21 (29)	1/6 (17)	10 (48)	16
Irani et al,[39] 2009	R	102	17 (17)	86/102 (84)	8 (8)	8 (8)	32 (incidental) 48 (FAP)
Jung et al,[40] 2009	R	22		12/22 (55)	2/12 (17)	10 (45)	169 d, median
Hooper et al,[41] 2010	P	10 (LST-P) 15 (C)		10/10 (100) 11/13 (85)	1/10 (10) 3/13 (23)	0 2 (13)	12
Hwang et al,[42] 2010	P, p	11		11/11 (100)	0	0	299 d, median
Igarashi et al,[43] 2010	R	36		—	0/24 (0) (adenoma) 1/4 (25) (adenocarcinoma in adenoma) 2/5 (40) (adenocarcinoma)	12 (33) (adenoma) 12 (33) (adenocarcinoma in adenoma)	—
Yamao et al,[44] 2010	R	36	3 (8)	29/36 (81)	1/36 (3)	8 (22)	14, median
Harano et al,[45] 2011	R	28		26/28 (93)	0	11 (39)	17-172
Jeanniard-Malet et al,[46] 2011	R	42	5 (12)	29/33 (88)	4/33 (12)	3 (7)	15, median
Patel et al,[47] 2011	R	38	8/47 (17)	31/38 (81)	6/38 (16)	0	17
Ito et al,[48] 2012	R	28 16 (MT) 12 (PT)		24/28 (86) 13/16 (81) 11/12 (92)	4/28 (14) 3 (19) 1 (8)	12 (43) 8 (50) 4 (33)	15 41[c]
Salmi et al,[49] 2012	P	61	6 (10)	37/45 (82)	3/34	13 (21)	36
Total		1012		714/903 (79)	90/761 (12)		

Abbreviations: A, abstract only; C, conventional adenoma; IDG(−), negative intraductal growth; IDG(+), positive intraductal growth; LST-P, giant laterally spreading tumors of the papilla; M, multicenter; MT, modified technique; NR, not reported; P, prospective; p, pilot; PT, previous technique; R, retrospective.

[a] P<.05 in comparison of age between IDG(−) and IDG(+) groups.

[b] P<.001 in comparison of endoscopic success between IDG(−) and IDG(+) groups.

[c] P = .016 in comparison of follow-up period between MT and PT groups.

Table 8
Complications related to EP

Reference	Patients	Total Complication Rate (%)	Pancreatitis (%)	Bleeding (%)	Perforation (%)	Cholangitis (%)	Papillary Stricture (%)	Mortality (%)
Binmoeller et al,[21] 1993	25	5/25 (20)	3 (12)	2 (8)	0	0	0	0
Greenspan et al,[22] 1997	8	1/8 (13)	0	0	0	1 (13)		
Martin et al,[23] 1997	14	2/14 (14)	1 (7)	1 (7)	0	0	0	1 (7)
Park et al,[24] 2000	6	2/6 (33)	2 (33)	0				0
Vogt et al,[25] 2000	18	5/18 (28)	2 (11)	2 (11)	0	0	0	0
Desilets et al,[26] 2001	13	1/13 (8)	1 (8)	0	0	0	0	0
Zadorova et al,[27] 2001	16		2 (13)	2 (13)	0	0	0	0
Norton et al,[28] 2002	26		4 (15)	2(8)	1 (4)	0	2 (10)	0
Saurin et al,[29] 2003	24	7/24 (29)	1 (4)					0
Catalano et al,[30] 2004	103	10/103 (10)	5 (5)	2 (2)	0	0	3 (3)	0
Cheng et al,[31] 2004	55	8/55 (15)	5 (9)	4 (7)	1 (2)	0	2 (4)	0

Study							
Kahaleh et al,[32] 2004	56	7/56 (13)	4 (7)	2 (4)	0	1 (2)		1 (2)
Bohnacker et al,[33] 2005	106; 75; IDG(−); 31; IDG(+)	40/206 (19)	13 (6), 10 (13), 3 (10)	27 (13)[d], 20, 4[e]			0	0
Harewood et al,[34] 2005	19	NR	3 (16)[b]	NR	NR		NR	NR
Eswaran et al,[35] 2006	29 (>3 cm), 22 (1–3 cm)	4/29 (14), 1/22 (5)	1 (3), 0	3, 1	0, 0		0, 0	0, 0
Katsinelos et al,[36] 2006	14	2/14 (14)	1 (7)	1 (7)	0		NR	0
Yoon et al,[37] 2007	16							0
Boix et al,[38] 2009	21	5/21 (24)	4 (19)	1	0	0	0	0
Irani et al,[39] 2009	102	21/102 (21)	10 (10)	5	2	1 (1)	3	0
Jung et al,[40] 2009	22	5/22 (23)	4 (18)	1	1 (5)			0
Hooper et al,[41] 2010	10 (LST-P), 15 (C)	4/10 (40), 1/15 (7)	0, 0	3 (30), 1 (7.7)	0, 0		1 (10)	0, 0
Hwang et al,[42] 2010	11	5/11 (45)	0	4	0		1	0
Igarashi et al,[43] 2010	36	20/36 (56)	11 (30)	6 (17)	0	0	2 (6)	0

(continued on next page)

Table 8
(continued)

Reference	Patients	Total Complication Rate (%)	Pancreatitis (%)	Bleeding (%)	Perforation (%)	Cholangitis (%)	Papillary Stricture (%)	Mortality (%)
Yamao et al,[44] 2010	36	7/36 (19)	3 (8)	3 (8)	0	0	1 (3)	0
Harano et al,[45] 2011	28	9/28 (32)	2 (7)	5 (18)	0	2 (7)		0
Jeanniard-Malet et al,[46] 2011	42	10/42 (24)	6 (14)	3 (7)		1 (2)		0
Patel et al,[47] 2011	38	6/38 (16)	3 (8)	2 (5)	0	1 (3)[f]	0	0
Ito et al,[48] 2012	28	10 (36) early/5 (18) late	1 (late)	7 (early)/1 (late)	2 (7)	3 (11)		
	16 (MT)	1 (6)/3 (19)	0	1 (early)/1 (late)				
	12 (PT)	9 (75)[a]/2 (17)	1 (late)	6	2 (17)	3		
Salmi et al,[49] 2012	61	11/61 (18)	6 (10)[c]	3 (5)	2 (3)			
Total		414/2148 (19)	224 (10)	94 (4)	9 (0.4)	13 (0.6)	30 (1.4)	2 (0.09)

Abbreviations: C, conventional adenoma; IDG(−), negative intraductal growth; IDG(+), positive intraductal growth; LST-P, giant laterally spreading tumors of the papilla; MT, modified technique; PD, pancreatic duct; PT, previous technique.

[a] 24 (12) Procedural bleeding/3(1) Delayed bleeding.

[b] $P<.05$ in comparison of bleeding between IDG(−) and IDG(+) groups.

[c] This was recorded as 1 infection in the original paper.

[d] $P = .00078$, odds ratio = 0.022 in comparison of early complication between MT and PT groups.

[e] $P = .02$ in comparison of pancreatitis between PD stent and no PD stent groups.

[f] $P<.05$ in comparison of pancreatitis between PD stent and no PD stent groups.

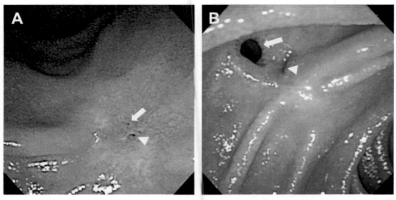

Fig. 12. Duodenoscopic examination shows typical postpapillectomy site during the postpapillectomy surveillance. White arrow indicates the biliary orifice and white arrowhead indicates the pancreatic orifice in (*A*) and (*B*).

that for patients with flat colonic polyps[110] by incorporating the degree of dysplasia and evidence of intraductal involvement into the decision-making process.[90]

SUMMARY AND FUTURE DIRECTIONS

Advances in diagnostic modality including EUS and IDUS have provided useful information to aid in diagnosing and managing for ampullary lesions. It is generally accepted that EP can be a curative therapy for localized ampullary adenoma and has a role in the diagnosis of indeterminate ampullary lesions that may contain a hidden malignancy. As techniques and equipment improve, the indications for EP will likely expand. Future randomized, long-term follow-up studies are required to address many unresolved issues brought up in this article and to provide the evidence for future consensus in this field.

REFERENCES

1. Scarpa A, Capelli P, Zamboni G, et al. Neoplasia of the ampulla of Vater. Ki-ras and p53 mutations. Am J Pathol 1993;142:1163–72.
2. Rosenberg J, Welch JP, Pyrtek LJ, et al. Benign villous adenomas of the ampulla of Vater. Cancer 1986;58:1563–8.
3. Grobmyer SR, Stasik CN, Draganov P, et al. Contemporary results with ampullectomy for 29 "benign" neoplasms of the ampulla. J Am Coll Surg 2008;206: 466–71.
4. Seifert E, Schulte F, Stolte M. Adenoma and carcinoma of the duodenum and papilla of Vater: a clinicopathologic study. Am J Gastroenterol 1992;87:37–42.
5. Spigelman AD, Talbot IC, Penna C, et al. Evidence for adenoma-carcinoma sequence in the duodenum of patients with familial adenomatous polyposis. The Leeds Castle Polyposis Group (Upper Gastrointestinal Committee). J Clin Pathol 1994;47:709–10.
6. Hirota WK, Zuckerman MJ, Adler DG, et al. ASGE guideline: the role of endoscopy in the surveillance of premalignant conditions of the upper GI tract. Gastrointest Endosc 2006;63:570–80.
7. Yamaguchi K, Enjoji M, Kitamura K. Endoscopic biopsy has limited accuracy in diagnosis of ampullary tumors. Gastrointest Endosc 1990;36:588–92.

8. Di Giorgio A, Alfieri S, Rotondi F, et al. Pancreatoduodenectomy for tumors of Vater's ampulla: report on 94 consecutive patients. World J Surg 2005;29:513–8.

9. Grobmyer SR, Pieracci FM, Allen PJ, et al. Defining morbidity after pancreatico-duodenectomy: use of a prospective complication grading system. J Am Coll Surg 2007;204:356–64.

10. Lowy AM, Lee JE, Pisters PW, et al. Prospective, randomized trial of octreotide to prevent pancreatic fistula after pancreaticoduodenectomy for malignant disease. Ann Surg 1997;226:632–41.

11. Aranha GV, Hodul PJ, Creech S, et al. Zero mortality after 152 consecutive pan-creaticoduodenectomies with pancreaticogastrostomy. J Am Coll Surg 2003; 197:223–31 [discussion: 31–2].

12. Winter JM, Cameron JL, Olino K, et al. Clinicopathologic analysis of ampullary neoplasms in 450 patients: implications for surgical strategy and long-term prognosis. J Gastrointest Surg 2010;14:379–87.

13. Branum GD, Pappas TN, Meyers WC. The management of tumors of the ampulla of Vater by local resection. Ann Surg 1996;224:621–7.

14. Grobmyer SR, Rivadeneira DE, Goodman CA, et al. Pancreatic anastomotic failure after pancreaticoduodenectomy. Am J Surg 2000;180:117–20.

15. Heidecke CD, Rosenberg R, Bauer M, et al. Impact of grade of dysplasia in villous adenomas of Vater's papilla. World J Surg 2002;26:709–14.

16. Suzuki K, Kantou U, Murakami Y. Two cases with ampullary cancer who under-went endoscopic excision. Prog Dig Endosc 1982;23:236–9.

17. van Stolk R, Sivak MV Jr, Petrini JL, et al. Endoscopic management of upper gastrointestinal polyps and periampullary lesions in familial adenomatous poly-posis and Gardner's syndrome. Endoscopy 1987;19(Suppl 1):19–22.

18. Lambert R, Ponchon T, Chavaillon A, et al. Laser treatment of tumors of the papilla of Vater. Endoscopy 1988;20(Suppl 1):227–31.

19. Shemesh E, Nass S, Czerniak A. Endoscopic sphincterotomy and endoscopic fulguration in the management of adenoma of the papilla of Vater. Surg Gynecol Obstet 1989;169:445–8.

20. Ponchon T, Berger F, Chavaillon A, et al. Contribution of endoscopy to diagnosis and treatment of tumors of the ampulla of Vater. Cancer 1989;64:161–7.

21. Binmoeller KF, Boaventura S, Ramsperger K, et al. Endoscopic snare excision of benign adenomas of the papilla of Vater. Gastrointest Endosc 1993;39: 127–31.

22. Greenspan AB, Walden DT, Aliperti G. Endoscopic management of ampullary adenomas: a report of eight patients [abstract]. Gastrointest Endosc 1997;45: AB133.

23. Martin JA, Haber GB, Kortan PP, et al. Endoscopic snare ampullectomy for resection of benign ampullary neoplasm [abstract]. Gastrointest Endosc 1997; 45:AB139.

24. Park SW, Song SY, Chung JB, et al. Endoscopic snare resection for tumors of the ampulla of Vater. Yonsei Med J 2000;41:213–8.

25. Vogt M, Jakobs R, Benz C, et al. Endoscopic therapy of adenomas of the papilla of Vater. A retrospective analysis with long-term follow-up. Dig Liver Dis 2000;32: 339–45.

26. Desilets DJ, Dy RM, Ku PM, et al. Endoscopic management of tumors of the major duodenal papilla: refined techniques to improve outcome and avoid complications. Gastrointest Endosc 2001;54:202–8.

27. Zadorova Z, Dvofak M, Hajer J. Endoscopic therapy of benign tumors of the papilla of Vater. Endoscopy 2001;33:345–7.

28. Norton ID, Gostout CJ, Baron TH, et al. Safety and outcome of endoscopic snare excision of the major duodenal papilla. Gastrointest Endosc 2002;56:239–43.
29. Saurin JC, Chavaillon A, Napoleon B, et al. Long-term follow-up of patients with endoscopic treatment of sporadic adenomas of the papilla of Vater. Endoscopy 2003;35:402–6.
30. Catalano MF, Linder JD, Chak A, et al. Endoscopic management of adenoma of the major duodenal papilla. Gastrointest Endosc 2004;59:225–32.
31. Cheng CL, Sherman S, Fogel EL, et al. Endoscopic snare papillectomy for tumors of the duodenal papillae. Gastrointest Endosc 2004;60:757–64.
32. Kahaleh M, Shami VM, Brock A, et al. Factors predictive of malignancy and endoscopic resectability in ampullary neoplasia. Am J Gastroenterol 2004;99:2335–9.
33. Bohnacker S, Seitz U, Nguyen D, et al. Endoscopic resection of benign tumors of the duodenal papilla without and with intraductal growth. Gastrointest Endosc 2005;62:551–60.
34. Harewood GC, Pochron NL, Gostout CJ. Prospective, randomized, controlled trial of prophylactic pancreatic stent placement for endoscopic snare excision of the duodenal ampulla. Gastrointest Endosc 2005;62:367–70.
35. Eswaran SL, Sanders M, Bernadino KP, et al. Success and complications of endoscopic removal of giant duodenal and ampullary polyps: a comparative series. Gastrointest Endosc 2006;64.925–32.
36. Katsinelos P, Paroutoglou G, Kountouras C, et al. Safety and long-term follow-up of endoscopic snare excision of ampullary adenomas. Surg Endosc 2006;20:608–13.
37. Yoon SM, Kim MH, Kim MJ, et al. Focal early stage cancer in ampullary adenoma: surgery or endoscopic papillectomy? Gastrointest Endosc 2007;66:701–7.
38. Boix J, Lorenzo-Zuniga V, Moreno de Vega V, et al. Endoscopic resection of ampullary tumors: 12-year review of 21 cases. Surg Endosc 2009;23:45–9.
39. Irani S, Arai A, Ayub K, et al. Papillectomy for ampullary neoplasm: results of a single referral center over a 10-year period. Gastrointest Endosc 2009;70:923–32.
40. Jung MK, Cho CM, Park SY, et al. Endoscopic resection of ampullary neoplasms: a single-center experience. Surg Endosc 2009;23:2568–74.
41. Hopper AD, Bourke MJ, Williams SJ, et al. Giant laterally spreading tumors of the papilla: endoscopic features, resection technique, and outcome (with videos). Gastrointest Endosc 2010;71:967–75.
42. Hwang JC, Kim JH, Lim SG, et al. Endoscopic resection of ampullary adenoma after a new insulated plastic pancreatic stent placement: a pilot study. J Gastroenterol Hepatol 2010;25:1381–5.
43. Igarashi Y, Okano N, Ito K, et al. Endoscopic snare excision of a major duodenal papillary tumor. Dig Surg 2010;27:119–22.
44. Yamao T, Isomoto H, Kohno S, et al. Endoscopic snare papillectomy with biliary and pancreatic stent placement for tumors of the major duodenal papilla. Surg Endosc 2010;24:119–24.
45. Harano M, Ryozawa S, Iwano H, et al. Clinical impact of endoscopic papillectomy for benign-malignant borderline lesions of the major duodenal papilla. J Hepatobiliary Pancreat Sci 2011;18:190–4
46. Jeanniard-Malet O, Caillol F, Pesenti C, et al. Short-term results of 42 endoscopic ampullectomies: a single-center experience. Scand J Gastroenterol 2011;46:1014–9.

47. Patel R, Davitte J, Varadarajulu S, et al. Endoscopic resection of ampullary adenomas: complications and outcomes. Dig Dis Sci 2011;56:3235–40.
48. Ito K, Fujita N, Noda Y, et al. Impact of technical modification of endoscopic papillectomy for ampullary neoplasm on the occurrence of complications. Dig Endosc 2012;24:30–5.
49. Salmi S, Ezzedine S, Vitton V, et al. Can papillary carcinomas be treated by endoscopic ampullectomy? Surg Endosc 2012;26:920–5.
50. Sobol S, Cooperman AM. Villous adenoma of the ampulla of Vater. An unusual cause of biliary colic and obstructive jaundice. Gastroenterology 1978;75:107–9.
51. Huibregtse K, Tytgat GN. Carcinoma of the ampulla of Vater: the endoscopic approach. Endoscopy 1988;20(Suppl 1):223–6.
52. Allgaier HP, Schwacha H, Kleinschmidt M, et al. Ampullary hamartoma: a rare cause of biliary obstruction. Digestion 1999;60:497–500.
53. Beger HG, Staib L, Schoenberg MH. Ampullectomy for adenoma of the papilla and ampulla of Vater. Langenbecks Arch Surg 1998;383:190–3.
54. Alexander JR, Andrews JM, Buchi KN, et al. High prevalence of adenomatous polyps of the duodenal papilla in familial adenomatous polyposis. Dig Dis Sci 1989;34:167–70.
55. Jagelman DG, DeCosse JJ, Bussey HJ. Upper gastrointestinal cancer in familial adenomatous polyposis. Lancet 1988;1:1149–51.
56. Walsh DB, Eckhauser FE, Cronenwett JL, et al. Adenocarcinoma of the ampulla of Vater. Diagnosis and treatment. Ann Surg 1982;195:152–7.
57. Tarazi RY, Hermann RE, Vogt DP, et al. Results of surgical treatment of periampullary tumors: a thirty-five-year experience. Surgery 1986;100:716–23.
58. Izumi Y, Teramoto K, Ohshima M, et al. Endoscopic resection of duodenal ampulla with a transparent plastic cap. Surgery 1998;123:109–10.
59. Kim MH, Lee SK, Seo DW, et al. Tumors of the major duodenal papilla. Gastrointest Endosc 2001;54:609–20.
60. Emory RE Jr, Emory TS, Goellner JR, et al. Neuroendocrine ampullary tumors: spectrum of disease including the first report of a neuroendocrine carcinoma of non-small cell type. Surgery 1994;115:762–6.
61. Nassar H, Albores-Saavedra J, Klimstra DS. High-grade neuroendocrine carcinoma of the ampulla of Vater: a clinicopathologic and immunohistochemical analysis of 14 cases. Am J Surg Pathol 2005;29:588–94.
62. Cheng SP, Yang TL, Chang KM, et al. Large cell neuroendocrine carcinoma of the ampulla of Vater with glandular differentiation. J Clin Pathol 2004;57:1098–100.
63. Zamboni G, Franzin G, Bonetti F, et al. Small-cell neuroendocrine carcinoma of the ampullary region. A clinicopathologic, immunohistochemical, and ultrastructural study of three cases. Am J Surg Pathol 1990;14:703–13.
64. Nishimori I, Morita M, Sano S, et al. Endosonography-guided endoscopic resection of duodenal carcinoid tumor. Endoscopy 1997;29:214–7.
65. Albores-Saavedra J, Hart A, Chable-Montero F, et al. Carcinoids and high-grade neuroendocrine carcinomas of the ampulla of Vater: a comparative analysis of 139 cases from the surveillance, epidemiology, and end results program–a population based study. Arch Pathol Lab Med 2010;134:1692–6.
66. Ricci JL. Carcinoid of the ampulla of Vater. Local resection or pancreaticoduodenectomy. Cancer 1993;71:686–90.
67. Roggin KK, Yeh JJ, Ferrone CR, et al. Limitations of ampullectomy in the treatment of nonfamilial ampullary neoplasms. Ann Surg Oncol 2005;12:971–80.

68. Elek G, Gyori S, Toth B, et al. Histological evaluation of preoperative biopsies from ampulla vateri. Pathol Oncol Res 2003;9:32–41.
69. Menzel J, Poremba C, Dietl KH, et al. Tumors of the papilla of Vater–inadequate diagnostic impact of endoscopic forceps biopsies taken prior to and following sphincterotomy. Ann Oncol 1999;10:1227–31.
70. Sakorafas GH, Friess H, Dervenis CG. Villous tumors of the duodenum: biologic characters and clinical implications. Scand J Gastroenterol 2000;35:337–44.
71. Bourgeois N, Dunham F, Verhest A, et al. Endoscopic biopsies of the papilla of Vater at the time of endoscopic sphincterotomy: difficulties in interpretation. Gastrointest Endosc 1984;30:163–6.
72. Seewald S, Omar S, Soehendra N. Endoscopic resection of tumors of the ampulla of Vater: how far up and how deep down can we go? Gastrointest Endosc 2006;63:789–91.
73. Uchiyama Y, Imazu H, Kakutani H, et al. New approach to diagnosing ampullary tumors by magnifying endoscopy combined with a narrow-band imaging system. J Gastroenterol 2006;41:483–90.
74. Itoi T, Tsuji S, Sofuni A, et al. A novel approach emphasizing preoperative margin enhancement of tumor of the major duodenal papilla with narrow-band imaging in comparison to indigo carmine chromoendoscopy (with videos). Gastrointest Endosc 2009;69:136–41.
75. Rosch T, Braig C, Gain T, et al. Staging of pancreatic and ampullary carcinoma by endoscopic ultrasonography. Comparison with conventional sonography, computed tomography, and angiography. Gastroenterology 1992;102:188–99.
76. Yasuda K, Mukai H, Cho E, et al. The use of endoscopic ultrasonography in the diagnosis and staging of carcinoma of the papilla of Vater. Endoscopy 1988; 20(Suppl 1):218–22.
77. Mitake M, Nakazawa S, Tsukamoto Y, et al. Endoscopic ultrasonography in the diagnosis of depth invasion and lymph node metastasis of carcinoma of the papilla of Vater. J Ultrasound Med 1990;9:645–50.
78. Tio TL, Sie LH, Kallimanis G, et al. Staging of ampullary and pancreatic carcinoma: comparison between endosonography and surgery. Gastrointest Endosc 1996;44:706–13.
79. Itoh A, Goto H, Naitoh Y, et al. Intraductal ultrasonography in diagnosing tumor extension of cancer of the papilla of Vater. Gastrointest Endosc 1997;45: 251–60.
80. Cannon ME, Carpenter SL, Elta GH, et al. EUS compared with CT, magnetic resonance imaging, and angiography and the influence of biliary stenting on staging accuracy of ampullary neoplasms. Gastrointest Endosc 1999;50:27–33.
81. Kubo H, Chijiiwa Y, Akahoshi K, et al. Pre-operative staging of ampullary tumours by endoscopic ultrasound. Br J Radiol 1999;72:443–7.
82. Menzel J, Hoepffner N, Sulkowski U, et al. Polypoid tumors of the major duodenal papilla: preoperative staging with intraductal US, EUS, and CT–a prospective, histopathologically controlled study. Gastrointest Endosc 1999; 49:349–57.
83. Chen CH, Tseng LJ, Yang CC, et al. The accuracy of endoscopic ultrasound, endoscopic retrograde cholangiopancreatography, computed tomography, and transabdominal ultrasound in the detection and staging of primary ampullary tumors. Hepatogastroenterology 2001;48:1750–3.
84. Skordilis P, Mouzas IA, Dimoulios PD, et al. Is endosonography an effective method for detection and local staging of the ampullary carcinoma? A prospective study. BMC Surg 2002;2:1.

85. Ito K, Fujita N, Noda Y, et al. Preoperative evaluation of ampullary neoplasm with EUS and transpapillary intraductal US: a prospective and histopathologically controlled study. Gastrointest Endosc 2007;66:740–7.
86. Artifon EL, Couto D Jr, Sakai P, et al. Prospective evaluation of EUS versus CT scan for staging of ampullary cancer. Gastrointest Endosc 2009;70:290–6.
87. Menees SB, Schoenfeld P, Kim HM, et al. A survey of ampullectomy practices. World J Gastroenterol 2009;15:3486–92.
88. Baillie J. Endoscopic ampullectomy: does pancreatic stent placement make it safer? Gastrointest Endosc 2005;62:371–3.
89. Lim GJ, Devereaux BM. EUS in the assessment of ampullary lesions prior to endoscopic resection. Tech Gastrointest Endosc 2010;12:49–52.
90. Standards of Practice Committee, Adler DG, Qureshi W, Davila R, et al. The role of endoscopy in ampullary and duodenal adenomas. Gastrointest Endosc 2006; 64:849–54.
91. Aiura K, Imaeda H, Kitajima M, et al. Balloon-catheter-assisted endoscopic snare papillectomy for benign tumors of the major duodenal papilla. Gastrointest Endosc 2003;57:743–7.
92. Jung S, Kim MH, Seo DW, et al. Endoscopic snare papillectomy of adenocarcinoma of the major duodenal papilla. Gastrointest Endosc 2001;54:622.
93. Ito K, Fujita N, Noda Y. Case of early ampullary cancer treated by endoscopic papillectomy. Dig Endosc 2004;16:157–61.
94. Yoon YS, Kim SW, Park SJ, et al. Clinicopathologic analysis of early ampullary cancers with a focus on the feasibility of ampullectomy. Ann Surg 2005;242: 92–100.
95. Lee SY, Jang KT, Lee KT, et al. Can endoscopic resection be applied for early stage ampulla of Vater cancer? Gastrointest Endosc 2006;63:783–8.
96. Woo SM, Ryu JK, Lee SH, et al. Feasibility of endoscopic papillectomy in early stage ampulla of Vater cancer. J Gastroenterol Hepatol 2009;24:120–4.
97. Han J, Kim MH. Endoscopic papillectomy for adenomas of the major duodenal papilla (with video). Gastrointest Endosc 2006;63:292–301.
98. Charton JP, Deinert K, Schumacher B, et al. Endoscopic resection for neoplastic diseases of the papilla of Vater. J Hepatobiliary Pancreat Surg 2004;11:245–51.
99. Feitoza AB, Gostout CJ, Burgart LJ, et al. Hydroxypropyl methylcellulose: a better submucosal fluid cushion for endoscopic mucosal resection. Gastrointest Endosc 2003;57:41–7.
100. Baillie J. Endoscopic ampullectomy. Am J Gastroenterol 2005;100:2379–81.
101. Hernandez LV, Catalano MF. Endoscopic papillectomy. Curr Opin Gastroenterol 2008;24:617–22.
102. Bassan M, Bourke M. Endoscopic ampullectomy: a practical guide. J Interv Gastroenterol 2012;2:23–30.
103. Patel R, Varadarajulu S, Wilcox CM. Endoscopic ampullectomy: techniques and outcomes. J Clin Gastroenterol 2012;46:8–15.
104. Mehdizadeh S, Sadda M, Lo SK. Mucosectomy-cap assisted ampullectomy (MCAA) is an effective technique in removing residual tissue after snare ampullectomy. Gastrointest Endosc 2006;63:AB242.
105. Smith MT, Sherman S, Ikenberry SO, et al. Alterations in pancreatic ductal morphology following polyethylene pancreatic stent therapy. Gastrointest Endosc 1996;44:268–75.
106. Zolotarevsky E, Fehmi SM, Anderson MA, et al. Prophylactic 5-Fr pancreatic duct stents are superior to 3-Fr stents: a randomized controlled trial. Endoscopy 2011;43:325–30.

107. Lee SK, Kim MH, Seo DW, et al. Endoscopic sphincterotomy and pancreatic duct stent placement before endoscopic papillectomy: are they necessary and safe procedures? Gastrointest Endosc 2002;55:302–4.
108. Kim JH, Han JH, Yoo BM, et al. Is endoscopic papillectomy safe for ampullary adenomas with high-grade dysplasia? Ann Surg Oncol 2009;16:2547–54.
109. Meneghetti AT, Safadi B, Stewart L, et al. Local resection of ampullary tumors. J Gastrointest Surg 2005;9:1300–6.
110. Davila RE, Rajan E, Baron TH, et al. ASGE guideline: colorectal cancer screening and surveillance. Gastrointest Endosc 2006;63:546–57.

Prevention and Management of Adverse Events of Endoscopic Retrograde Cholangiopancreatography

Bryan Balmadrid, MD, Richard Kozarek, MD*

KEYWORDS

- ERCP • Endoscopic retrograde cholangiopancreatography • Prevention
- Management • Adverse events • Complications • Pancreatitis • Perforation

KEY POINTS

- Recognize preprocedure and intraprocedure risks for post-ERCP pancreatitis to perform effective risk-reducing modalities, which include prophylactic pancreatic stent placement and rectal indomethacin.
- Endoscopic options for the management of luminal and pancreaticobiliary duct perforations exist, so it is important to recognize these adverse events early.
- Intraprocedural bleeding occurs commonly, but most cases spontaneously resolve. For unresolved bleeding, standard endoscopic therapy modalities can be used through the duodenoscope with good efficacy.
- With increased knowledge about adverse events and the different modalities of treatment, endoscopists practicing ERCP should have the necessary volume and experience to maintain these skills.

INTRODUCTION

Endoscopic retrograde cholangiopancreatography (ERCP) has been a classic modality to evaluate the biliary and pancreatic ducts. Because of its invasive nature and significant rate of complication, ERCP is no longer used as an initial diagnostic procedure but instead has become a therapeutic option. In general, endoscopies share similar complications, such as perforation, bleeding, and issues with sedation. However, ERCP adds other unique complications, such as acute pancreatitis, cholangitis, and cholecystitis, in addition to increased risk of bleeding and perforation, depending on the initial goal and indication of the ERCP. To compare, colonoscopies have a 0.1% rate of perforation and 1% to 4% postpolypectomy rate of bleeding [1,2]

Virginia Mason Medical Center Digestive Disease Institute, 3rd Floor Buck Pavillion, 1100 9th Street, Seattle, WA 98101, USA
* Corresponding author.
E-mail address: gasrak@vmmc.org

Gastrointest Endoscopy Clin N Am 23 (2013) 385–403
http://dx.doi.org/10.1016/j.giec.2012.12.007
1052-5157/13/$ – see front matter © 2013 Elsevier Inc. All rights reserved.

compared with ERCPs with 0.34% rate of perforation and 2% postsphincterotomy rate of bleeding.[3] Other noninvasive modalities used in evaluating the pancreaticobiliary ducts, such as cross-sectional imaging and transabdominal ultrasound (US), are usually readily available and should be the primary diagnostic modalities. Diagnostic endoscopic ultrasound (EUS) has a lower rate of complications than ERCP and can be considered among the primary diagnostic approaches. However, EUS requires sedation and is more invasive in nature than the other imaging modalities. ERCP should now be considered a therapeutic option and, with the exception of a patient with potential sphincter of Oddi dysfunction (SOD), is not a diagnostic option. ERCP should be performed if there is a reasonable probability that therapy (ie, stone extraction) is required, and as always, the benefits of the procedure need to be weighed against the risks and potential complications.

The most common complication and untoward event when performing ERCP is post-ERCP pancreatitis (PEP). Other complications to consider are perforations, including those of the duodenal wall, as well as the biliary and pancreatic ducts. Sphincterotomies are often performed simultaneously and thus postsphincterotomy bleeding is also of concern. Overall, there may be a 5% to 10% risk of short-term complications after ERCP, but this varies greatly depending on the patient's risk factors.[4] For example, patients with SOD have up to a 40% risk of developing PEP in some studies.

INDICATIONS

An effective way to reduce complications is to limit or avoid ERCP, and as noted above, there has been more focus placed on the indications to perform an ERCP as it has moved away from the realm of diagnostic procedures. Classic indications include choledocholithiasis and cholangitis. Clinical criteria are available to estimate the likelihood of these diagnoses and the suggested management protocols based on their likelihood. Thus, even with classic indications, ERCP may not necessarily be the first modality of choice.[5] For example, the American Society of Gastrointestinal Endoscopy recommends that only patients meeting the criteria for high suspicion undergo an ERCP for choledocholithiasis. The high suspicion group includes a common bile duct (CBD) stone on visible on US, total bilirubin greater than 4 mg/dL, or clinical ascending cholangitis.[6] In addition, a dilated CBD greater than 6 mm on US and total bilirubin 1.8 to 4.0 mg/dL are also highly suspicious (**Table 1**). Otherwise, EUS or magnetic resonance cholangiopancreatography is recommended for the initial evaluation, or simply proceeding with a cholecystectomy with intraoperative cholangiogram.[5] There are many reasonable indications for an ERCP that may fall outside of the classic indications. It is then important to have a detailed patient discussion, preferably with patient's friends and family participating, and that this be clearly documented.

Operator Experience

Increased operator experience also seems to reduce the risk of overall complications slightly, but more importantly, reduces risk of major complications.[4] The role of experience is difficult to quantify because the more experienced centers tend to perform more complicated procedures and thus may have an increased risk for complications. The patients may also be in poorer health or have more difficult anatomy. For example, community gastrointestinal groups often refer patients who have had unsuccessful ERCP cannulations or patients with altered anatomy to tertiary centers. It is intuitively obvious that the number and frequency of ERCPs performed by the endoscopist

Table 1
Predictors of likelihood of ongoing choledocholithiasis

Very Strong	Strong	Moderate
CBD stone on US	Dilated CBD on US >6 mm (with gallbladder in situ)	Other abnormal liver biochemical levels
Clinical ascending cholangitis	Bilirubin 1.8–4 mg/dL	Age >55 y
Bilirubin >4 mg/dL		Clinical gallstone pancreatitis
Likelihood based on predictors		**Suggested management**
Presence of any very strong predictor	High	Preoperative ERCP
Presence of both strong predictors	High	Preoperative ERCP
No predictors present	Low	Laparoscopic cholecystectomy (no cholangiography)
All other patients	Intermediate	Laparoscopic IOC or preoperative EUS or MRCP

Abbreviations: IOC,   intraoperative   cholangiogram;   MRCP,   magnetic   resonance cholangiopancreatography.

correlates inversely with rates of complication. However, determining the number of completed procedures that are required to achieve proficiency is difficult because of all the variables involved. The British Society of Gastroenterology has recommended a minimum of 75 ERCPs performed yearly.[6] There is also evidence that the number of ERCP sphincterotomies performed in a week makes a difference in the rate of bleeding complications.[4] Finally, undertaking a dedicated ERCP/EUS (advanced endoscopy) fellowship reduces the risk, but controversy remains and it is still unclear how many procedures need to be performed to gain even the basic competencies. Less than 200 cases does not seem to be adequate,[7] but how many remains a question.

POST-ERCP PANCREATITIS

PEP is the most common complication of ERCP with an average rate of 5%, but the incidence varies widely depending on risk factors.[8] For example, SOD carries with it a 10% to 40% chance of PEP (**Table 2**).[4] The diagnosis of PEP is similar to other acute pancreatitis: the combination of new onset abdominal pain along with an amylase and lipase elevation at least 3 times the upper limits of normal. The onset is usually within 24 hours of the procedure, often occurring within 2 to 4 hours. Because of the varying rates of PEP, it is important to risk stratify patients based on their preprocedure and intraprocedure risk.

Preprocedure Risk Factors

Patients with SOD carry the highest risk for PEP, ranging from 10% to 40%, and, therefore, it is important to assess this special population of patients carefully (see **Table 2**).[4,8] SOD is often suspected in younger women with abdominal pain and it seems women, in general, have a higher likelihood of PEP (odds ratio [OR], 2.23). Simply being evaluated for SOD dysfunction can raise the PEP likelihood to 10% to 30%.[4] It was initially thought that biliary and pancreatic sphincter manometry added

Table 2
Preprocedure and intraprocedure risk factors to develop post-ERCP pancreatitis

Increased Risk (Pre-ERCP)	Protective for PEP (Pre-ERCP)	Intraprocedure Risk for PEP
Evaluation for SOD	Chronic pancreatitis	Pancreatic sphincterotomy
Female	Pancreatic malignancy	Repeated cannulation (>8 cannulation attempts)
Age <60–70 y	Age >80 y	Pneumatic dilation of biliary sphincter
Normal caliber bile duct	Increased bilirubin levels	Precut sphincterotomy (depending on context)
History of alcohol use		Ampullectomy
Pancreas divisum (usually associated with dorsal duct cannulation)		Multiple or excessive injections into the pancreatic duct (ie, injection to the tail, pancreatic acini opacification)
Previous history of PEP		Cytologic brushing of the pancreatic duct

to this risk factor. Cotton and colleagues[8] retrospectively analyzed 11,497 ERCPs and found biliary and pancreatic manometry to have ORs of 1.16 and 1.43, respectively, neither of which were statistically significant. Other risk factors usually attributed, but not exclusive, to this population, include an age less than 60 to 70 years and normal caliber bile duct. History of alcohol use has been shown to be a significant risk factor (2 to 3 relative risk). Pancreas divisum has shown some increased risk in some studies but the data are not uniform. A more recent retrospective review showed that there is a low PEP rate of 1.2% if dorsal duct cannulation is not attempted, but with dorsal duct cannulation attempts, the risk of PEP is 8.2% and goes up to 10.6% when a minor duct sphincterotomy is performed.[9] A previous history of PEP also puts patients at risk to develop PEP with future ERCPs.

There are also factors that are protective of PEP. Patients with chronic pancreatitis and pancreatic malignancy have lower risk, which is likely because of the atrophy of the upstream pancreatic parenchyma from the chronic obstruction.[10] Because younger age and normal total levels of bilirubin are risk factors for PEP, ages greater than 80 years and increased total bilirubin have been shown to be protective.[8]

Intraprocedure Risk of PEP

Ampullary trauma plays an important role in the pathophysiology of PEP. This trauma can be caused by prolonged cannulation attempts, which reflects the difficulty of cannulation or the experience level of the endoscopist. Initially, it was thought that alternate ways of accessing the duct after difficult cannulation, such as precut sphincterotomy or needle-knife access, increased the risk for PEP. However, there has been growing evidence that early precut access, after only 4 to 10 attempts for cannulation, actually decreases the risk for PEP compared with persistent attempts at cannulation, which can traumatize the papilla further. Two meta-analyses (6 randomized controlled trials) published in 2010 showed relative risks of 0.46 (95% confidence interval [CI]: 0.23–0.92)[11] and 0.47 (95% CI: 0.24–0.91)[12] when early precut access was obtained, which supports the concept of ampullary trauma after multiple attempts. Precut sphincterotomy performed early by an experienced endoscopist before significant trauma results is most likely helpful in preventing PEP. However, precut papillotomy is considered an advanced technique and may be better suited for more experienced endoscopists. It is often difficult to determine how many attempts can be tried until precut is considered. One suggestion would be to consider this after 10 cannulation attempts.[13]

Contrast dye injection into the pancreatic duct has been shown, in multivariate analysis, to be a PEP risk factor, and avoidance or minimization of contrast injection with guidewire cannulation has been shown to decrease PEP. This is somewhat controversial, because there are many trials with mixed results and a most recent prospective comparison trial by Mariani and colleagues[14] showed no difference in rates of PEP. However, a recent meta-analysis[15] evaluated 7 randomized controlled trials and showed a significant difference of 3.2% versus 8.7% PEP with guidewire cannulation compared with contrast-guided biliary cannulation, with a statistically significant relative risk reduction of 0.38 (95% CI, 0.19–0.76). Although guidewire cannulation seems to have a lower risk of PEP than contrast dye injection, another study found a significantly high rate (34.6%) of PEP when pancreatic guidewire was left in place to achieve selective biliary cannulation.[16] It is reasonable to theorize that any pancreatic duct manipulation is, in itself, a risk for PEP, and that if the endoscopist resorts to leaving a guidewire in the pancreatic duct, it was likely a difficult cannulation, further increasing the risk for PEP.

Balloon dilation sphincteroplasty is often used instead of electrocautery sphincterotomy to reduce the risk of postsphincterotomy bleeding. However, this may increase the risk of PEP in certain patient groups; thus, assessing risks before deciding which modality to use is important.

There is some controversy as to whether self-expanding metal stents (SEMS) placed in the biliary tree for malignant biliary obstruction potentially increases the risk of PEP. Theoretically, the greater diameter and radial expansion of the SEMS has the potential to obstruct or distort the pancreatic orifice or common channel, thus increasing the risk of PEP. A recent, large prospective trial[17] showed that SEMS were associated with a 7.3% incidence of PEP and plastic stents were associated with a 1.3% incidence of PEP, which conflicts with previous preliminary studies of safety using SEMS, in which PEP occurred in approximately 1% of the cases.[10,18–21] More studies are needed to determine the true risk.

An intraductal ultrasound probe, inserted through the working channel of the duodenoscope, has been used for investigating suspected malignancies and strictures of the biliary duct. However, intraductal ultrasound has been shown to increase the risk of PEP with a hazard ratio of 2.41 (P = .004). It is likely that the rigid probe causes mechanical irritation of the papilla as it enters the bile duct.[22]

There are additional methods variably used to reduce the risk of PEP. The use of guidewire cannulation instead of contrast dye injection has already been discussed. Another important technique is the use of prophylactic, plastic, pancreatic stents (**Box 1**). It is theorized that outflow tract obstructions of the pancreatic duct can occur from edema and inflammation during manipulation of the papilla. This obstruction can trigger iatrogenic pancreatitis. By placing a small (3F or 5F) temporary, plastic stent

---

Box 1
Mechanical prevention and risk reduction for post-ERCP pancreatitis

Guidewire cannulation

Pancreatic stent placement

Precut access (after only minimal attempts)

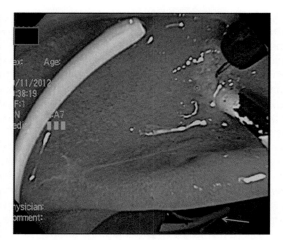

Fig. 1. Needle knife sphincterotomy of the minor papilla over a prophylactic, plastic, pancreatic stent. Note a plastic, biliary stent coming out of the major papilla in the background (*arrow*).

into the pancreatic duct, flow can be maintained (**Figs. 1** and **2**). Several studies have shown the benefits of pancreatic stents, and 3 meta-analyses have been published on this subject.[23–25] The most recent, published in 2011, pooled data from 8 randomized controlled trials and showed an OR of 0.22 (95% CI: 0.12–0.38) with an impressive absolute risk reduction of 13.3%, giving the number of patients needed to treat as 8 patients to prevent a single episode of pancreatitis. This risk reduction was true for both mild and moderate PEP.[23] Although this meta-analysis did not show a decrease in frequency of severe PEP, a previous meta-analysis did.[24] With this overwhelming evidence derived from randomized controlled trials, it has become the standard of care to place prophylactic plastic stents in patients at high risk for PEP (see **Table 2** for risk of PEP). The effects of diameter, length, and presence of flanges have also been studied. There does not seem to be a difference in flanged versus unflanged

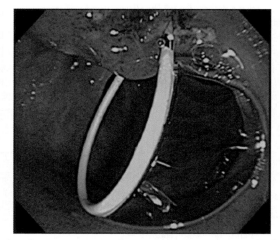

Fig. 2. Examples of a plastic, pancreatic duct stent in the major papilla for PEP Prophylaxis.

stents, or shorter (<3 cm) versus longer (>3 cm) stents,[23,24] although the studies focusing on these factors are small. Intuitively, it makes sense that smaller unflanged stents may fall out of the pancreatic orifice more quickly, thus limiting their efficacy in mitigating outflow obstructions. In contrast, longer, flanged stents have a higher retention risk and may require a separate procedure to remove. The data continue to be mixed, and it is still unclear what the perfect length of time that a stent should remain in place to balance out the reduction of risk for PEP with the risk of damaging the pancreatic orifice. However, it seems that 3-F or 5-F short plastic stents are just as effective as large-diameter stents. In the authors' practice, 1-sided pigtail stents to prevent proximal migration are used. Abdominal plain film radiographs should be performed after 2 weeks to assess for spontaneous passage of these stents, as retained stents have the potential for scarring and damage to the pancreatic duct and parenchyma. Because failed attempts of pancreatic duct stent placement have been associated with increased risk of PEP, an intention-to-treat analysis was conducted and it was found that there is a strong trend toward benefit; however, the study was likely not powered enough to reach statistical significance. In this group, the pancreatic duct placement rate of success was 88%.[16] Despite its ability to decrease PEP incidence in high-risk patients, prophylactic pancreatic duct stent placement does not seem, based on a survey of community and tertiary care practices, to have disseminated to the endoscopy community. Although more than 75% of cases were identified as high risk, fewer than 50% of endoscopists reported attempting pancreatic duct stent placement in this setting. Importantly, 21% did not place prophylactic pancreatic duct stents in any circumstance.[25] This results in the debate of requiring that endoscopists who perform ERCPs to be proficient in pancreatic duct stent placement or whether all high-risk ERCP patients should be referred to appropriate care centers with endoscopists who possess the necessary expertise.

Pharmacologic Strategies for the Prevention of Post-ERCP Pancreatitis

Given the frequency of PEP, pharmacologic agents to reduce PEP have been sought. Although some show promise, most agents either had mixed results or fared no better than placebo in rigorous trials. Nonsteroidal anti-inflammatory drugs (NSAIDs) have most recently been in the spotlight for their potential to reduce the frequency of PEP substantially. NSAIDs are potent inhibitors of the phospholipase A2 and other inflammatory mediators. Phospholipase A2 is believed to play a critical role in the initial inflammatory cascade of acute pancreatitis. Early studies of rectal diclofenac showed some efficacy in preventing acute pancreatitis.[26–28] Most recently, rectal indomethacin has shown promise. Earlier studies of rectal indomethacin looked at treated patients with average or varying risk factors for PEP. In one of the first large studies, there was a trend toward statistical significance (PEP in 3.2% with rectal indomethacin vs 6.8% with placebo; n = 490; P = .06).[29] Earlier studies showed trends that did not meet statistical significance.[30] Another study showed significant hyperamylasemia differences in patients treated with rectal indomethacin versus placebo.[30] The earlier studies used rectal indomethacin either 2 hours before or immediately before ERCP on the premise that it takes 30 to 90 minutes to achieve a therapeutic level.[31] A recent, large, randomized controlled study that received considerable press showed an absolute difference of 7.7% in patients receiving rectal indomethacin versus placebo (9.2%–6.9%) with the number needed to treat as 13. However, the difference from the previous study was the inclusion of only patients considered to be at high risk of PEP, who were given either rectal indomethacin or placebo immediately after ERCP.[32] Importantly, there were no significant increases in bleeding or renal failure in the indomethacin group when compared with the placebo group. Rectal indomethacin (100 mg) seems to be a safe, effective, prophylactic treatment in patients who are at high risk for PEP. It also has the potential to reduce the risk of PEP for average-risk patients, but further investigation is needed. The timing of administration is still questioned, but the authors' personal perspective is that it is reasonable to administer rectal indomethacin before the procedure in patients with significant preprocedure risk for PEP. For patients who move into the high-risk group only during ERCP (ie, difficult cannulation, multiple pancreatic duct injections, precut sphincterotomy, and so on), rectal indomethacin can be administered immediately afterward. The potential for an indomethacin suppository may be included in the informed consent for the ERCP.

Various other pharmaceutical agents targeting various components of the pathophysiologic process of acute pancreatitis have been studied, including pretreatment to induce papillary dilation with agents such as nifedipine, lidocaine, epinephrine, and glyceryl trinitrate, on the premise that manipulating the pancreatic orifice causes spasms and temporary duct obstruction, leading to acute pancreatitis. The first 3 agents did not show any efficacy, but glyceryl trinitrate (GTN) showed the most promise, although, again, data are mixed.[33] The most recent meta-analysis of 7 randomized controlled studies comprising 1841 patients showed an OR of 0.56 (0.40–0.79; 95% CI) PEP reduction compared with placebo.[34] Adverse events included hypotensive episodes (systolic blood pressure <100 mm Hg) in 50% of the GTN group compared with 5% of the placebo group, but all responded to intravenous colloid infusions. The GTN group also had more headaches.[34] The best route of GTN administration is not completely clear, although a recent meta-analysis suggests the sublingual approach is more effective than the transdermal approach.[34] An intravenous approach has also been used. Interestingly, centers with a higher baseline incidence of PEP had a higher risk reduction with GTN than centers with a lower PEP at baseline. This difference in risk reduction can be viewed in the following 2 ways: if it is assumed that a higher baseline incidence of PEP is because the center undertook more complicated, high-risk procedures, then, much like indomethacin, GTN should perhaps be reserved for the higher risk cases. Alternatively, if it is assumed that the higher incidence of PEP is because of a lack of expertise in these centers, then GTN may be more protective in cases where there is difficulty in cannulating. Another meta-analysis in the same year reviewed 8 randomized controlled trials and showed a risk reduction with an OR of 0.60 (0.39–0.92; 95% CI).[35] However, using sensitivity analysis, in which they removed the trial that did not use standard diagnostic criteria for PEP, the OR range crossed 1.0 with an OR 0.68 (0.41–1.11; 95% CI). Because of mixed results and the question of the ideal route of administration, recommendations about nitroglycerin remain inconsistent.

Protease inhibitors, including Gabexate, Ulinastatin, and Nafamostat mesylate, have been used extensively to manage acute pancreatitis and are part of the standard of care in Japan. Protease inhibitors inactivate the proteolytic enzymes that are thought to play in important role in pancreatic injury. In the most recent meta-analysis in 2011, in which 19 cohort studies were pooled, the overall results showed a modest but significant risk reduction with a pooled risk difference of −0.029 (95% CI, −0.051 to −0.008).[36] This difference yielded nonsignificant results when only high-quality studies in the analysis were included. Most recently, in a study that compared the use of Gabexate, Ulinastatin, and placebo, the Gabexate group had a 3.5% incidence of PEP compared with the Ulinastatin group with 7.0% and placebo group with 7.3%, a statistically significant difference.[37] Thus, Gabexate, but not Ulnistatin, showed efficacy in preventing PEP. Aside from the mixed data and the cost of these agents, another limiting factor is the administration schedule. The infusion of

Gabexate and Ulnistatin begins 30 minutes before the procedure and continues for 24 hours. The newer Nafamostat mesylate infusion is started 1 hour before the procedure and is continued for 6 hours after ERCP.[38] Although their use is a common practice in Japan, protease inhibitors have not been adopted in western countries because of these limitations.

Secretin is a gastrointestinal peptide endocrine hormone that primarily stimulates the secretion of bicarbonate-rich fluid from the pancreas. In 1 study, 869 patients were randomly administered 16 ug (8 mL) of synthetic secretin (equivalent to 80 clinical units of biologic activity) or placebo at the start of the ERCP or the start of pancreaticobiliary manometry. The secretin group had an 8.7% incidence of PEP compared with 15.1% in the placebo group ($P = .004$).[39] In this study, secretin was highly effective in reducing PEP in patients undergoing biliary sphincterotomy in subgroup analysis. Although this seems promising, further studies are needed.

Somatostatin and octreotide function by inhibiting the exocrine secretion of the pancreas, which theoretically prevents pancreatitis and autodigestion. Meta-analyses of many randomized trials have not shown any efficacy with these modalities.[40–42] Other agents, such as low-molecular-weight heparin (based on animal models of inhibition of pancreatic damage),[43] allopurinol, and n-acetyl cysteine, have not shown efficacy in preventing PEP.[44]

Prophylactic corticosteroids, in turn, have also been used to decrease the inflammatory response of acute pancreatitis. The most recent meta-analysis showed an OR of 1.13 (95% CI, 0.88–1.46) with subsequent sensitivity and subgroup analysis confirming no statistical difference in risk reduction.[41]

PERFORATIONS

Perforations at the time of ERCP occur less than 1% (0.35%–0.6%) of the time.[3] When recognized early and for certain types of perforations, many of these cases can be managed conservatively, avoiding surgery. This conservative management is especially true because closure devices, which can be applied through the scope, have been in use.

There are 3 types of perforations (**Table 3**). Type 1 perforations affect the luminal wall and include esophageal perforations in a difficult intubation, gastric perforations, and more commonly, duodenal perforations. Duodenal perforations can occur when too much pressure is applied to the sweep of the thin-walled duodenum, or as is often the case, when the ampulla is near a duodenal diverticulum and the scope tip directly perforates the diverticulum. Most of these perforations are force and angle related.

Type 2 perforations are sphincterotomy-induced or precut, needle-knife–induced perforations of the periampullary region of the duodenum. The classic "zipper cut" falls into this category. With more frequent use of the microprocessor-controlled ERBE generator (New Marietta, GA), cautery settings, these occur less frequently.

Classically, these perforations required surgical repair, but more attempts have been made to close these perforations endoscopically. SEMS have been used to

Table 3 Type of perforation	
Type 1	Luminal wall perforation by the scope (ie, duodenal, gastric, esophageal wall perforation)
Type 2	Sphincterotomy-induced perforation of the periampullary region
Type 3	Guidewire perforation of the pancreatic or biliary duct

close esophageal and, more specifically, ERCP-induced duodenal perforations successfully.[45,46] SEMS have been shown to be effective with both scope perforations through the luminal wall as well as sphincterotomy-induced duodenal wall perforations. Through-the-scope clips have also been used with success.[45] Newer over-the-scope clips are larger sets of clips attached over the scope in a fashion similar to a banding cap, and there are now multiple reports of successful closure of esophageal, gastric, and duodenal perforations. Closure has been consistently successful in defects up to 20 to 30 mm in size.[47] Regardless of the method selected to close perforations, the endoscopist requires the appropriate level of training and comfort before undertaking endoscopic closure. Availability of equipment is also a consideration. Although through-the-scope clips are readily available, SEMS, over-the-scope clips, and CO_2 insufflation may not be immediately available. In particular, attempts to close perforations should be performed using CO_2 to minimize the risk of tension pneumothorax or pneumoperitoneum.

Finally, type 3 perforations originate while cannulating the bile and pancreatic duct. They usually involve guidewire perforations through a side branch of the pancreatic duct or hepatic capsule (**Fig. 3**). The former leak tends to be a controlled, retroperitoneal perforation, but recognizing the leak quickly and placing plastic stents, allowing appropriate drainage from the area of perforation, are important. Imaging demonstrates a blush of contrast outside a side branch. If contrast is not used, it can be difficult to recognize this complication; thus, it is important to understand the general path of the main pancreatic duct and biliary intrahepatic ducts and to be wary of resistance. It is important to monitor the guidewire frequently and only advance the wire under fluoroscopic guidance. Management of type 3 perforations is usually conservative because they tend to respond well to intraductal stent drainage and antibiotics.[48] Further, an abdominal computed tomography is usually required to assess the degree of fluid collection and inflammation.

Regardless of the type of perforation, early recognition is important. One review found that only 27% of duodenal perforations were discovered during ERCP.[3] The endoscopist must also be aware of the risk factors for this complication, which include sphincterotomy (OR 9.0), biliary stricture dilation (OR 7.2), a dilated common bile duct (OR 4.07), and SOD (OR 3.8). Historically, approximately 20% of perforations have required surgery, with more needed in type 1 perforations. There are multiple management algorithms available; however, in summary, if peritoneal signs are present, then a surgical approach is often required. Aggressive drainage (nasogastric tubes, nasobiliary tubes, or pancreaticobiliary stents) coupled with broad-spectrum antibiotics may be adequate to avoid surgery and prevent retroperitoneal and intraperitoneal contamination with gastric or pancreaticobiliary secretions. If the appropriate expertise and equipment are available, the addition of endoscopic closure has been shown to preclude surgical intervention effectively.

BLEEDING

Bleeding complications are usually related to sphincterotomy. Not all bleeding seen endoscopically is considered clinically significant or an adverse event, although attempts have been made to more clearly define clinically significant bleeding with the timing and severity of bleeding as defining features. The incidence of bleeding is about 1%, with most cases classified as mild.[49] However, because of the lack of a standard definition of bleeding, the rates vary depending on the source. Oozing immediately after an intervention is not considered clinically significant. Thus, a certain amount of elapsed time is required to consider the bleeding significant. Immediate

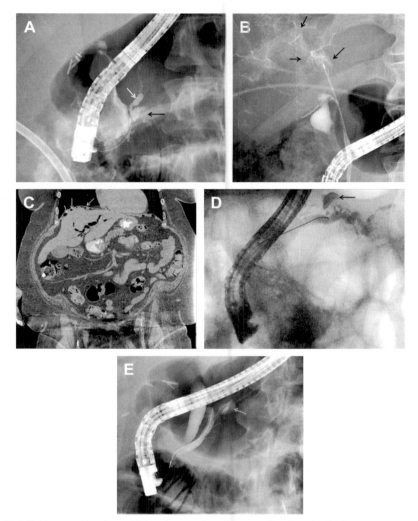

Fig. 3. (A) Pancreatic duct (PD) wire perforation at the head of the pancreas. Note extravasation (*lower arrow*) from the PD (*upper arrow*). There is a collection of contrast also within the duodenal lumen left of the PD. (B) Ei e duct wire perforation. Irregular contrast extravasation at the area of the bifurcation (*see arrows*). (C) Follow-up computed tomographic coronal images of a guidewire perforation of the bile duct. Free air under the diaphragm (*arrows*). Pneumobilia is also noted. (D) Pancreatic duct (body) guidewire perforation. Guidewire in a dilated pancreatic duc. Arrow points to contrast extravasation from a side branch. (E) Pancreatic duct guidewire perforation. Guidewire in the pancreatic duct. There is contrast extravasation from a side branch of the pancreatic duct (*see arrows*).

bleeding is defined as continued bleeding 2 to 3 minutes after the initial sphincterotomy. Delayed bleeding is defined as occurring after the completion of ERCP, which can happen hours or up to several weeks after the procedure. The severity of bleeding is based on the drop of hemoglobin and the need for transfusions (**Table 4**).

Being aware of the risk factors that predispose patients for bleeding allows possible risk reduction measures to be taken before the procedure and alerts the operator for

Table 4
Risk factors for hemorrhage after endoscopic sphincterotomy in multivariate analysis

Definite	Maybe	No
Coagulopathy	Cirrhosis	Aspirin or NSAIDs
Anticoagulation <3 d after ERCP	Dilated common bile duct	Ampullary tumor
Cholangitis before ERCP	Common bile duct stone	Longer sphincterotomy
Bleeding during sphincterotomy	Periampullary diverticulum	Extension of previous sphincterotomy
Lower ERCP case volume	Precut sphincterotomy	

Adapted from Freeman ML. Adverse outcomes of ERCP. Gastrointest Endosc 2002;56:S273–82; and Howard TJ, Tan T, Lehman GA, et al. Classification and management of perforations complicating endoscopic sphincterotomy. Surgery 1999;126(4):658–63; with permission. *Data from* Freeman ML. Adverse outcomes of ERCP. Gastrointest Endosc 2002;56:S273–82; and Howard TJ, Tan T, Lehman GA, et al. Classification and management of perforations complicating endoscopic sphincterotomy. Surgery 1999;126(4):658–63.

the potential of complications. Through multivariate analysis, Freeman[50] has developed criteria labeled as "definite," "maybe," and "no" (**Table 5**). Patients with any underlying coagulopathy, patients with ongoing cholangitis, or patients who have started anticoagulation therapy fewer than 3 days before sphincterotomy have a definite risk of procedural or postprocedural hemorrhage. Definite risks have also been noted if there is bleeding during sphincterotomy and if the endoscopist has lower ERCP case volume. Other potential risk factors include cirrhosis, dilated common bile duct, common bile duct stone, periampullary diverticulum, and precut sphincterotomy. Aspirin and NSAID use, along with longer sphincterotomy and extension of previous sphincterotomy, have not shown any definitive risk (see **Table 4**). Using aspirin, NSAIDs, and other platelet inhibitors in the setting of high-risk endoscopies has been greatly debated and is covered in detail in guidelines published by the American Society for Gastrointestinal Endoscopy.

Intraprocedurally, the use of pure-cut cautery has been shown to increase the risk of bleeding. Blended current reduces the bleeding risk, but as mentioned before, will increase the risk for PEP.[50] It is common practice to use pure-cut cautery when performing pancreatic duct sphincterotomy and using blended currents for biliary sphincterotomies. However, the risk of bleeding is greatly reduced by avoiding sphincterotomy altogether. Balloon sphincteroplasty is an alternative to sphincterotomy, but it is variably associated with a higher risk for PEP.

When bleeding does occur (**Fig. 4**A, B), most cases will resolve spontaneously, but it is important to monitor the site. For continued bleeding, the same modalities available

Table 5
Grading system for post-ERCP bleeding

Mild	Moderate	Severe
Clinical bleeding (ie, hemoglobin drop <3 g, and no need for transfusion)	Transfusion of 4 units or less and no angiographic or surgical intervention	Transfusions of 5 units or more, or intervention (angiographic or surgical)

Data from Cotton PB, Lehman G, Vennes J, et al. Endoscopic sphincterotomy complications and their management: an attempt at consensus. Gastrointest Endosc 1991;37:383–93; and Kapral C, Duller C, Wewalka F, et al. Case volume and outcome of endoscopic retrograde cholangiopancreatography: results of a nationwide Austrian benchmarking project. Endoscopy 2008;40(8):625–30.

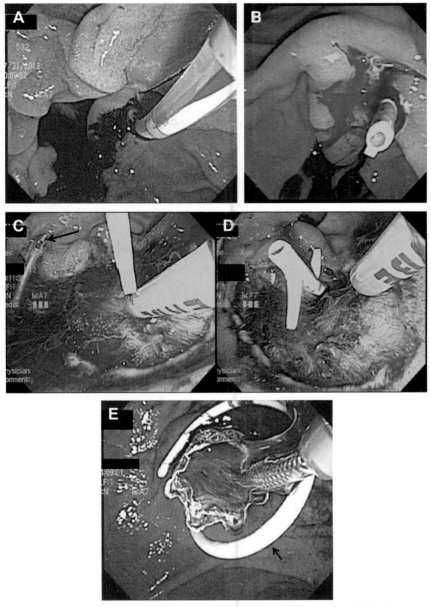

Fig. 4. (*A*) Postsphincterotomy bleed of the major papilla. (*B*) Continued bleeding despite plastic stent in place. Plastic stents have the potential to create a tamponade effect for postsphincterotomy bleeding. In this situation, bleeding did not cease with stent placement. (*C, D*) Argon plasma coagulation of postsphincterotomy bleeding site. Continued bleeding despite clip placement (*arrow*). Note that PD has been stented to prevent injury to the pancreatic orifice. (*E*) SEMS placement for control of postsphincterotomy bleeding. Note a prophylactic, pancreatic, pigtail stent in place (*arrow*).

for other upper gastrointestinal bleeding sources can be applied. With delayed bleeding, repeat endoscopic evaluation is recommended before using other modalities such as angiographic embolization, which is effective for refractory bleeding.

Epinephrine injection is the most common approach and has shown good efficacy for hemostasis in multiple studies. A recent study showed equal efficacy of epinephrine monotherapy compared with the combination of epinephrine and thermal therapy, with rates of success of 96.2% and 100%, respectively. Moreover, there were similar rates of recurrent hemorrhage (16% vs 12.1%) and other procedural complications (1 case of pancreatitis in the combination group).[51] Varying amounts are injected at a targeted site or in the apex of the sphincterotomy site if bleeding obscures visualization. With standard sclerotherapy needles, it is important to advance the sheath out of the channel and advance the needle with the elevator relaxed.

Thermal coaptive coagulation can be performed with either multipolar probes or heater probes. Larger diameter probes have been shown to have better coagulative efficacy, but this must be balanced against their increased stiffness and decreased maneuverability. The endoscopist must also avoid the pancreatic orifice because inadvertent cauterization can cause PEP. Argon plasma coagulation has been used with some success, but the endoscopist must consider that the path of the energy delivered is not always predictable. Thus, thermal treatment can potentially cause damage to the pancreatic orifice. The cutting wire of the sphincterotome using coagulation settings can also be used to apply thermal therapy to bleedings sites.

Metallic clips have also been used, but care is required to make sure the clips are not prematurely deployed, because the elevator's action can prematurely deliver the clip (see **Fig. 4**C, D).

As in sphincterotomy perforation, SEMS have been used with success as a rescue technique if other methods have failed (see **Fig. 4**E). Expanding a 10-mm-diameter stent creates a tamponade effect at the area of bleeding.[52,53]

CARDIOPULMONARY COMPLICATIONS AND SEDATION

Often underemphasized, cardiopulmonary concerns are a common and potentially devastating complication of ERCP and are often associated with sedation. Complications include myocardial infarctions, strokes, respiratory failure, other thromboembolic events, as well as other analgesia-related complications. According to 1 study, the aforementioned events occur in as many as 5% of all ERCP procedures.[54] A meta-analysis of prospective studies showed the rate to be 1.33% for "cardiovascular and/or analgesia-related complications,"[55] which is also in line with an Austrian study using their country's centralized database for ERCP benchmarking. This study showed a cardiopulmonary rate of complication of 0.9%.[56] Interestingly, only 3.2% of patients had general anesthesia and propofol was rarely used in the Austrian study. The details of sedation were not given in the other studies.

It has become more common over the past decade to use propofol for ERCP sedation.[57,58] A recent Cochrane database systematic review compared cardiopulmonary complications among patients who received conscious sedation with those among patients who received propofol and found no significant difference. There was, however, a possible trend toward higher ERCP rates of completion and faster and better recovery in patients with propofol sedation, which led to the author's conclusion that propofol is the generally preferred method of sedation.[57]

Aspiration is a general concern in patients undergoing any type of sedation. However, patients undergoing ERCP may be at higher risk for 2 reasons. First, because of the discomfort of a larger diameter scope in the oropharynx and longer procedure time, patients normally require deeper sedation than they do for upper endoscopies and colonoscopies. Second, the population of patients undergoing ERCP may be predisposed by their condition. Patients with malignant obstructions of the biliary tree may be at risk or already have concomitant gastric outlet obstruction and are at risk for retention of gastric contents and thus an increased risk for aspiration. Appropriate risk assessment should be performed and a decision about the use of endotracheal intubation and general anesthesia for patients in this population should be made.

CHOLANGITIS/CHOLECYSTITIS

Cholangitis and cholecystitis are potential complications that are usually caused by introducing gut flora into the biliary system without subsequent draining or clearing. Thus, a risk factor for these complications is failed or incomplete drainage. If cannulation of the biliary system is achieved but there is not complete resolution of the biliary blockage, then prophylactic, broad-spectrum antibiotics with gram-negative coverage are usually started during the procedure and continued for 3 to 5 days. It is important to assess the success of drainage by monitoring the clearance of contrast fluoroscopically through the bile ducts. Antibiotics are not recommended for procedures with successful drainage in patients without antecedent cholangitis. Less commonly, insertion of a covered SEMS, which may occlude the cystic duct, has been associated with cholecystitis.[18]

SUMMARY

ERCP is a therapeutic procedure that should rarely be used as an initial diagnostic tool because of its invasive nature and risk for complications. Avoiding unnecessary ERCP is the first step in risk management. When ERCP is appropriate, the goals and risk of the procedure should be discussed clearly with the patient. The endoscopist's experience plays a large role in procedural risk and thus it is recommended that individuals performing ERCPs have consistently adequate volume to maintain the appropriate skills.

There are many factors before and during the procedure that can help the endoscopist assess the patient's risk of developing complications. Thus, it is important to be aware of these risks and attempt to moderate them. For example, when a young woman is being evaluated for SOD, it is prudent to administer rectal indomethacin and place a plastic pancreatic duct stent.

Early recognition is the key in managing perforations, because most can be managed conservatively if detected quickly. Significant bleeding during the procedure can be successfully managed with standard endoscopic therapies, despite the added difficulty in manipulating these devices over the elevator of the scope.

As important as recognizing and mitigating risk factors and knowing the appropriate management for adverse events, the ability to perform the interventions effectively, if the need arises, is equally important. The endoscopist must be prepared to place a pancreatic stent in high-risk cases, which may account for up to one-third of all cases, depending on the patient and procedure. For patients at high risk of bleeding, the endoscopist should be comfortable using all the available hemostatic devices through the duodenoscope. ERCP is a therapeutic procedure with higher risk than other gastrointestinal endoscopic procedures, but most risks can be anticipated and appropriate steps can be taken to reduce the risks and control the adverse events as they arise.

REFERENCES

1. Ginsberg GG. Risk of colonoscopy and polypectomy. Tech Gastrointest Endosc 2008;10:7–13.
2. Panteris V, Haringsma J, Kuipers EJ. Colonoscopy perforation rate, mechanisms and outcome: from diagnostic to therapeutic colonoscopy. Endoscopy 2009; 41(11):941–51.
3. Enns R, Eloubeidi MA, Mergener K, et al. ERCP-related perforations: risk factors and management. Endoscopy 2002;34(4):293–8.
4. Freeman ML. Complications of endoscopic retrograde cholangiopancreatography: avoidance and management. Gastrointest Endosc Clin N Am 2012;22(3): 567–86.
5. Maple JT, Ben-Menachem T, Anderson MA, et al. The role of endoscopy in the evaluation of suspected choledocholithiasis. Gastrointest Endosc 2010;71(1):1–9.
6. Available at: www.thejag.org.uk. Accessed September 15, 2012.
7. Jowell PS, Baillie J, Branch MS, et al. Quantitative assessment of procedural competence. A prospective study of training in endoscopic retrograde cholangiopancreatography. Ann Intern Med 1996;125(12):983–9.
8. Cotton PB, Garrow DA, Gallagher J, et al. Risk factors for complications after ERCP: a multivariate analysis of 11,497 procedures over 12 years. Gastrointest Endosc 2009;70(1):80–8.
9. Moffatt DC, Cote GA, Avula H, et al. Risk factors for ERCP-related complications in patients with pancreas divisum: a retrospective study. Gastrointest Endosc 2011;73(5):963–70.
10. Banerjee N, Hilden K, Baron TH, et al. Endoscopic biliary sphincterotomy is not required for transpapillary SEMS placement for biliary obstruction. Dig Dis Sci 2011;56(2):591–5.
11. Gong B, Hao L, Bie L, et al. Does precut technique improve selective bile duct cannulation or increase post-ERCP pancreatitis rate? A meta-analysis of randomized controlled trials. Surg Endosc 2010;24(11):2670–80.
12. Cennamo V, Fuccio L, Zagari RM, et al. Can early precut implementation reduce endoscopic retrograde cholangiopancreatography-related complication risk? Meta-analysis of randomized controlled trials. Endoscopy 2010;42(5):381–8.
13. Testoni PA, Giussani A, Vailati C, et al. Precut sphincterotomy, repeated cannulation and post-ERCP pancreatitis in patients with bile duct stone disease. Dig Liver Dis 2011;43(10):792–6.
14. Mariani A, Giussani A, Di Leo M, et al. Guidewire biliary cannulation does not reduce post-ERCP pancreatitis compared with the contrast injection technique in low-risk and high-risk patients. Gastrointest Endosc 2012;75(2):339–46.
15. Cheung J, Tsoi KK, Quan WL, et al. Guidewire versus conventional contrast cannulation of the common bile duct for the prevention of post-ERCP pancreatitis: a systematic review and meta-analysis. Gastrointest Endosc 2009;70(6):1211–9.
16. Sofuni A, Maguchi H, Mukai T, et al. Endoscopic pancreatic duct stents reduce the incidence of post-endoscopic retrograde cholangiopancreatography pancreatitis in high-risk patients. Clin Gastroenterol Hepatol 2011;9(10):851–8 [quiz: e110].
17. Cote GA, Kumar N, Ansstas M, et al. Risk of post-ERCP pancreatitis with placement of self-expandable metallic stents. Gastrointest Endosc 2010;72(4):748–54.
18. Isayama H, Komatsu Y, Tsujino T, et al. A prospective randomised study of "covered" versus "uncovered" diamond stents for the management of distal malignant biliary obstruction. Gut 2004;53(5):729–34.

19. Moss AC, Morris E, Mac Mathuna P. Palliative biliary stents for obstructing pancreatic carcinoma. Cochrane Database Syst Rev 2006;(2):CD004200.
20. Schmassmann A, von Gunten E, Knuchel J, et al. Wallstents versus plastic stents in malignant biliary obstruction: effects of stent patency of the first and second stent on patient compliance and survival. Am J Gastroenterol 1996; 91(4):654–9.
21. Yoon WJ, Lee JK, Lee KH, et al. A comparison of covered and uncovered Wallstents for the management of distal malignant biliary obstruction. Gastrointest Endosc 2006;63(7):996–1000.
22. Meister T, Heinzow H, Heinecke A, et al. Post-ERCP pancreatitis in 2364 ERCP procedures: is intraductal ultrasonography another risk factor? Endoscopy 2011;43(4):331–6.
23. Choudhary A, Bechtold ML, Arif M, et al. Pancreatic stents for prophylaxis against post-ERCP pancreatitis: a meta-analysis and systematic review. Gastrointest Endosc 2011;73(2):275–82.
24. Mazaki T, Masuda H, Takayama T. Prophylactic pancreatic stent placement and post-ERCP pancreatitis: a systematic review and meta-analysis. Endoscopy 2010;42(10):842–53.
25. Cote GA, Keswani RN, Jackson T, et al. Individual and practice differences among physicians who perform ERCP at varying frequency: a national survey. Gastrointest Endosc 2011;74(1):65–73.e12.
26. Makela A, Kuusi T, Schroder T. Inhibition of serum phospholipase-A2 in acute pancreatitis by pharmacological agents in vitro. Scand J Clin Lab Invest 1997; 57(5):401–7.
27. Wildenhain PM, Melhem MF, Birsic WI, et al. Acute hemorrhagic pancreatitis in mice: improved survival after indomethacin administration. Digestion 1989; 44(1):41–51.
28. Murray B, Carter R, Imrie C, et al. Diclofenac reduces the incidence of acute pancreatitis after endoscopic retrograde cholangiopancreatography. Gastroenterology 2003;124(7):1786–91.
29. Montano Loza A, Garcia Correa J, Gonzalez Ojeda A, et al. Prevention of hyperamilasemia and pancreatitis after endoscopic retrograde cholangiopancreatography with rectal administration of indomethacin. Rev Gastroenterol Mex 2006; 71(3):262–8 [in Spanish].
30. Montano Loza A, Rodriguez Lomeli X, Garcia Correa JE, et al. Effect of the administration of rectal indomethacin on amylase serum levels after endoscopic retrograde cholangiopancreatography, and its impact on the development of secondary pancreatitis episodes. Rev Esp Enferm Dig 2007;99(6):330–6 [in Spanish].
31. Sotoudehmanesh R, Khatibian M, Kolahdoozan S, et al. Indomethacin may reduce the incidence and severity of acute pancreatitis after ERCP. Am J Gastroenterol 2007;102(5):978–83.
32. Elmunzer BJ, Scheiman JM, Lehman GA, et al. A randomized trial of rectal indomethacin to prevent post-ERCP pancreatitis. N Engl J Med 2012;366(15): 1414–22.
33. Feurer ME, Adler DG. Post-ERCP pancreatitis: review of current preventive strategies. Curr Opin Gastroenterol 2012;28(3):280–6.
34. Chen B, Fan T, Wang CH. A meta-analysis for the effect of prophylactic GTN on the incidence of post-ERCP pancreatitis and on the successful rate of cannulation of bile ducts. BMC Gastroenterol 2010;10:85.
35. Shao LM, Chen QY, Chen MY, et al. Nitroglycerin in the prevention of post-ERCP pancreatitis: a meta-analysis. Dig Dis Sci 2010;55(1):1–7.

36. Seta T, Noguchi Y. Protease inhibitors for preventing complications associated with ERCP: an updated meta-analysis. Gastrointest Endosc 2011;73(4):700–6.

37. Yoo YW, Cha SW, Kim A, et al. The use of gabexate mesylate and ulinastatin for the prevention of post-endoscopic retrograde cholangiopancreatography pancreatitis. Gut Liver 2012;6(2):256–61.

38. Yoo KS, Huh KR, Kim YJ, et al. Nafamostat mesilate for prevention of post-endoscopic retrograde cholangiopancreatography pancreatitis: a prospective, randomized, double-blind, controlled trial. Pancreas 2011;40(2):181–6.

39. Jowell PS, Branch MS, Fein SH, et al. Intravenous synthetic secretin reduces the incidence of pancreatitis induced by endoscopic retrograde cholangiopancreatography. Pancreas 2011;40(4):533–9.

40. Andriulli A, Leandro G, Federici T, et al. Prophylactic administration of somatostatin or gabexate does not prevent pancreatitis after ERCP: an updated meta-analysis. Gastrointest Endosc 2007;65(4):624–32.

41. Bai Y, Gao J, Shi X, et al. Prophylactic corticosteroids do not prevent post-ERCP pancreatitis: a meta-analysis of randomized controlled trials. Pancreatology 2008;8(4–5):504–9.

42. Bai Y, Gao J, Zou DW, et al. Prophylactic octreotide administration does not prevent post-endoscopic retrograde cholangiopancreatography pancreatitis: a meta-analysis of randomized controlled trials. Pancreas 2008;37(3):241–6.

43. Li S, Cao G, Chen X, et al. Low-dose heparin in the prevention of post endoscopic retrograde cholangiopancreatography pancreatitis: a systematic review and meta-analysis. Eur J Gastroenterol Hepatol 2012;24(5):477–81.

44. Pande H, Thuluvath P. Pharmacological prevention of post-endoscopic retrograde cholangiopancreatography pancreatitis. Drugs 2003;63(17):1799–812.

45. Vezakis A, Fragulidis G, Nastos C, et al. Closure of a persistent sphincterotomy-related duodenal perforation by placement of a covered self-expandable metallic biliary stent. World J Gastroenterol 2011;17(40):4539–41.

46. Canena J, Liberato M, Horta D, et al. Short-term stenting using fully covered self-expandable metal stents for treatment of refractory biliary leaks, postsphincterotomy bleeding, and perforations. Surg Endosc 2013;27(1):313–24.

47. Gubler C, Bauerfeind P. Endoscopic closure of iatrogenic gastrointestinal tract perforations with the over-the-scope clip. Digestion 2012;85(4):302–7.

48. Howard TJ, Tan T, Lehman GA, et al. Classification and management of perforations complicating endoscopic sphincterotomy. Surgery 1999;126(4):658–63 [discussion: 664–55].

49. Anderson MA, Fisher L, Jain R, et al. Complications of ERCP. Gastrointest Endosc 2012;75(3):467–73.

50. Freeman ML. Adverse outcomes of ERCP. Gastrointest Endosc 2002;56(6 Suppl): S273–82.

51. Tsou YK, Lin CH, Liu NJ, et al. Treating delayed endoscopic sphincterotomy-induced bleeding: epinephrine injection with or without thermotherapy. World J Gastroenterol 2009;15(38):4823–8.

52. Shah JN, Marson F, Binmoeller KF. Temporary self-expandable metal stent placement for treatment of post-sphincterotomy bleeding. Gastrointest Endosc 2010; 72(6):1274–8.

53. Itoi T, Yasuda I, Doi S, et al. Endoscopic hemostasis using covered metallic stent placement for uncontrolled post-endoscopic sphincterotomy bleeding. Endoscopy 2011;43(4):369–72.

54. Christensen M, Matzen P, Schulze S, et al. Complications of ERCP: a prospective study. Gastrointest Endosc 2004;60(5):721–31.

55. Andriulli A, Loperfido S, Napolitano G, et al. Incidence rates of post-ERCP complications: a systematic survey of prospective studies. Am J Gastroenterol 2007;102(8):1781–8.
56. Kapral C, Duller C, Wewalka F, et al. Case volume and outcome of endoscopic retrograde cholangiopancreatography: results of a nationwide Austrian benchmarking project. Endoscopy 2008;40(8):625–30.
57. Garewal D, Powell S, Milan SJ, et al. Sedative techniques for endoscopic retrograde cholangiopancreatography. Cochrane Database Syst Rev 2012;(6):CD007274.
58. Cotton PB, Lehman G, Vennes J, et al. Endoscopic sphincterotomy complications and their management: an attempt at consensus. Gastrointest Endosc 1991; 37(3):383–93.

Endoscopic Approach to the Patient with Motility Disorders of the Bile Duct and Sphincter of Oddi

Wesley D. Leung, MD, Stuart Sherman, MD*

KEYWORDS

- Sphincter of Oddi dysfunction • Manometry • Sphincterotomy • Sphincteroplasty
- Recurrent pancreatitis

KEY POINTS

- Sphincter of Oddi dysfunction (SOD) is a clinical syndrome with variable presentation that is characterized by pancreatobiliary pain and biochemical and radiographic abnormalities.
- The optimal method to diagnose SOD in symptomatic type II and III patients is manometry.
- Manometry should be conducted using standardized techniques.
- Therapeutic options for SOD include medical, surgical, and endoscopic modalities.
- If an endoscopic approach is chosen for suspected SOD, patients should be informed of the risk/benefit ratio, and the endoscopist should minimize the risk of complications.

DEFINITION

Sphincter of Oddi dysfunction (SOD) refers to a clinical syndrome that occurs because of abnormal sphincter of Oddi (SO) contractility. As a result, flow of biliary or pancreatic juice is obstructed through a dyskinetic or stenotic SO. Pancreatobiliary pain, pancreatitis, abnormal liver function tests, or abnormal pancreatic enzymes are common characteristics of SOD. SO dyskinesia refers to a motor abnormality that is more commonly caused by a hypertonic than a hypotonic sphincter. In contrast, SO stenosis is a structural abnormality, probably from inflammation and subsequent fibrosis. These abnormalities are clinically indistinguishable and are grouped together as SOD. The Hogan-Geenen SOD classification system was designed to classify

Disclosures: None.
Division of Gastroenterology/Hepatology, Indiana University Medical Center, 550 North University Boulevard, Suite 4100, Indianapolis, IN 46202, USA
* Corresponding author.
E-mail address: ssherman@iupui.edu

Gastrointest Endoscopy Clin N Am 23 (2013) 405–434
http://dx.doi.org/10.1016/j.giec.2012.12.006
1052-5157/13/$ – see front matter © 2013 Elsevier Inc. All rights reserved.

giendo.theclinics.com

biliary-type pain (**Table 1**). A pancreatic classification system has also been developed, but is less commonly used (**Box 1**). Both systems have been modified since their initial design, because the measurements of biliary and pancreatic drainage times, which were originally criteria, have generally been abandoned. A variety of less accurate terms, such as papillary stenosis, biliary dyskinesia, and postcholecystectomy syndrome, are listed in the literature to describe this entity. However, postcholecystectomy syndrome is a misnomer, because SOD may occur with the gallbladder in situ.[1]

ANATOMY

The SO is a complex of smooth muscles approximately 4 to 10 mm in length that surrounds the terminal common bile duct, main (ventral) pancreatic duct (of Wirsung), and common channel (ampulla of Vater) (**Fig. 1**). The basal pressure of the SO regulates the flow of bile and pancreatic exocrine juice into the duodenum, and the phasic contractions prevent duodenal content reflux, maintaining a sterile intraductal milieu. Phasic wave activity of the sphincter is closely tied to the migrating motor complex of the duodenum. Innervation of the bile duct does not seem to be essential, because sphincter function has been reported to be preserved after liver transplantation.[2] Control of SO motility is complex and involves both hormonal and neural pathways. Cholecystokinin (CCK) and secretin seem to be the most important hormones involved in sphincter relaxation. Nonadrenergic, noncholinergic neurons,

Table 1
Hogan-Geenen biliary SO classification system (postcholecystectomy) related to the frequency of abnormal SO manometry and pain relief by biliary sphincterotomy

Patient Group Classifications	Approximate Frequency of Abnormal Sphincter Manometry (%)	Probability of Pain Relief by Sphincterotomy if Manometry (%)		Manometery Before Sphincter Ablation
		Abnormal	Normal	
Biliary Type I				
Patients with biliary-type pain, abnormal AST or alkaline phosphatase >2 times normal documented on 2 or more occasions, delayed drainage of ERCP contrast agent from the biliary tree >45 min, and dilated CBD >12 mm diameter	75–95	90–95	90–95	Unnecessary
Biliary Type II				
Patients with biliary-type pain and only 1 or 2 of the previous criteria	55–65	85	35	Highly recommended
Biliary Type III				
Patients with only biliary-type pain and none of the 3 previous criteria	25–60	55–65	<10	Mandatory

Abbreviations: AST, aspartate aminotransferase; CBD, common bile duct; ERCP, endoscopic retrograde cholangiopancreatography.

> **Box 1**
> **Pancreatic SO classification system: patient group classification**
>
> *Pancreatic Type I*
>
> Patients with pancreatic-type pain, abnormal amylase or lipase 1.5 times normal on any occasion, delayed drainage of endoscopic retrograde cholangiopancreatography (ERCP) contrast agent from the pancreatic duct greater than 9 minutes, and dilated pancreatic duct greater than 6 mm diameter in the head or 5 mm in the body
>
> *Pancreatic Type II*
>
> Patients with pancreatic-type pain but only 1 or 2 of criteria for type I
>
> *Pancreatic Type III*
>
> Patients with pancreatic-type pain only and no other abnormalities

which at least partially transmit vasoactive intestinal peptide and nitric oxide, also relax the sphincter.[3] The mechanism by which cholecystectomy alters these neural pathways is unclear. Luman and colleagues[4] reported that cholecystectomy, at least in the short-term, suppresses the normal inhibitory effect of pharmacologic doses of CCK on the SO.

The pathophysiology of SOD is also unclear. Processes such as pancreatitis, gallstone passage, intraoperative trauma, infection (ie, cytomegalovirus or *Cryptosporidium*) and adenomyosis may result in SO stenosis. Wedge specimens of the SO obtained at surgical sphincteroplasty from patients with SOD show evidence of

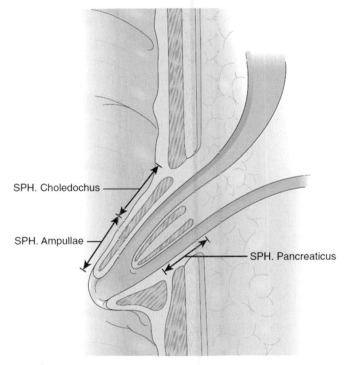

Fig. 1. Anatomy of SO.

inflammation, muscular hypertrophy, fibrosis, or adenomyosis within the papillary zone in approximately 60% of patients.[5] In the remaining 40% with normal histology, symptoms may be explained by SO dyskinesia. Functional intermittent biliary obstruction caused by SO dyskinesia is not well understood. SO dyskinesia may occur as a result of a dysregulated hormonal or neural mechanism that has not been elucidated, because SO motility is influenced by agents such as nitroglycerin.

Several theories potentially explain how SOD causes pain. The SO may impede flow of bile and pancreatic juice, resulting in ductal hypertension. Alternatively, spastic contractions of the SO may induce ischemia. Patients may also be hypersensitive to SO contractions. Patients with SOD have been shown to have lower perception thresholds in the referred pain area. Therefore, visceral and referred hyperalgesia may be important features in the pathogenesis of pain in patients with SOD.[6]

In addition, there is evidence that SOD may cause acute pancreatitis. This theory was suggested in an animal model in which topical carbachol given to possums abolished transsphincteric flow. Carbachol also increased pancreatic exocrine secretion and pancreatic duct pressure to levels comparable with those seen in pancreatic duct ligation models, causing transient sphincter obstruction. Stimulating pancreatic secretion with CCK and secretin in addition to the carbachol caused pancreatic tissue damage and an increase in serum amylase levels.[7]

EPIDEMIOLOGY

SOD occurs in children or adults of any age; however, it typically affects middle-aged women.[8,9] SOD also is most common after cholecystectomy, but, as mentioned earlier, it may occur with the gallbladder in situ. Patients with SOD have an impaired quality of life, manifested by increased absenteeism from work, disability, health care use, and high levels of somatic complaints.[10,11]

SOD can involve abnormalities of the biliary sphincter, pancreatic sphincter, or both.[12,13] The prevalence of SOD is difficult to estimate because of different potential sources of bias: variable definitions of SOD, inconsistent patient selection criteria, different manometry systems, study of biliary or pancreatic sphincters, variable investigation of other causes of symptoms, and potential referral bias, because most studies were performed at tertiary medical centers.

In 1 series of 454 patients who had undergone cholecystectomy, the prevalence of SOD was estimated to be less than 1%.[14] However, among patients with symptoms after cholecystectomy, the prevalence was 14%. Sherman and colleagues[15] used SO manometry (SOM) to evaluate 115 patients with pancreaticobiliary pain. Patients with both normal and abnormal liver function tests were included, but patients with bile duct stones and tumors were excluded. Fifty-nine (51%) of 115 patients showed abnormal basal SO pressure, which is typically defined as greater than 40 mm Hg. These patients were further categorized by the Hogan-Geenen SOD classification system into 3 types based on clinical presentation, laboratory results, imaging tests, and ERCP findings. Abnormal manometry was seen in at least 1 sphincter segment in 86%, 55%, and 28% for biliary type I, II, and III patients, respectively.

Abnormalities can be seen in the biliary sphincter, pancreatic sphincter, or both. Therefore, the frequency of SOD depends on whether 1 or both sphincters are studied. In a large series, Eversman and colleagues[12] performed manometry of the biliary and pancreatic sphincter segments in 360 patients with pancreatobiliary pain and intact sphincters. The overall frequency of SOD was 65%; 11% had abnormal biliary basal sphincter pressure alone, 19% had abnormal pancreatic sphincter basal sphincter pressure alone, and 31% had abnormal basal sphincter pressure in both segments. In 123 type II patients, SOD was diagnosed in 65%, with 11%, 22%, and 32% having increased basal sphincter pressure in the biliary, pancreatic, or both sphincter segments, respectively. In the 214 type III patients, overall frequency of SOD was 59%, with 11%, 17%, and 31% having increased basal sphincter pressure in the biliary, pancreatic, or both segments, respectively. Similar findings were reported by Aymerich and colleagues.[16] In a series of 73 patients with suspected SOD, basal pressures were normal in both segments in 19%, abnormal in only 1 segment in 41%, and abnormal in both segments in 40%. Although SOM has traditionally been believed to be reproducible,[17] 2 recent studies have shown abnormal sphincter pressures in 42% and 60% in symptomatic patients restudied about 1 year after a normal study.[18,19]

Pancreatic SOD is one of the most common diagnoses in patients with unexplained acute recurrent pancreatitis. Manometrically documented SOD has been reported in 15% to 72% of patients with recurrent pancreatitis, previously labeled as idiopathic.[15,20,21] This subject is discussed later in this article.

CLINICAL MANIFESTATIONS OF SOD

Abdominal pain is the most common presenting symptom for patients with SOD. The pain, which is usually epigastric or right upper quadrant, may be disabling and lasts for 30 minutes to hours. The pain often recurs at different time intervals, but in some people, it may be continuous, with episodic flares. Pain may radiate to the back or shoulder and be accompanied by nausea and vomiting. Food or narcotics may precipitate the pain. The pain may awaken the patient from sleep, interrupt a patient's daily activities, or lead to an emergency room visit. The pain is not relieved by bowel movements, postural changes, or trial medications for acid suppression or irritable bowel syndrome.

The pain may begin several years after a cholecystectomy has been performed for a gallbladder dysmotility or stone disease and is similar in character to the pain leading to the cholecystectomy. Alternatively, patients may have continuous pain that was not relieved by a cholecystectomy.

Jaundice, fever, and chills are rarely observed. Physical examination is typically characterized only by mild epigastric or right upper quadrant tenderness. Laboratory abnormalities consisting of transient increase of liver function tests, typically during episodes of pain, are present in less than 50% of patients. Other patients with SOD may present with typical pancreatic pain (epigastric or left upper quadrant radiating to the back) with or without pancreatic enzyme increase and recurrent pancreatitis. The pain is often indistinguishable from biliary pain.[22] As mentioned, SOD may exist in the presence of an intact gallbladder.[23–25] Because the symptoms of SOD and gallbladder dysfunction cannot be reliably separated, the diagnosis of SOD is commonly made after cholecystectomy or, less often, after gallbladder abnormalities have been excluded.[22]

A symposium on functional disorders of the pancreas and biliary tree established the Rome III diagnostic criteria[22] for SOD. Criteria include episodes of severe abdominal pain located in the epigastrum or right upper quadrant, and all of the following: (1) symptom episodes lasting 30 minutes or more with pain-free intervals, (2) recurrent symptoms occurring at different intervals (not daily), (3) pain that builds up to a steady level, (4) pain that is moderate or severe enough to interrupt the patient's daily activities or lead to an emergency department visit, (5) pain not relieved by bowel movements, (6) pain not relieved by postural change, (7) pain not relieved by antacids, (8) exclusion of other structural disease that would explain the symptoms. Supportive criteria are nausea and vomiting, pain radiating to the back or right subscapular region, and pain awakening the patient from sleep.

GENERAL INITIAL EVALUATION

For patients with suspected SOD, accurate diagnosis depends on a thorough history and exclusion of structural abnormalities. However, the clinical manifestations of SOD may not always be easily distinguishable from organic causes (eg, common bile duct stones) or other functional nonpancreaticobiliary disorders (eg, irritable bowel syndrome), and there may be considerable overlap between disorders. Evaluating patients with suspected SOD should begin with standard liver chemistries, serum amylase or lipase, and abdominal imaging (abdominal ultrasonography, magnetic resonance imaging/magnetic resonance cholangiopancreatography (MRCP), or computed tomography (CT) scan).

Tests of liver biochemistries and pancreatic enzymes should be obtained during bouts of pain, if possible. In SOD, mild increases (<2 times upper limits of normal) are frequent, whereas greater abnormalities are more suggestive of stones, tumors, and liver parenchymal disease. Evidence suggests that although the diagnostic sensitivity and specificity of abnormal serum liver chemistries are low,[1] the presence of abnormal liver tests in patients with type II biliary SOD may predict a favorable response to endoscopic sphincterotomy (ES).[26]

CT scans and abdominal ultrasonography usually have normal results, but occasionally a dilated bile duct or pancreatic duct may be found, particularly in patients with type I SOD. MRCP and endoscopic ultrasonography (EUS) are more commonly used to look for structural and parenchymal disease of the pancreas, pancreatic duct, and biliary tree. Standard evaluation and treatment of more common gastrointestinal (GI) conditions, such as peptic ulcer disease, irritable bowel syndrome, and gastroesophageal reflux, should be performed simultaneously. When mass lesions, stones, or response to medical therapy trials are absent, the suspicion of SOD is increased.

DIAGNOSTIC METHODS (NONINVASIVE)

Many consider SOM to be the gold standard for diagnosing SOD. However, SOM is invasive, difficult to perform, not widely available, and associated with relatively high morbidity; therefore, numerous noninvasive and provocative tests have been designed to diagnose SOD and predict response to sphincterotomy.

Morphine-Prostigmin Provocative Test (Nardi Test)

Morphine has been shown to stimulate SO contraction. A morphine-prostigmin challenge test involves administering 1 mg subcutaneous neostigmine (prostigmin), a vigorous cholinergic secretory stimulant, and 10 mg subcutaneous morphine. The reproduction of the patient's typical pain along with a 4-fold increase in liver or pancreatic enzymes is considered a positive response. Five studies have investigated the efficacy of this test. The usefulness of this test is limited by its low sensitivity and specificity in predicting the presence of SOD and its poor correlation with outcome after sphincter ablation.[27,28] This test has largely been replaced by tests believed to be more sensitive.

Radiographic Assessment of Bile and Pancreatic Duct Diameter After Secretory Stimulation

After a lipid-rich meal or CCK administration, the gallbladder contracts, bile flow from the hepatocytes increases, and the SO relaxes, resulting in bile entry into the duodenum. Similarly, after a lipid-rich meal or secretin administration, pancreatic exocrine juice flow is stimulated, and the SO relaxes. If the SO is dysfunctional and obstructs the flow, secretory pressure may trigger pain or cause dilation of the bile or pancreatic duct that can be seen on abdominal ultrasonography. Sphincter and terminal duct obstruction from other causes (stones, tumors, strictures) may similarly cause ductal dilation and, therefore, need to be excluded. Six studies that compared ultrasonography after secretory stimulation with SOM revealed sensitivities and specificities ranging from 21% to 88% and 82% to 100%, respectively. One study[29] reported symptom improvement with sphincterotomy in 29% of patients with a negative test, whereas another[30] reported that 87% (n = 13) patients had symptomatic improvement after sphincterotomy with an abnormal test. One limitation of this test is that overlying bowel gas may prevent the pancreatic duct from being visualized.

Despite the superiority of EUS in visualizing the pancreas, Catalano and colleagues[31] reported the sensitivity of secretin-stimulated EUS in detecting SOD to be only 57%, suggesting little value of EUS in diagnosing SOD. However, EUS may have a role in assessing alternative diagnoses, such as microlithiasis, and for assessing ampullary morphology.[32] EUS is superior to transcutaneous ultrasonography and similar in accuracy to MRCP in diagnosing causes of biliary obstruction,[33,34] but it is invasive and requires specialized equipment and expertise that are not widely available.

MRCP is commonly regarded as the best noninvasive test to evaluate for structural causes of pancreatobiliary symptoms. Four studies compared MRCP after secretin stimulation (ss-MRCP) with SOM for diagnosing SOD. One study showed that ss-MRCP results were no different in people with SOD compared with normal volunteers.[35] Pereira and colleagues[36] and Baillie and Kimberly[37] also found ss-MRCP to be insensitive in predicting abnormal manometry and to have low specificity. Testoni and colleagues,[38] investigating 37 patients with intact gallbladders and idiopathic pancreatitis, reported sensitivities and specificities of 57.1% and 100%, respectively, and disappointing clinical success of sphincter ablation. Aisen and colleagues[39] showed that the pancreatic duct diameter increased significantly after secretin injection, as monitored by MRCP, but the magnitude and duration of increase were similar for patients with normal and abnormal basal sphincter pressure.

Quantitative Hepatobiliary Scintigraphy

Hepatobiliary scintigraphy (HBS) assesses bile flow of a radionucleotide through the biliary tract. Bile flow can be impaired from sphincter disease, tumors, or stones (and parenchymal liver disease). The criteria of an abnormal study are controversial, but prolonged duodenal arrival time, prolonged hepatic hilum-to-duodenal transit time, and high Johns Hopkins scintigraphic score (JHSS) are the most widely used.[40,41]

Four studies[42–44] showed a correlation between HBS and SOM. However, these promising results have not been reproduced by others. Using SOM as the gold standard in 29 patients with suspected SOD, independent reviewers[45] found the JHSS to have a sensitivity of 25% to 38%, specificity of 85% to 90%, positive predictive value of 40% to 60%, and negative predictive value of 75% to 79%. Pineau and colleagues[46] performed CCK-stimulated HBS in 20 asymptomatic postcholecystectomy volunteers and calculated the JHSS. The investigators reported that 8 patients (specificity of 60%) had an abnormal study, which suggests that the test is of questionable value for excluding patients with suspected SOD.

In another study, the hilum-to-duodenal transit time had a sensitivity of 13%, specificity of 95%, positive predictive value of 50%, and negative predictive value of 74%.

The duodenal arrival time mirrored the hilum-to-duodenal transit time findings.[40] The value of adding morphine provocation to HBS was studied in 34 patients with a clinical diagnosis of type II and type III SOD.[44] Scintigraphy with and without morphine and subsequent biliary manometry were performed. The standard HBS scan did not distinguish between patients with normal and abnormal SOM. However, after provocation with morphine, there were significant differences in the time to maximal activity and the percentage of excretion at 45 minutes and 60 minutes. With a cutoff value of 15% excretion at 60 minutes, the use of morphine during HBS increased the sensitivity and specificity for SOD detection to 83% and 81%.[26]

The Milwaukee group[30] reported their retrospective review of fatty meal sonography and HBS as potential predictors of SOD. In this study, 304 postcholecystectomy patients suspected of having SOD were evaluated by SOM, fatty meal sonography, and HBS. A diagnosis of SOD was made in 73 patients (24%), using SOM as the reference standard. The sensitivity of fatty meal sonography and HBS were 21% and 49%, respectively, whereas specificities were 97% and 78%.

Most studies assessing the value of HBS compare it with SOM only for diagnosing SOD but do not assess whether HBS can select patients who are likely to respond to sphincterotomy. Roberts and colleagues[47] investigated 17 patients with suspected SOD; 9 were labeled type III. Among the 11 patients who had a positive HBS and underwent sphincterotomy, 10 patients had an improvement in symptoms.

In another study, Cicala and colleagues[48] compared HBS (hilum-to-duodenal transit time) with manometry for outcomes after sphincterotomy in 30 postcholecystectomy patients with type I and II SOD. Although HBS was not as sensitive as manometry in people with type II disease, it successfully predicted outcomes of sphincterotomy in 93% of patients, compared with 57% by manometry. However, in this study, 40% of the enrolled patients were men, which is unusually high in the SOD population, and the frequency of abnormal maximal basal sphincter pressures in biliary type II patients was exceedingly low (36%). If the investigators had used the mean basal sphincter pressure, the more commonly recommended manometric parameter for diagnosing SOD, the frequency of an abnormal SOM would likely have been even lower. These factors call into question the investigators' SOM technique and interpretation.

In the absence of more definitive data, we and others[46] conclude that the use of HBS as a screening tool for SOD should not be recommended for general clinical use. Abnormal results seem frequent in asymptomatic controls. Moreover, HBS does not address the pancreatic sphincter, which may be dysfunctional and responsible for patients' symptoms. However, in situations in which more manometry is unsuccessful or unavailable, HBS or other noninvasive methods may be appropriate.

DIAGNOSTIC METHODS (INVASIVE)

Because of the associated risks, invasive testing with ERCP and manometry should be reserved for patients with clinically significant or disabling symptoms, and in cases in which definitive therapy (sphincter ablation) is planned if an abnormal sphincter is found.

ERCP

Cholangiography can be obtained in a variety of ways. Noninvasive cholangiographic studies, such as MRCP, are very sensitive in assessing biliary obstructive processes, and direct cholangiography can be obtained by percutaneous and intraoperative methods, but is more conventionally obtained during ERCP.

Cholangiography is essential to rule out stones, tumors, or other obstructing processes of the biliary tree that may cause symptoms identical to those of SOD. When such lesions are ruled out by a good-quality cholangiographic study but ducts are dilated or slow to drain, obstruction at the level of the sphincter is suggested. Extrahepatic ducts with a diameter greater than 12 mm (postcholecystectomy) are considered dilated in ERCP, although some controversy exists. Definitive normal supine drainage times have not been well defined, but a postcholecystectomy biliary tree that fails to empty all contrast media by 45 minutes is generally considered abnormal.

Endoscopic evaluation of the papilla and peripapillary area can yield important information that can influence the diagnosis and treatment of patients with suspected SOD. For example, ampullary cancer may occasionally simulate SOD. If endoscopy is performed, the papilla should be biopsied, preferably after sphincterotomy, in suspicious cases.[49]

ERCP alone (without manometry) is not indicated in the evaluation of abdominal pain of obscure origin in the absence of objective findings that suggest a biliary or pancreas disease. It was shown in 1 study that ERCP without manometry led to a finding that affected treatment plan in less than 3% of 265 patients with pancreatobiliary pain and normal findings in liver function tests, serum amylase, upper GI tract evaluation, and abdominal ultrasound or CT scan.[50] Because of the high procedure-related complication rate in these patients, the investigators concluded that ERCP alone could not be justified, but when it is performed, it should be combined with SOM. These findings were corroborated in the National Institutes of Health State-of-the-Science Conference on ERCP.[51]

SOM

Manometry, the gold standard for diagnosis and prediction of response to sphincterotomy, is the only method that directly measures SO motor activity, and can be performed intraoperatively and percutaneously, but is most commonly performed during ERCP. However, it should be reserved for cases in which sphincterotomy for an abnormal sphincter is considered. Further, although not well studied, the results of SOM may predict outcome of sphincter ablation.

Indications for the use of SOM have also been developed according to the Hogan-Geenen SOD classification system. In type I patients, there is a general consensus that a structural disorder of the sphincter (ie, sphincter stenosis) exists. Some authorities do not advocate manometry in patients with type I SOD, citing high rates of improvement with sphincterotomy regardless of manometry findings. However, normal manometry has been encountered in up to 35% of patients with type I SOD.[15,44,52] Type II patients show SOD in 55% to 65% of cases. In these patients, SOM is highly recommended, because the results of the study predict outcome from sphincter ablation. Type III patients have pancreaticobiliary pain without other objective evidence of sphincter outflow obstruction.

Sedation

All drugs that relax (anticholinergics, nitrates, calcium channel blockers, glucagon) or stimulate (most narcotics, cholinergic agents) the sphincter should be avoided beginning at least 8 to 12 hours before and throughout SOM. Current data indicate that benzodiazepines, droperidol,[53] propofol,[54] and ketamine[55] do not affect sphincter pressure and are acceptable sedatives for SOM. Meperidine, at a dose of 1 mg/kg or less, does not affect the basal sphincter pressure but does alter phasic wave characteristics.[56] Because the basal sphincter pressure is generally the only manometric criterion used to diagnose SOD and determine therapy, it was suggested that meperidine could be used to facilitate conscious sedation for manometry. If glucagon must be used to achieve cannulation, an 8-minute to 15-minute waiting period is required to restore the sphincter to its basal condition.

Equipment

Various triple-lumen catheters are available from several manufacturers. Most standards have been established using 5-F catheters. Long intraductal tip catheters may help secure the catheter within the bile duct, but may hinder pancreatic manometry. Over-the-wire (monorail) catheters can be passed after first securing the position within the duct with a guidewire, but it is unclear whether these wires influence basal sphincter pressure. Some triple-lumen catheters accommodate a 0.46-mm to 0.53-mm (0.018-inch to 0.021-inch) diameter guidewire passed through the entire length of the catheter and can be used to facilitate cannulation or maintain position in the duct. However, in our published experience,[57] stiffer shafted nitinol core guidewires commonly increase basal sphincter pressure by 50% to 100% and should be avoided. To avoid artifacts, such wires need to be pulled back into the catheter during the recording period, or guidewires with a soft core need to be used. Using aspiration catheters with 1 recording port sacrificed to permit both end and side hole aspiration of intraductal juice is recommended (**Fig. 2**) for pancreatic sphincter manometry. Most centers prefer to perfuse the catheters at 0.25 mL/channel using a low-compliance pump. Lower perfusion rates give accurate basal sphincter pressures but do not give accurate phasic wave information. A new water-perfused sleeve system, similar to that used in the lower esophageal sphincter, awaits further study for use in the SO.[58] The perfusate is generally distilled water, although physiologic saline needs further evaluation. Saline may crystallize in the capillary tubing of perfusion pumps and must be flushed out often.

Technique

During endoscopy, the papilla and surrounding area should be examined. A cholangiogram and pancreatogram should be obtained to rule out structural abnormalities. SOM requires selective cannulation of the bile duct or pancreatic duct, which can be confirmed by aspirating on any port. The appearance of yellow fluid indicates entry

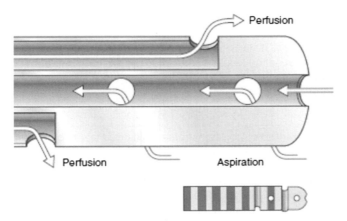

Fig. 2. Modified triple-lumen aspirating catheter.

into the bile duct, whereas clear fluid indicates entry into the pancreatic duct. Blaut and colleagues[59] showed that injection of contrast material into the biliary tree before SOM does not significantly alter characteristics of sphincter pressure. A similar study in the pancreatic duct has not been published. Extrahepatic ducts greater than 10 mm diameter postcholecystectomy on ultrasonography are considered dilated. Dilation of the pancreatic duct (>6 mm in the pancreatic head and >5 mm in the body) and delayed contrast agent drainage time (9 minutes in the prone position) may give indirect evidence for the presence of SOD.

To ensure accurate pressure readings, the endoscopist must ensure that the catheter is not impacted against the duct wall. The catheter is then withdrawn across the sphincter at 1-mm to 2-mm intervals by standard station pull-through technique. Good communication between endoscopist and manometrist is essential for optimal results. Alternatively, electronic manometry systems with a television screen mounted near the endoscopic image screen permit the endoscopist to view the manometry tracing during endoscopy.

Abnormalities of the basal sphincter pressure ideally should be observed for at least 30 seconds in each lead and be seen on 2 or more separate pull-throughs, but practically, 1 pull-through from each duct is generally sufficient if the readings are clearly normal or abnormal.

Ideally, both the pancreatic and the bile ducts should be studied. Sphincter dysfunction may be limited to only 1 of the sphincters in 35% to 65% of patients with abnormal SOM.[12,16,60–62] Raddawi and colleagues[62] reported that an abnormal basal sphincter was more likely to be confined to the pancreatic duct segment in patients with pancreatitis and to the bile duct segment in patients with biliary-type pain and increased liver function tests.

After the baseline study is performed, provocative agents (ie, CCK) to relax or stimulate the sphincter can be given, and manometric or pain response can be monitored. However, the value of these provocative maneuvers for everyday use needs further study.

Interpretation of SOM

The interpretation of SOM tracings has been standardized but there are some areas of disagreement between centers: the required duration of basal SO pressure increase, the number of leads in which basal pressure increase is required, and the role of averaging pressures from the 3 (or 2 in an aspirating catheter) recording ports.[63] Our recommended method for reading the manometry tracings is first to define the zero duodenal baseline before and after the pull-through. Alternatively, intraduodenal pressure can be continuously recorded from a separate intraduodenal catheter attached to the endoscope. The highest basal pressure, defined as the pressure above the zero duodenal baseline (**Fig. 3**) that is sustained for at least 30 seconds, is identified. The mean of the readings from the 4 lowest amplitude points in this zone is taken as the basal sphincter pressure for that lead for that pull-through. The basal sphincter pressure for all interpretable observations is averaged; this is the final basal sphincter pressure. The amplitude of phasic wave contractions is measured from the beginning of the slope of the pressure increase from the basal pressure to the peak of the contraction wave. Four representative waves are taken for each lead, and the mean pressure is determined. The number of phasic waves per minute and the duration of the phasic waves can also be determined.

Most authorities read only the basal sphincter pressure as an indicator of disease of the SO. However, data from Kalloo and colleagues[64] suggest that intraductal biliary pressure, which is easier to measure than SO pressure, correlates with SO basal

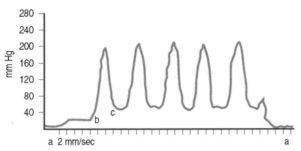

Fig. 3. One lead of abnormal station pull-through at SOM. Baseline duodenal 0 reference (a). Intraductal (pancreatic) pressure of 20 mm Hg (abnormal) (b). Basal pancreatic sphincter pressure is 45 mm Hg (abnormal) (c). Phasic waves are 155 to 175 mm Hg in amplitude and 6 seconds in duration (normal).

pressure. In this study, intrabiliary pressure was significantly higher in patients with SOD than in patients with normal SO pressure (20 mm Hg vs 10 mm Hg; $P<.01$). Similar findings were found by Fazel and colleagues[65] for intrapancreatic pressures. These studies support the theory that increased intrabiliary or intrapancreatic pressures may cause pain in SOD. The best study establishing normal values for SOM evaluated 50 asymptomatic control patients[66] and established normal values for intraductal pressure, basal sphincter pressure, and phasic wave parameters (**Table 2**). Various authorities interchangeably use 35 mm Hg or 40 mm Hg, 3 standard deviations above the mean, as the upper limits of normal for mean basal SO pressure. Although all authorities diagnose SOD when the basal sphincter pressure is 35 to 40 mm Hg or greater, some also make this diagnosis when there are greater than 50% retrograde contractions, tachyoddia (phasic wave frequency >7/min), or a paradoxic contraction response after an intravenous dose of CCK.[67]

Minimizing Complications

The most common major complication after SOM is post-ERCP pancreatitis (PEP), occurring in 31% of patients in whom standard perfused catheters were used. Rolny and colleagues[68] found that patients with chronic pancreatitis were at higher risk of PEP after pancreatic duct manometry (26%) versus those patients without chronic pancreatitis (11%). Methods to decrease the incidence of PEP include (1) use of an

Table 2
Suggested standard abnormal values for endoscopic SOM obtained from 50 volunteers without abdominal symptoms

Basal sphincter pressure[a]	>35 mm Hg
Basal ductal pressure	>13 mm Hg
Phasic contractions	
Amplitude	>220 mm Hg
Duration	>8 s
Frequency	>10/min

Values were obtained by adding 3 standard deviations to the mean (means were obtained by averaging the results on 2–3 station pull-throughs). Data combine pancreatic and biliary studies.
    [a] Basal pressures determined by (1) reading the peak basal pressure (ie, the highest single lead as obtained using a 3-lumen catheter) and (2) obtaining the mean of these peak pressures from multiple station pull-throughs.

aspiration catheter; (2) gravity drainage of the pancreatic duct after manometry; (3) decrease in the perfusion rate to 0.05 to 0.1 mL/lumen/min; (4) limitation of pancreatic duct manometry time to less than 2 minutes (or avoid pancreatic manometry); (5) use of the microtransducer (nonperfused) or sleeve SOM system[69–73]; (6) placement of a pancreatic stent after manometry, sphincterotomy, or both; (7) indomethacin suppositories in all patients with suspected SOD.[74,75] In a prospective randomized study, Sherman and colleagues[15] found that using an aspirating catheter, which allows for aspiration of the perfused fluid from end and side holes and accurately records pressure from the 2 remaining side ports, reduced the frequency of PEP from 31% to 4%. In a prospective randomized trial, Wehrmann and colleagues[76] found that microtransducer manometry was associated with a significantly lower incidence of PEP than standard (nonaspirating) perfusion manometry (13.8% vs 3.1%; $P = .04$). A sleeve SOM catheter-based system was shown more recently to have similar accuracy as the standard triple-lumen SOM catheter with less artifact[77] and potentially lower rates of PEP, because the sleeve assembly is reverse-perfused and no fluid enters the ducts. In another prospective randomized trial, Tarnasky and colleagues[78] showed that placement of a stent in the pancreatic duct decreased PEP from 26% to 6% in a group of patients with pancreatic sphincter hypertension undergoing biliary sphincterotomy alone. In a recent prospective randomized trial,[74] our group reported that administering rectal indomethacin decreased PEP from 16.9% to 9.2% ($P = .005$) in a group in which 82% of patients had SOM for suspected SOD.

Intraductal Ultrasonography

Intraductal ultrasonography allows SO morphology to be observed during endoscopy. The sphincter appears as a thin hypoechoic circular structure on intraductal ultrasonography.[79] Limited studies so far reveal no correlation between the basal sphincter pressures, as detected at SOM, and the thickness of the hypoechoic layer.[69] Although intraductal ultrasonography may provide additional information at the level of the sphincter, it cannot be used as a substitute for SOM.

TREATMENT OF SOD
Medical Therapy

There are limited data assessing the value of medical therapy for suspected or documented SOD. Available studies have focused on medications that aim to reduce the resistance of or relax the SO. In theory, pharmaceutical agents would be expected to have more of a role in SO dyskinesia compared with stenosis.

Vardenafil (Levitra), an inhibitor of phosphodiesterase type 5 and a smooth muscle relaxant used most commonly for male erectile dysfunction, was found to reduce basal sphincter pressure and phasic wave amplitude.[80,81] However, this drug has not been investigated in clinical trials. Sublingual nifedipine and nitrates have been shown to reduce basal sphincter pressures in asymptomatic volunteers and symptomatic patients with SOD.[82] Khuroo and colleagues[83] evaluated the clinical benefit of nifedipine in a placebo-controlled crossover trial. Of 28 patients with manometrically documented SOD, 21 (75%) had a reduction in pain scores, emergency department visits, and use of oral analgesics during short-term follow-up. In a similar study, Sand and colleagues[84] found that 9 (75%) of 12 patients with type II SOD (suspected; SOM was not performed) improved with nifedipine. In a study of 59 patients with postcholecystectomy pain and suspected SOD treated with medical therapy for 1 year (nitrates or an antispasmodic or both), 30 (51%) reported complete relief and 8 (14%) reported partial relief, including 45%, 67%, and 71% type I, type II, and type III patients.[85] In a pilot randomized controlled trial, Craig and Toouli[86] found no benefit for extended-release nifedipine. A prospective case series by Vitton and colleagues[85] investigating the efficacy of trimebutine or a nitrate derivative reported that 50.8% improved with therapy. Both agents were tolerated by 71.1% of patients. Complete or partial symptomatic relief per Milwaukee classification was 45%, 67%, and 71% for type I, II, and III, respectively. The study was not blinded and therefore placebo effect cannot be excluded. Other agents that have been shown to reduce basal sphincter pressures in SOD and asymptomatic volunteers during SOM include hyoscine butylbromide, octreotide, and nitrates.[80,83,85,87] None of these drugs is specific to the SO and, therefore, systemic side effects and tachyphylaxis may limit the long-term use of these agents. Long-term data for outcomes from regular medical therapy are lacking.

Although medical therapy may be an attractive initial approach in patients with SOD, several drawbacks exist. First, side effects of medication may be seen in one-third of patients.[1] Second, smooth muscle relaxants are unlikely to be of any benefit in patients with SO stenosis, and the response is incomplete in patients with SO dyskinesia. Long-term outcome from medical therapy has not been reported. Nevertheless, because of the relative safety of medical therapy and the benign, although painful, character of SOD, this approach should be considered before more aggressive sphincter ablation therapy in all patients with type III SOD, and in patients with type II SOD who have less severe symptoms.

Transcutaneous electrical nerve stimulation was shown by Guelrud and colleagues[88] to reduce the basal sphincter pressure in patients with SOD by a mean of 38%, although generally not into the normal range. This stimulation was associated with an increase in serum vasoactive intestinal peptide levels. Electroacupuncture applied at acupoint GB 34, which affects the hepatobiliary system, was shown to relax the SO in association with increased plasma CCK levels.[89] The long-term role of these modalities in the management of SOD has not been investigated.

Surgical Therapy

The traditional management for SOD had been surgical, most commonly transduodenal biliary sphincteroplasty with a transampullary septoplasty (pancreatic septoplasty). During a 1-year to 10-year follow-up, 60% to 70% of patients were reported to have benefited from this therapy.[70,71,90,91] Patients with an increased basal sphincter pressure, determined by intraoperative SOM, were more likely to improve from surgical sphincter ablation than patients with a normal basal pressure.[91] Some reports have suggested that patients with biliary-type pain have a better outcome than patients with idiopathic pancreatitis, whereas others suggested no difference.[90,91] However, some studies have found that symptom improvement after surgical sphincter ablation was uncommon in patients who were young or had established chronic pancreatitis.[71,91]

The surgical approach for SOD has largely been replaced by endoscopic therapy in many centers for several reasons, including high patient tolerance, reduced cost of care, lower morbidity and mortality, and favorable cosmetic results. Surgical therapy is reserved for patients with restenosis after ES and when endoscopic evaluation or therapy is unavailable or technically difficult because of altered anatomy (eg, Roux-en-Y gastrojejunostomy). Among 68 surgical sphincteroplasties performed at Medical University of South Carolina over a 5-year period, 51 had previous ES, and 17 had endoscopically inaccessible papillae because of previous gastric surgery. There was a trend toward improved outcome after surgical sphincteroplasty ($P = .06$) in patients who had previous gastric surgery and no previous ERCP compared with patients who had ES before surgery.[71]

ENDOSCOPIC THERAPY
ES

ES is the standard therapy for patients with SOD.[72] Variable rates of clinical improvement have been reported in studies, ranging from 55% to 95%. These variable outcomes are reflective of the different criteria used to document SOD, the degree of obstruction (type I biliary patients seem to have a better outcome than type II and type III patients), the methods of data collection (retrospective vs prospective), and the techniques used to determine benefit.

Rolny and colleagues[52] studied 17 patients with type I SOD by biliary SOM and found 65% to have abnormal SOM but with 100% clinical improvement after a mean follow-up of 2.3 years (**Table 3**). Several other case series have reported symptom improvement in 75% to 100% of patients with type I undergoing biliary sphincterotomy.[48,73,92–94] These studies suggest that SOM in this group not only may be unnecessary but also may be misleading.

In contrast, SOM is highly recommended in type II and III patients, because the results may predict benefit from ES. Three key randomized trials have been reported in these groups (**Table 4**).

In a landmark study, Geenen and colleagues[95] randomly assigned 47 postcholecystectomy type II biliary patients to biliary sphincterotomy or sham sphincterotomy. SOM was performed in all patients, but the results of SOM were not used as a criterion for randomization. During a 4-year follow-up, 95% of patients with an increased basal sphincter pressure benefited from sphincterotomy. In contrast, only 30% to 40% of patients with an increased sphincter pressure treated by sham sphincterotomy or with a normal sphincter pressure treated by ES or sham sphincterotomy benefited from this therapy. Thus, SOM predicted the outcome from ES and that the benefits of ES in type II patients were durable.

Similarly, in a 2-year follow-up study by Toouli and colleagues,[96,97] postcholecystectomy patients with biliary-type pain (mostly type II) were prospectively randomly assigned to ES or sham after stratification according to SOM. At 2 years after the intervention, 85% (11 of 13) of patients with increased basal pressure undergoing ES improved, whereas 38% (5 of 13) of patients improved after a sham procedure (P = .041). Patients with normal SOM were also randomly assigned to sphincterotomy or sham. The outcome was similar for both groups (8 of 13 improved after sphincterotomy, and 8 of 19 improved after sham; P = .47).

Sherman and colleagues[98] reported their preliminary results of a randomized study comparing ES and surgical biliary sphincteroplasty with pancreatic septoplasty (with or without cholecystectomy) with sham sphincterotomy for type II and type III biliary

---

Table 3
Biliary sphincter ablation in type I SOD (28-month follow-up)[a]

Basal SO Pressure	N (%)	Asymptomatic or Improved After ES or SS (N) (%)
<40 mm Hg	6 (35)	6 (100)
>40 mm Hg	11 (65)	11 (100)

Abbreviations: ES, endoscopic sphincterotomy; SS, surgical sphincterotomy.
[a] 15 ES, 2 SS.
Data from Rolny P, Geenen JE, Hogan WJ: Post-cholecystectomy patients with 'objective signs' of partial bile outflow obstruction: Clinical characteristics, sphincter of Oddi manometry findings, and results of therapy. Gastrointest Endosc 1993;39:778–81.

Table 4
Biliary sphincter ablation in type II and III SOD documented by SOM

Reference	Clinical Benefit	
	Type II (N) (%)	Type III (N) (%)
Choudhry et al,[25,a] 1993	10/18 (56)	9/16 (56)
Botoman et al,[152] 1994	13/19 (68)	9/16 (56)
Bozkurt et al,[153] 1996	14/19 (78)	5/5 (100)
Wehrmann et al,[154] 1996	12/20 (60)	1/13 (8)
Rosenblatt et al,[30] 2001	22/30 (73)	11/32 (34)

[a] Six had cholecystectomy.

patients with manometrically documented SOD (see **Table 4**). During a 3-year follow-up period, 69% of patients undergoing endoscopic or surgical sphincter ablation improved compared with 24% in the sham sphincterotomy group ($P = .009$). There was a trend for type II patients to benefit more often from sphincter ablation than type III patients (13 of 16 [81%] vs 11 of 19 [58%]; $P = .14$).

The recommended Rome III committee approach for therapy for type I, II, and III biliary SOD is summarized in **Fig. 4**.

Multiple studies suggest that the addition of pancreatic sphincterotomy to biliary sphincterotomy in patients with pancreatic sphincter disease improves outcomes. In a study from our unit,[99] we examined the outcome of endoscopic therapy in patients with SOD with initial pancreatic sphincter hypertension, with or without biliary sphincter hypertension. Patients were followed for a mean of 43.1 months (range 11–77 months); reintervention was offered for sustained or recurrent symptoms at a median of 8 months after initial therapy. Performance of initial dual pancreatobiliary sphincterotomy was associated with a lower reintervention rate (70 of 285 [24.6%]) than biliary sphincterotomy alone (31 of 95 [33%]; $P<.05$).

Many authorities argue that the current SOD classification systems might not be a good predictor of outcome.[67,100–102] In a study of 121 patients with SOD treated by biliary sphincterotomy with (49) or without (72) pancreatic sphincterotomy, Freeman and colleagues[100] reported a good to excellent response in 69%. The response was not significantly different between biliary types I, II, and III. The investigators found that significant predictors of a poor response to therapy were normal pancreatic manometry, delayed gastric emptying, daily opioid use, and age younger than 40 years. Abnormal liver function tests or dilated bile duct were not significant predictors of outcome. These results indicate that proceeding with ERCP in patients with suspected SOD should consider the patient presentation as well as Milwaukee classification type and be balanced against the high complication rates reported for endoscopic therapy for SOD. As previously discussed, patients with suspected SOD have up to a 30% chance of PEP, and suspected SOD has been found to be an independent risk factor for PEP in several prospective studies. These studies have also shown that the risk of pancreatitis is intrinsic to the patient group and events occurring during the procedure rather than the SOM when the SOM is performed with an aspirating catheter.[68,74,75,77–79] In multivariate analysis, SOM has not been shown to be a risk factor for pancreatitis.[103,104]

BOTULINUM TOXIN (BOTOX) INJECTION

Botulinum toxin (Botox), a potent inhibitor of acetylcholine release from nerve endings, has been successfully applied to smooth muscle disorders of the GI tract such as

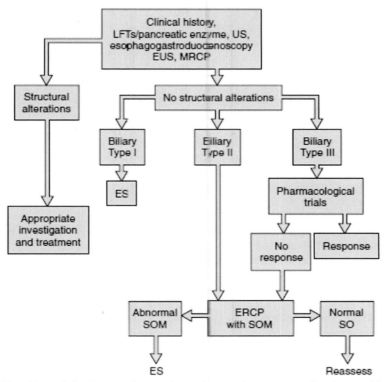

Fig. 4. Algorithm of the history, diagnostic workup, and treatment of patients with types I, II, and III biliary SOD.

achalasia and anal fissures. In a case report, Botox injection into the SO in 2 patients with SOD resulted in a 50% reduction in the basal biliary sphincter pressure and improved bile flow, which was sustained for 4 months.[105] Despite these findings, neither patient reported sustained improvement in pain even after subsequent sphincterotomy. In contrast, a case series of 22 type III postcholecystectomy patients with manometric evidence of SOD suggested that Botox injection might serve as a therapeutic trial for people with SOD. Eleven of 12 who responded to Botox later benefited from ES, whereas 2 of 10 patients who did not benefit from Botox injection later responded to sphincter ablation ($P<.01$).[106] No complications from the use of Botox have been reported. Although the response to Botox may predict the benefit from sphincterotomy, such an approach requires 2 endoscopies to achieve symptom relief. Patients must have relatively frequent episodes of pain to assess the benefit from Botox. Further studies are needed before this technique can be recommended.

STENT TRIAL AND BALLOON DILATION

Placement of a pancreatic or biliary stent on a trial basis in hope of achieving pain relief and predicting the response to more definitive therapy (ie, sphincter ablation) has received only limited application. Pancreatic stent trials, especially in patients with normal pancreatic ducts, are strongly discouraged, because serious ductal and parenchymal injury may occur if stents are left in place for more than a few days.[107,108]

Goff[109] reported a biliary stent trial in 21 patients with normal biliary manometry suspected to have type II and type III SOD. Stents (7 F) were left in place for at least

2 months if symptoms resolved and were removed sooner if they were judged to be ineffective. Relief of pain with the stent was predictive of long-term pain relief after biliary sphincterotomy. Pancreatitis developed in 38% of the patients (severe in 14%) after stent placement. Because of this high complication rate, biliary stent trials are strongly discouraged.

Rolny[110] also reported a series of bile duct stent placement as a predictor of outcome after biliary sphincterotomy in 23 postcholecystectomy patients (7 type II and 16 type III). Similar to the study by Goff, resolution of pain during at least 12 weeks of stent placement predicted a favorable outcome from sphincterotomy regardless of SO pressure. In this series, there were no complications related to stent placement. The reasons for such discrepancy in complications have not been examined. It is known that the nature of the patient and activity of the sphincter (in particular, sphincter hypertension) is relevant to PEP. All of the patients reported by Rolny and Goff had suspected SOD but most had normal manometry, although it is not stated if this was restricted to the biliary orifice.

Biliary stent placement might offer short-term symptom benefit in patients with SOD and predict outcome from sphincter ablation; however, it too has an unacceptably high complication rate and cannot be advocated in this setting.[109] Further studies on the role of biliary stenting with prophylactic pancreatic duct stents are needed.

Balloon dilation of strictures in the GI tract has become a common procedure. In an attempt to be less invasive and possibly to preserve sphincter function, adaptation of this technique to treat SOD has been described. Similar to stent placement, balloon dilation has an unacceptably high complication rate, primarily pancreatitis, and this technology has little role in the primary management of SOD.[111]

REASONS FOR FAILURE OF BILIARY SPHINCTEROTOMY TREATMENT

There are many potential reasons why patients may fail to experience symptom relief or only experience transient relief after biliary sphincterotomy for well-documented SOD. First, biliary sphincterotomy may be inadequate, because the biliary sphincter is not commonly totally ablated.[112] Over time, restenosis after biliary sphincterotomy may occur; however, clinically significant biliary restenosis is believed to occur infrequently.[113] If no cutting space remains for biliary sphincterotomy, an alternative is balloon dilation to 8 to 10 mm, but long-term outcome from such therapy is unknown. In addition, the increased risk of PEP warrants prophylactic pancreatic stenting to reduce this risk.[79] Second, as noted earlier, the importance of coexisting pancreatic sphincter hypertension and need for pancreatic sphincter ablation is being increasingly recognized. Third, patients with chronic pancreatitis may not respond to ES. Tarnasky and colleagues[114] reported that patients with SOD were 4 times more likely to have evidence of chronic pancreatitis than patients without SOD ($P = .01$). Although there seems to be an association between SOD and chronic pancreatitis, no causal relationship has been definitively shown. These patients may or may not have abnormal pancreatograms. More subtle chronic pancreatitis, not seen on pancreatogram, can be diagnosed by intraductal pancreatic juice aspiration after secretin stimulation[115] or EUS.[116] Fourth, some patients may have pain from altered gut motility of the stomach, small bowel, or colon (irritable bowel or pseudo-obstruction variants). There is increasing evidence that upper GI motility disorders may masquerade as pancreatobiliary-type pain (ie, discrete right upper quadrant pain). Multiple preliminary studies show disordered duodenal motility in such patients.[117–119] Soffer and Johli[120] found that small bowel dysmotility occurred with greater frequency in patients with type II and type III SOD who failed to benefit from sphincterotomy than in patients who did respond. This area needs more study to determine the frequency, significance, and coexistence of these motor disorders along with SOD. DeSautels and colleagues[121] suggested that type III patients have duodenal specific visceral hyperalgesia with pain reproduction by duodenal distention. These patients were also shown to have high levels of somatization, depression, obsessive-compulsive behavior, anxiety, and history of sexual or physical abuse compared with control individuals.[122,123] Patients with SOD seem to have a higher than expected prevalence of irritable bowel syndrome[124] and SOD may occur as part of a more generalized functional disorder of the gut. Wald[125] suggested that selective treatment of the SO cannot be expected to provide symptom resolution in such patients, and this may account for the high failure rate of sphincterotomy in many patients with type III SOD.

SOD IN IDIOPATHIC RECURRENT ACUTE PANCREATITIS

Disorders of the pancreatic sphincter may give rise to idiopathic pancreatitis or episodic pain suggestive of a pancreatic origin.[67] Although the pathogenesis of acute pancreatitis in SOD is uncertain, it is thought that the combination of pancreatic duct obstruction and increased exocrine juice flow are required elements.[126] SOD is a frequent cause of recurrent pancreatitis previously labeled as idiopathic acute recurrent pancreatitis (IARP), and has been documented with manometry in 15% to 72% of such patients (**Table 5**).[127–136] Pancreatic sphincter manometry should be performed in patients with IARP, particularly patients with normal biliary manometry and patients who have recurrent attacks after a biliary sphincterotomy. Isolated pancreatic sphincter hypertension is common among patients with IARP found to have SOD.[62,137] In addition, pancreatic sphincter hypertension may explain recurrent pancreatitis despite biliary sphincterotomy or surgical biliary sphincteroplasty.[137] Biliary sphincterotomy alone has been reported to prevent further pancreatitis episodes in more than 50% of patients in some series. From a scientific, but not practical, view point, care must be taken to separate out subtle biliary pancreatitis,[138] which would similarly respond to biliary sphincterotomy. Because IARP is an episodic illness, long-term follow-up is necessary to conclude that a patient is cured. Sphincter ablation is the recommended therapy for patients with IARP resulting from SOD.

Table 5 Manometrically documented SOD causing idiopathic acute pancreatitis	
Reference	Frequency (N) (%)
Toouli et al,[130] 1985	16/26 (62)
Guelrud et al,[131] 1986	17/42 (40)
Gregg,[132] 1989	38/125 (30)
Venu et al,[129] 1989	17/116 (15)
Raddawi et al,[62] 1991	7/24 (29)
Sherman et al,[133] 1993	18/55 (33)
Toouli et al,[96] 1996	24/33 (73)
Choudari et al,[128] 1998	79/225 (35)
Testoni et al,[146] 2000	14/40 (35)
Coyle et al,[135] 2002	28/90 (31)
Kaw and Brodmerkel,[134] 2002	67/126 (53)
Fischer et al,[136] 2010	418/952 (44)
Total	743/1854 (40)

Historically, ablation has been accomplished surgically[91]; however, with increasing experience, ES has become the treatment of choice.

Controversy continues to exist about the type of sphincterotomy that should be performed in patients with IARP.[139] Many patients benefit from biliary sphincterotomy alone and thus may have subtle gallstone pancreatitis.[133]

The value of ERCP, SOM, and sphincter ablation therapy was studied in 51 patients with idiopathic pancreatitis.[140] Twenty-four patients (47.1%) had an increased basal sphincter pressure. Thirty were treated by biliary sphincterotomy (n = 20), or surgical sphincteroplasty with septoplasty (n = 10). Fifteen of 18 patients (83%) with an increased basal sphincter pressure had long-term benefit (mean follow-up, 38 months) from sphincter ablation therapy (including 10 of 11 treated by biliary sphincterotomy) in contrast to only 4 of 12 (33.3%; $P<.05$) with a normal basal sphincter pressure (including 4 of 9 treated by biliary sphincterotomy). However, Guelrud and colleagues[141] found that the severance of the pancreatic sphincter was necessary to resolve the pancreatitis. In this series, 69 patients with idiopathic pancreatitis caused by SOD underwent treatment by standard biliary sphincterotomy (n = 18), biliary sphincterotomy with pancreatic sphincter balloon dilation (n = 24), biliary sphincterotomy followed by pancreatic sphincterotomy in separate sessions (n = 13), or combined pancreatic and biliary sphincterotomy in the same session (n = 14). Eighty-one percent of patients undergoing pancreatic and biliary sphincterotomy had resolution of their pancreatitis compared with 28% of patients undergoing biliary sphincterotomy alone ($P<.005$). Sherman and colleagues[133] reported that only 44% of patients with SOD with IARP had no further attacks during a 5-year follow-up interval after biliary sphincterotomy alone. These data are consistent with the theory that many such patients who benefit from biliary sphincterotomy alone may have subtle gallstone pancreatitis, or perhaps the follow-up has not been long enough to detect another attack of pancreatitis. A recent article by Wehrmann[142] attempted to help clarify the issue by studying patients with a longer follow-up of (11.5 ± 1.6 years) after endoscopic therapy in SOD for IARP. In this study, 5 of 37 (14%) had a recurrent attack of pancreatitis over a mean duration of 32.4 months (range 24–53) and this increased to 19 of 37 (51%) at 11.5 years. However, the frequency of pancreatitis episodes was lower than before endoscopic therapy. The investigator suggests that endoscopic sphincter ablation may slow the progress of the natural course of the disease.

The results of Guelrud and colleagues[141] also support the anatomic findings of separate biliary and pancreatic sphincters, and the manometry findings of residual pancreatic sphincter hypertension in more than 50% of persistently symptomatic patients who undergo biliary sphincterotomy alone. Kaw and colleagues[134] reported that among patients with idiopathic pancreatitis secondary to SOD, 78% had persistent manometric evidence of pancreatic sphincter hypertension despite a biliary sphincterotomy. Toouli and colleagues[143] showed the importance of pancreatic and biliary sphincter ablation in patients with idiopathic pancreatitis. In this series, 23 of 26 patients (88%) undergoing surgical ablation of both the biliary and pancreatic sphincter were either asymptomatic or had minimal symptoms at a median follow-up of 24 months (range 9–105 months). Okolo and colleagues[144] retrospectively evaluated the long-term results of endoscopic pancreatic sphincterotomy in 55 patients with manometrically documented or presumed pancreatic sphincter hypertension, based on recurrent pancreatitis with pancreatic duct dilation and contrast medium drainage time from the pancreatic duct greater than 10 minutes. During a median follow-up of 16 months (range 3–52 months), 34 patients (62%) reported significant pain improvement. Patients with normal pancreatograms were more likely to respond to therapy than those with pancreatographic evidence of chronic pancreatitis (73% vs 58%).

Jacob and colleagues[145] postulated that SOD might cause recurrent episodes of pancreatitis, even although SOM was normal, and placement of a pancreatic duct stent might prevent further attacks. In a randomized trial in 34 patients with IARP, normal pancreatic duct SOM, ERCP, secretin testing, and no biliary crystals were treated with pancreatic stents or conservative therapy. During a 3-year follow-up period, pancreatitis recurred in 53% of the control group and 11% of the stented group (P<.02). This study suggests that SOM may be an imperfect test because patients may have SOD that is not detected at SOM. However, long-term studies are needed to evaluate the outcome after removal of stents, and concern remains regarding stent-induced pancreatic injury.[107, 108] Thus, trial of pancreatic duct stent placement to predict outcome from pancreatic sphincterotomy is not recommended.[146] Wehrmann and colleagues[147] showed that injection of Botox into the papilla is safe, may be effective in the short-term, and may predict the outcome from pancreatic sphincter ablation in patients having frequent episodes of pancreatitis, but the need for definitive sphincter ablation in most patients limits its clinical use.

These data show that SOD is the most common cause of IARP when detailed endoscopic evaluation is performed. SOM should be considered the gold standard for diagnosing SOD. Complete sphincter evaluation requires manometric assessment of both the biliary and pancreatic sphincters. Although the best endoscopic therapy for SOD is not definitively determined, there is mounting evidence that pancreatic sphincter ablation is necessary in most patients to achieve the best long-term results. However, controversy persists as to the appropriateness of performing SOM in patients with IARP.[148] In a recent editorial, Tan and Sherman[149] stated that although the studies described earlier suggest that endoscopic therapy may benefit most patients with IARP caused by SOD, there are many limitations that need to be emphasized. (1) Most published studies are retrospective and suffer from incomplete follow-up, lack homogeneity of patient selection for therapy, and are not blinded or compared with an untreated group. (2) Uncontrolled prospective studies are prone to bias. (3) Length of follow-up of most studies is less than 3 years. Short follow-up may result in an underestimate of the true recurrence rates. (4) Differences exist in defining study outcomes; investigators have used different outcomes, including documented recurrent pancreatitis, need for reintervention, or a grading system. (5) There is a lack of a homogeneous population of treated patients with IARP. (6) Variable interventions have been used, with different studies performing biliary sphincterotomy, pancreatic sphincterotomy, or dual sphincterotomy, with unclear reasons as to why the particular therapy was chosen. Completeness of sphincter ablation was also often not determined. In the absence of well-conducted randomized controlled trials and long-term patient follow-up, many authorities consider the benefits of sphincter ablation therapy to be unproved.[102,149,150]

A seminal randomized study was recently published addressing the effectiveness of endoscopic therapy for patients with IARP found to have pancreatic SOD.[151] Among 139 eligible patients, 89 (64%) had no identifiable cause after ductography. Of these patients, 69 (78%) had SOD. Among patients with SOD, the frequency of recurrent pancreatitis during follow-up was similar among patients randomized to biliary sphincterotomy (48.5%) and dual biliary and pancreatic sphincterotomy (47.2%) (difference 1.2%) (95% confidence interval, −22.3, 24.9], P = 1.0). In patients with normal SOM, subsequent recurrent pancreatitis was similar among patients with sham (11.1%) and biliary sphincterotomy (27.3%), (difference −16.2% [−49.5, 17.2], P = .59). In all, 16.9% developed chronic pancreatitis during follow-up (median 78 months, interquartile range 35, 108). The odds of recurrent pancreatitis during follow-up were significantly higher among patients with SOD versus normal SOM (unadjusted hazard ratio [HR] 3.5

[1.07, 11.4], $P<.04$), and remained so after adjusting for potential confounders (HR 4.3 [1.3, 14.5], $P<.02$). The investigators concluded that among patients with SOD, pancreatic sphincterotomy has no incremental benefit over biliary sphincterotomy alone in eliminating future episodes of recurrent pancreatitis. Pancreatic SOD is an independent, negative prognostic marker for future episodes of acute pancreatitis. Although SOD seems to be the most common cause of IARP, the results of this trial question whether endoscopic therapy is indicated. Further confirmatory studies are warranted, and attempts to identify those patients with SOD with IARP who will benefit from intervention are desperately needed.

SUMMARY

Knowledge of SOD and manometric techniques to assist in this diagnosis is evolving. Successful endoscopic SOM requires good general ERCP skills and careful attention to the main details summarized in this article. Type I SOD should be managed by ES without SOM. If SOD is suspected in a patient with type III or type II SOD with mild to moderate pain level, medical therapy should generally be tried. If medical therapy fails, ERCP and SOM evaluation should be considered when expertise is available. An alternative to SOM in these patients may be a trial of Botox or stenting, after careful patient counseling. Abnormal manometry or a positive outcome from Botox/stenting may be used to select patients for ES. Although the role of less invasive studies is uncertain, current evidence does not support their routine use because of their low sensitivities and specificities. Symptom relief from ES ranges from 55% to 95%, depending on the patient presentation and selection. Initial nonresponders after biliary sphincterotomy alone may benefit from thorough pancreatic sphincter and pancreatic parenchymal evaluation at expert centers, particularly in type III patients, to achieve optimal outcome. Patients with suspected SOD are at high risk for complications from SOM and ES. Therefore, the risk/benefit ratio of invasive tests should be reviewed extensively with these patients, and risk reduction methods, as outlined in this article, should be undertaken to minimize risks to these patients.

REFERENCES

1. Steinberg WM. Sphincter of Oddi dysfunction: a clinical controversy. Gastroenterology 1988;95:1409–15.
2. Richards RD, Yeaton P, Shaffer HA, et al. Human sphincter of Oddi motility and cholecystokinin response following liver transplantation. Dig Dis Sci 1993;38: 462–8.
3. Becker JM, Parodi JM. Basic control mechanisms of sphincter of Oddi motor function. Gastrointest Endosc Clin North Am 1993;3:41–66.
4. Luman W, Williams AJ, Pryde A, et al. Influence of cholecystectomy on sphincter of Oddi motility. Gut 1997;41:371–4.
5. Anderson TM, Pitt HA, Longmire WP Jr. Experience with sphincteroplasty and sphincterotomy in pancreatobiliary surgery. Ann Surg 1985;201:399–406.
6. Kurucsai G, Joo I, Fejes R, et al. Somatosensory hypersensitivity in the referred pain area in patients with chronic biliary pain and a sphincter of Oddi dysfunction: new aspects of an almost forgotten pathogenetic mechanism. Am J Gastroenterol 2008;103:2717–25.
7. Chen JW, Thomas A, Woods CM, et al. Sphincter of Oddi dysfunction produces acute pancreatitis in the possum. Gut 2000;47:539.
8. Corazziari E, Shaffer EA, Hogan W, et al. Functional disorders of the biliary tract and pancreas. Gut 1999;45:48–54.

9. Misra S, Treanor MR, Vegunta RK, et al. Sphincter of Oddi dysfunction in children with recurrent abdominal pain: 5-year follow-up after endoscopic sphincterotomy. J Gastroenterol Hepatol 2007;22:2246–50.

10. Drossman DA, Zhiming L, Andruzzi E, et al. US Householder Survey of functional gastrointestinal disorders. Prevalence, sociodemography, and health impact. Dig Dis Sci 1993;38:1569–80.

11. Winstead NJ, Wilcox CM. Health-related quality of life, somatization, and above in sphincter of Oddi dysfunction. J Clin Gastroenterol 2007;41:773–6.

12. Eversman D, Fogel EL, Rusche M, et al. Frequency of abnormal pancreatic and biliary sphincter manometry compared with clinical suspicion of sphincter of Oddi dysfunction. Gastrointest Endosc 1999;50:637–41.

13. Linder JD, Geels W, Wilcox CM. Prevalence of sphincter of Oddi dysfunction: can results from specialized centers be generalized? Dig Dis Sci 2002;47:2411–5.

14. Bar-Meir S, Halpern Z, Bardan E, et al. Frequency of papillary dysfunction among cholecystectomized patients. Hepatology 1984;4:328.

15. Sherman S, Troiano FP, Hawes RH, et al. Frequency of abnormal sphincter of Oddi manometry compared with the clinical suspicion of sphincter of Oddi dysfunction. Am J Gastroenterol 1991;86:586–90.

16. Aymerich RR, Prakash C, Aliperti G. Sphincter of Oddi manometry: is it necessary to measure both biliary and pancreatic sphincter pressure? Gastrointest Endosc 2000;52:183–6.

17. Thune A, Scicchitano J, Roberts-Thompson I, et al. Reproducibility of endoscopic sphincter of Oddi manometry. Dig Dis Sci 1991;36:1401–5.

18. Varadarajulu S, Hawes RH, Cotton PB. Determination of sphincter of Oddi dysfunction in patients with prior normal manometry. Gastrointest Endosc 2003;58:341–4.

19. Khashab MA, Watkins JL, McHenry L Jr, et al. Frequency of sphincter of Oddi dysfunction in patients with previously normal sphincter of Oddi manometry studies. Endoscopy 2010;42:369–74.

20. Lehman GA, Sherman S. Sphincter of Oddi dysfunction. Int J Pancreatol 1996;20:11–25.

21. Geenen JE, Nash JA. The role of sphincter of Oddi manometry and biliary microscopy in evaluating idiopathic recurrent pancreatitis. Endoscopy 1998;30:237–41.

22. Behar J, Corazziari E, Guelrud M, et al. Functional gallbladder and sphincter of Oddi disorders. Gastroenterology 2006;130:1498–509.

23. Guelrud M, Mendoza S, Mujica V, et al. Sphincter of Oddi (SO) motor function in patients with symptomatic gallstones. Gastroenterology 1993;104:A361.

24. Ruffolo TA, Sherman S, Lehman GA, et al. Gallbladder ejection fraction and its relationship to sphincter of Oddi dysfunction. Dig Dis Sci 1994;39:289–92.

25. Choudhry U, Ruffolo T, Jamidar P, et al. Sphincter of Oddi dysfunction in patients with intact gallbladder: therapeutic response to endoscopic sphincterotomy. Gastrointest Endosc 1993;39:492–5.

26. Lin OS, Soetikno RM, Young HS. The utility of liver function test abnormalities concomitant with biliary symptoms in predicting a favorable response to endoscopic sphincterotomy in patients with presumed sphincter of Oddi dysfunction. Am J Gastroenterol 1998;93:1833–6.

27. Steinberg WM, Salvato RF, Toskes PP. The morphine-prostigmin provocative test: is it useful for making clinical decisions? Gastroenterology 1980;78:728–31.

28. Lobo DN, Takhar AS, Thaper A, et al. The morphine prostigmine provocation (Nardi) test for sphincter of Oddi dysfunction: results in healthy volunteers and in patients before and after transduodenal sphincteroplasty and transampullary septectomy. Gut 2007;56:1472–3.

29. Warshaw AL, Simeone J, Schapiro RH, et al. Objective evaluation of ampullary stenosis with ultrasonography and pancreatic stimulation. Am J Surg 1985;149: 65–72.

30. Rosenblatt ML, Catalano MF, Alcocer E, et al. Comparison of sphincter of Oddi manometry, fatty meal sonography, and hepatobiliary scintigraphy in the diagnosis of sphincter of Oddi dysfunction. Gastrointest Endosc 2001;54:697–704.

31. Catalano MF, Lahoti S, Alcocer E, et al. Dynamic imaging of the pancreas using real-time endoscopic ultrasonography with secretin stimulation. Gastrointest Endosc 1998;48:580–7.

32. Corazziari E. Biliary tract imaging. Curr Gastroenterol Rep 1999;1:123–31.

33. Dancygier H, Nattermann C. The role of endoscopic ultrasound in biliary tract disease: obstructive jaundice. Endoscopy 1994;26:800–2.

34. Materne R, van Bees BE, Gigont SF, et al. Extrahepatic biliary obstruction: magnetic resonance imaging compared with endoscopic ultrasonography. Endoscopy 2000;32:3–9.

35. Gillams AR, Lees WR. Quantitative secretin MRCP (MRCPQ): results in 215 patients with known or suspected pancreatic pathology. Eur Radiol 2007; 17(11):2984–90.

36. Pereira SP, Gillams A, Sgouros SN, et al. Prospective comparison of secretin-stimulated magnetic resonance cholangiopancreatography with manometry in the diagnosis of sphincter of Oddi dysfunction types II and III. Gut 2007;56: 809–13.

37. Baillie J, Kimberly J. Prospective comparison of secretin-stimulated MRCP with manometry in the diagnosis of sphincter of Oddi dysfunction types II and III. Gut 2007;56:742–4.

38. Testoni PA, Mariani A, Curioni S, et al. MRCP-secretin test-guided management of idiopathic recurrent pancreatitis: long-term outcomes. Gastrointest Endosc 2008;67(7):1028–34.

39. Aisen A, Sherman S, Jennings SG, et al. Comparison of secretin-stimulated magnetic resonance pancreatography and manometry results in patients with suspected sphincter of Oddi dysfunction. Acad Radiol 2008;15:601–9.

40. Kalloo AN, Sostre S, Pasricha PJ. The Hopkins scintigraphic score: a non-invasive, highly accurate screening test for SOD. Gastroenterology 1994;106:A342.

41. Sostre S, Kalloo AN, Spiegler EJ, et al. A noninvasive test of sphincter of Oddi dysfunction in postcholecystectomy patients: the scintigraphic score. J Nucl Med 1992;33(6):1216–22.

42. Corazziari E, Cicala M, Habib FI, et al. Hepatoduodenal bile transit in cholecystectomized subjects: relationship with sphincter of Oddi dysfunction and diagnostic value. Dig Dis Sci 1994;39:1985–93.

43. Peng NJ, Lai KH, Tsay DG, et al. Efficacy of quantitative cholescintigraphy in the diagnosis of sphincter of Oddi dysfunction. Nucl Med Commun 1994;15: 899–904.

44. Thomas PD, Turner JG, Dobbs BR, et al. Use of 99m Tc-DISIDA biliary scanning with morphine provocation in the detection of elevated sphincter of Oddi basal pressure. Gut 2000;46:838–41.

45. Craig AG, Peter D, Saccone GT, et al. Scintigraphy versus manometry in patients with suspected biliary sphincter of Oddi dysfunction. Gut 2003;52:352–7.

46. Pineau BC, Knapple WL, Spicer KM, et al. Cholecystokinin-stimulated mebrofenin (99mTc-Choletec) hepatobiliary scintgraphy in asymptomatic postcholecystectomy individuals: assessment of specificity, interobserver reliability, and reproducibility. Am J Gastroenterol 2001;96:3106–9.

47. Roberts KJ, Ismail A, Coldham C, et al. Long-term symptomatic relief following surgical sphincteroplasty for sphincter of Oddi dysfunction. Dig Surg 2011; 28(4):304–8.

48. Cicala M, Habib FI, Vavassori P, et al. Outcome of endoscopic sphincterotomy in post cholecystectomy patients with sphincter of Oddi dysfunction as predicted by manometry and quantitative choledochoscintigraphy. Gut 2002;50(5):665–8.

49. Ponchon T, Aucia N, Mitchell R, et al. Biopsies of the ampullary region in patients suspected to have sphincter of Oddi dysfunction. Gastrointest Endosc 1995;42: 296–300.

50. Imler TD, Sherman S, McHenry L, et al. Low yield of significant findings on endoscopic retrograde cholangiopancreatography in patients with pancreatobiliary pain and no objective findings. Dig Dis Sci 2012;57(12):3252–7.

51. Cohen S, Bacon B, Berlin JA, et al. NIH state-of-the-science conference statement: ERCP for diagnosis and therapy, January 14–16, 2002. Gastrointest Endosc 2002;56:803–16.

52. Rolny P, Geenen JE, Hogan WJ. Post-cholecystectomy patients with "objective signs" of partial bile outflow obstruction: clinical characteristics, sphincter of Oddi manometry findings, and results of therapy. Gastrointest Endosc 1993; 39(6):778–81.

53. Fogel EL, Sherman S, Bucksot L, et al. Effects of droperidol on the pancreatic and biliary sphincter. Gastrointest Endosc 2003;58:488–92.

54. Goff JS. Effect of propofol on human sphincter of Oddi. Dig Dis Sci 1995;40: 2364–7.

55. Varadarajulu S, Tamhane A, Wilcox CM. Prospective evaluation of adjunctive ketamine on sphincter of Oddi motility in humans. J Gastroenterol Hepatol 2008;23:e405–9.

56. Sherman S, Gottlieb K, Uzer MF, et al. Effects of meperidine on the pancreatic and biliary sphincter. Gastrointest Endosc 1996;44:239–42.

57. Blaut U, Alazmi W, Sherman S, et al. The influence of variable-stiffness guide wires on basal biliary sphincter of Oddi pressure measured at endoscopic retrograde cholangiopancreatography. Endoscopy 2010;42(5):375–80.

58. Craig AG, Omari T, Lingenfelser T, et al. Development of a sleeve sensor for measurement of sphincter of Oddi motility. Endoscopy 2001;33:651–7.

59. Blaut U, Sherman S, Fogel E, et al. Influence of cholangiography on biliary sphincter of Oddi manometric parameters. Gastrointest Endosc 2000;52:624–9.

60. Rolny P, Arleback A, Funch-Jensen P, et al. Clinical significance of manometric assessment of both pancreatic duct and bile duct sphincter in the same patient. Scand J Gastroenterol 1989;24:751–4.

61. Silverman WB, Ruffolo TA, Sherman S, et al. Correlation of basal sphincter pressures measured from both the bile duct and pancreatic duct in patients with suspected sphincter of Oddi dysfunction. Gastrointest Endosc 1992;38:440–3.

62. Raddawi HM, Geenen JE, Hogan WJ, et al. Pressure measurements from biliary and pancreatic segments of sphincter of Oddi: comparison between patients with functional abdominal pain, biliary or pancreatic disease. Dig Dis Sci 1991;36:71–4.

63. Hogan W, Sherman S, Pasricha P, et al. Position paper on sphincter of Oddi manometry. Gastrointest Endosc 1997;45:342–8.

64. Kalloo AN, Tietjen TG, Pasricha PJ. Does intrabiliary pressure predict basal sphincter of Oddi pressure? A study in patients with and without gallbladders. Gastrointest Endosc 1996;44:696–9.
65. Fazel A, Geenen JE, MoezArdalan K, et al. Intrapancreatic ductal pressure in sphincter of Oddi dysfunction. Pancreas 2005;30:359–62.
66. Guelrud M, Mendoza S, Rossiter G, et al. Sphincter of Oddi manometry in healthy volunteers. Dig Dis Sci 1990;35:38–46.
67. McLoughlin MT, Mitchell RM. Sphincter of Oddi dysfunction and pancreatitis. World J Gastroenterol 2007;13:6333–43.
68. Rolny P, Anderberg B, Ihse I, et al. Pancreatitis after sphincter of Oddi manometry. Gut 1990;31:821–4.
69. Wehrmann T, Stergiou N, Riphaus A, et al. Correlation between sphincter of Oddi manometry and intraductal ultrasound morphology in patients with suspected sphincter of Oddi dysfunction. Endoscopy 2001;33:773–7.
70. Madura JA, Madura JA II, Sherman S, et al. Surgical sphincteroplasty in 446 patients. Arch Surg 2005;140:504–13.
71. Morgan KA, Romagnuolo J, Adams DB. Transduodenal sphincteroplasty in the management of sphincter of Oddi dysfunction and pancreas divisum in the modern era. J Am Coll Surg 2008;206:908–14.
72. Sherman S. What is the role of ERCP in the setting of abdominal pain of pancreatic or biliary origin (suspected sphincter of Oddi dysfunction)? Gastrointest Endosc 2002;56(Suppl):258–66.
73. Thatcher BS, Snak MV, Tedesco FJ, et al. Endoscopic sphincterotomy for suspected dysfunction of the sphincter of Oddi. Gastrointest Endosc 1987;33:91–5.
74. Sherman S, Troiano FP, Hawes RH, et al. Sphincter of Oddi manometry: decreased risk of clinical pancreatitis with the use of a modified aspirating catheter. Gastrointest Endosc 1990;36:462–6.
75. Elmunzer BJ, Scheiman JM, Lehman GA, et al. A randomized trial of rectal indomethacin to prevent post-ERCP pancreatitis. U.S. Cooperative for Outcomes Research in Endoscopy (USCORE). N Engl J Med 2012;366(15):1414–22.
76. Wehrmann T, Stergiou N, Schmitt T, et al. Reduced risk for pancreatitis after endoscopic microtransducer manometry of the sphincter of Oddi: a randomized comparison with perfusion manometry technique. Endoscopy 2003;35:472–7.
77. Kawamoto M, Geenen J, Omari T, et al. Sleeve sphincter of Oddi (SO) manometry: a new method for characterizing the motility of the sphincter of Oddi. J Hepatobiliary Pancreat Surg 2008;15:391–6.
78. Tarnasky PR, Palesch YY, Cunningham JT, et al. Pancreatic stenting prevents pancreatitis after biliary sphincterotomy in patients with sphincter of Oddi dysfunction. Gastroenterology 1998;115:1518–24.
79. Itoh A, Tsukamoto Y, Naitoh Y, et al. Intraductal ultrasonography for the examination of duodenal papillary region. J Ultrasound Med 1994;13:679–84.
80. Cheon YK, Cho YD, Moon JH, et al. Effects of vardenafil, a phosphodiesterase type-5 inhibitor, on sphincter of Oddi motility in patients with suspected biliary sphincter of Oddi dysfunction. Gastrointest Endosc 2009;69:1111–6.
81. Affronti J. Levitra for sphincter of Oddi dysfunction? Are you kidding? Gastrointest Endosc 2009;69:1117–9.
82. Guelrud M, Mendoza S, Rossiter G, et al. Effect of nifedipine on sphincter of Oddi motor activity: studies in healthy volunteers and patients with biliary dyskinesia. Gastroenterology 1988;95:1050–5.

83. Khuroo MS, Zargar SA, Yattoo GN. Efficacy of nifedipine therapy in patients with sphincter of Oddi dysfunction: a prospective, double-blind, randomized, placebo-controlled, cross over trial. Br J Clin Pharmacol 1992;33:477–85.

84. Sand J, Nordback I, Koskinen M, et al. Nifedipine for suspected type II sphincter of Oddi dyskinesia. Am J Gastroenterol 1993;88:530–5.

85. Vitton V, Delpy R, Gasmi M, et al. Is endoscopic sphincterotomy avoidable in patients with sphincter of Oddi dysfunction? Eur J Gastroenterol Hepatol 2008;20:15–21.

86. Craig AG, Toouli J. Slow release nifedipine for patients with sphincter of Oddi dysfunction: results of a pilot study. Intern Med J 2002;32:119–20.

87. Kalaitzakis E, Ambrose T. Phillips-Hughes J, et al. Management of patients with biliary sphincter of Oddi disorder without sphincter of Oddi manometry. BMC Gastroenterol 2010;10:124.

88. Guelrud M, Rossiter A, Souney P, et al. The effect of transcutaneous nerve stimulation on sphincter of Oddi pressure in patients with biliary dyskinesia. Am J Gastroenterol 1991;86:581–5.

89. Lee SK, Kim MH, Kim HJ, et al. Electroacupuncture may relax the sphincter of Oddi in humans. Gastrointest Endosc 2001;53:211–6.

90. Moody FG, Vecchio R, Calabuig R, et al. Transduodenal sphincteroplasty with transampullary septectomy for stenosing papillitis. Am J Surg 1991;161:213–8.

91. Sherman S, Hawes RH, Madura J, et al. Comparison of intraoperative and endoscopic manometry of the sphincter of Oddi. Surg Gynecol Obstet 1992;175:410–8.

92. Boender J, VanBlankenstein M, Nix GA, et al. Endoscopic papillotomy in biliary tract pain and fluctuating cholestasis with common bile duct dilation and small gallbladder stones. Endoscopy 1992;24:203–7.

93. Elmi F, Silverman WB. Biliary sphincter of Oddi dysfunction type I versus occult biliary microlithiasis in post-cholecystectomy patients: are they both part of the same clinical entity? Dig Dis Sci 2010;55:842–6.

94. Sgouros SN, Pereira SP. Systematic review: sphincter of Oddi dysfunction–noninvasive diagnostic methods and long-term outcome after endoscopic sphincterotomy. Aliment Pharmacol Ther 2006;24:237–46.

95. Geenen JE, Hogan WJ, Dodds WJ, et al. The efficacy of endoscopic sphincterotomy after cholecystectomy in patients with sphincter of Oddi dysfunction. N Engl J Med 1989;320:82–7.

96. Toouli J, Roberts-Thomson I, Kellow J, et al. Prospective randomized trial of endoscopic sphincterotomy for treatment of sphincter of Oddi dysfunction. J Gastroenterol Hepatol 1996;11:A115.

97. Toouli J, Roberts-Thomson IC, Kellow J, et al. Manometry based randomized trial of endoscopic sphincterotomy for sphincter of Oddi dysfunction. Gut 2000;46:98–102.

98. Sherman S, Lehman GA, Jamidar P, et al. Efficacy of endoscopic sphincterotomy and surgical sphincteroplasty for patients with sphincter of Oddi dysfunction (SOD): randomized, controlled study. Gastrointest Endosc 1994;40:A125.

99. Park SH, Watkins JL, Fogel EL, et al. Long-term outcome of endoscopic dual pancreatobiliary sphincterotomy in patients with manometry-documented sphincter of Oddi dysfunction and normal pancreatogram. Gastrointest Endosc 2003;57:483–91.

100. Freeman ML, Gill M, Overby C, et al. Predictors of outcomes after biliary and pancreatic sphincterotomy for sphincter of Oddi dysfunction. J Clin Gastroenterol 2007;41:94–102.

101. Petersen BT. An evidence-based review of sphincter of Oddi dysfunction, part I: presentations with "objective" biliary findings (types I and II). Gastrointest Endosc 2004;59:525–34.
102. Petersen BT. Sphincter of Oddi dysfunction, part 2: evidence-based review of the presentations, with "objective" pancreatic findings (types I and II) and of presumptive type III [review]. Gastrointest Endosc 2004;59:670–87.
103. Cheng CL, Sherman S, Watkins JL, et al. Risk factors for post-ERCP pancreatitis: a prospective multicenter study. Am J Gastroenterol 2006;101:139–47.
104. Singh P, Gurudu SR, Davidoff S, et al. Sphincter of Oddi manometry does not predispose to post-ERCP acute pancreatitis. Gastrointest Endosc 2004;59: 499–505.
105. Pasricha PJ, Miskovsky EP, Kalloo AN. Intrasphincteric injection of botulinum toxin for suspected sphincter of Oddi dysfunction. Gut 1994;35:1319–21.
106. Wehrmann T, Seifert H, Seipp M, et al. Endoscopic injection of botulinum toxin for biliary sphincter of Oddi dysfunction. Endoscopy 1998;30(8):702–7.
107. Kozarek RA. Pancreatic stents can induce ductal changes consistent with chronic pancreatitis. Gastrointest Endosc 1990;36:93–5.
108. Smith MT, Sherman S, Ikenberry S, et al. Alterations in pancreatic ductal morphology following polyethylene pancreatic duct stenting. Gastrointest Endosc 1996;44:268–75.
109. Goff JS. Common bile duct sphincter of Oddi stenting in patients with suspected sphincter of Oddi dysfunction. Am J Gastroenterol 1995;90:586–9.
110. Rolny P. Endoscopic bile duct stent placement as a predictor of outcome following endoscopic sphincterotomy in patients with suspected sphincter of Oddi dysfunction. Eur J Gastroenterol Hepatol 1997;9:467–71.
111. Kozarek RA. Balloon dilation of the sphincter of Oddi. Endoscopy 1988;20: 207–10.
112. Heinerman PM, Graf AH, Boeckl O. Does endoscopic sphincterotomy destroy the function of Oddi's sphincter? Arch Surg 1994;129:876–80.
113. Manoukian AV, Schmalz MJ, Geenen JE, et al. The incidence of postsphincterotomy stenosis in group II patients with sphincter of Oddi dysfunction. Gastrointest Endosc 1993;39:496–8.
114. Tarnasky PR, Hoffman B, Aabakken L, et al. Sphincter of Oddi dysfunction is associated with chronic pancreatitis. Am J Gastroenterol 1997;92:1125–9.
115. Gregg JA. The intraductal secretin test (IDST)–an adjunct to the diagnosis of pancreatic disease and pancreatic physiology. In: Sivak MV, editor. Gastroenterologic endoscopy. Philadelphia: Saunders; 1987. p. 794–807.
116. Wiersema MJ, Hawes RH, Lehman GA, et al. Prospective evaluation of endoscopic ultrasonography and endoscopic retrograde cholangiopancreatography in patients with chronic abdominal pain of suspected pancreatic origin. Endoscopy 1993;25:555–64.
117. Gottlieb K, Nowak T, Sherman S, et al. Sphincter of Oddi dysfunction (SOD) and abnormal small bowel motility: analysis of 32 patients. Gastrointest Endosc 1994;40:A109.
118. Evans PR, Bak YT, Dowsett JF, et al. Small bowel motor dysfunction occurs in patients with biliary dyskinesia. Gastroenterology 1994;106:A496.
119. Koussayer T, Ducker TE, Clench MH, et al. Ampulla of Vater/duodenal wall spasm diagnosed by antroduodenal manometry. Dig Dis Sci 1995;40:1710–9.
120. Soffer EE, Johlin FL. Intestinal dysmotility in patients with sphincter of Oddi dysfunction: a reason for failed response to sphincterotomy. Dig Dis Sci 1994; 39:1942–6.

121. DeSautels SG, Slivka A, Hutson WR, et al. Postcholecystectomy pain syndrome: pathophysiology of abdominal pain in sphincter of Oddi type III. Gastroenterology 1999;116:900–5.
122. Chun A, Desautels S, Slivka A, et al. Visceral algesia in irritable bowel syndrome, fibromyalgia, and sphincter of Oddi dysfunction, type III. Dig Dis Sci 1999;44:631–6.
123. Abraham HD, Anderson C, Lee D. Somatization disorder in sphincter of Oddi dysfunction. Psychosom Med 1997;59:553–7.
124. Evans PR, Dowsett JF, Kak YT, et al. Abnormal sphincter of Oddi response to cholecystokinin in post-cholecystectomy syndrome patients with irritable bowel syndrome: the "irritable sphincter". Dig Dis Sci 1995;40:1149–56.
125. Wald A. Functional biliary-type pain: update and controversies. J Clin Gastroenterol 2005;39:S217–22.
126. Chen JW, Saccone GT, Toouli J. Sphincter of Oddi dysfunction and acute pancreatitis. Gut 1998;43:305–8.
127. Kuo WH, Pasricha PJ, Kalloo AN. The role of sphincter of Oddi manometry in the diagnosis and therapy of pancreatic disease. Gastrointest Endosc Clin North Am 1998;8:79–85.
128. Choudari CP, Fogel EL, Sherman S, et al. Idiopathic pancreatitis: yield of ERCP correlated with patient age. Am J Gastroenterol 1998;93:1654A.
129. Venu RP, Geenen JE, Hogan W, et al. Idiopathic recurrent pancreatitis: an approach to diagnosis and treatment. Dig Dis Sci 1989;34:56–60.
130. Toouli J, Roberts-Thomson IC, Dent J, et al. Sphincter of Oddi motility disorders in patients with idiopathic recurrent pancreatitis. Br J Surg 1985;72:859–63.
131. Guelrud M, Mendoz S, Viera L. Idiopathic recurrent pancreatitis and hypercontractile sphincter of Oddi: treatment with endoscopic sphincterotomy and pancreatic duct dilation [abstract]. Gastroenterology 1986;90:1443.
132. Gregg JA. Function and dysfunction of the sphincter of Oddi. In: Jacobson IM, editor. ERCP: diagnostic and therapeutic applications. New York: Elsevier; 1989. p. 137–70.
133. Sherman S, Jamidar P, Reber H. Idiopathic acute pancreatitis (IAP): endoscopic diagnosis and therapy. Am J Gastroenterol 1993;88:1541A.
134. Kaw M, Brodmerkel GJ. ERCP, biliary crystal analysis, and sphincter of Oddi manometry in idiopathic pancreatitis. Gastrointest Endosc 2002;55:157–62.
135. Coyle WJ, Pineau BC, Tarnasky PR, et al. Evaluation of unexplained acute and acute recurrent pancreatitis using endoscopic retrograde cholangiopancreatography, sphincter of Oddi manometry, and endoscopic ultrasound. Endoscopy 2002;34:617–23.
136. Fischer M, Hassan A, Sipe BW, et al. Endoscopic retrograde cholangiopancreatography and manometry findings in 1,241 idiopathic pancreatitis patients. Pancreatology 2010;10:444–52.
137. Tarnasky PR, Hawes RH. Endoscopic diagnosis and therapy of unexplained (idiopathic) acute pancreatitis. Gastrointest Endosc Clin North Am 1998;8:13–37.
138. Ros E, Navarro S, Bru C, et al. Occult microlithiasis in "idiopathic" acute pancreatitis: prevention of relapses by cholecystectomy or ursodeoxycholic acid therapy. Gastroenterology 1991;101:1701–9.
139. Elta GH. Sphincter of Oddi dysfunction and bile duct microlithiasis in acute idiopathic pancreatitis. World J Gastroenterol 2008;14:1023–6.
140. Lans JL, Parikh NP, Geenen JE. Applications of sphincter of Oddi manometry in routine clinical investigations. Endoscopy 1991;23:139–43.
141. Guelrud M, Plaz J, Mendoza S, et al. Endoscopic treatment in Type II pancreatic sphincter dysfunction. Gastrointest Endosc 1995;41:A398.

142. Wehrmann T. Long-term results (≥ 10 years) of endoscopic therapy for sphincter of Oddi dysfunction in patients with acute recurrent pancreatitis. Endoscopy 2011;43(3):202–7.

143. Toouli J, Francesco V, Saccone G, et al. Division of sphincter of Oddi for treatment of dysfunction associated with recurrent pancreatitis. Br J Surg 1996;83:1205–10.

144. Okolo PI, Pasricha PJ, Kalloo AN. What are the long-term results of endoscopic pancreatic sphincterotomy. Gastrointest Endosc 2000;52:15–9.

145. Jacob L, Geenen JE, Catalano MF, et al. Prevention of pancreatitis in patients with idiopathic recurrent pancreatitis: a prospective nonblinded randomized study using endoscopic stents. Endoscopy 2001;33:559–62.

146. Testoni PA, Caporuscio S, Bagnolo F, et al. Idiopathic recurrent pancreatitis: long-term results after ERCP, endoscopic sphincterotomy, or ursodeoxycholic acid treatment. Am J Gastroenterol 2000;95:1702–7.

147. Wehrmann T, Schmitt TH, Arndt A, et al. Endoscopic injection of botulinum toxin in patients with recurrent acute pancreatitis due to pancreatic sphincter of Oddi dysfunction. Aliment Pharmacol Ther 2000;14:1469–77.

148. Steinberg WM. Controversies in clinical pancreatology: should the sphincter of Oddi be measured in patients with idiopathic recurrent acute pancreatitis, and should sphincterotomy be performed if the pressure is high? Pancreas 2003;27(2):118–21.

149. Tan D, Sherman S. After all these years of SOD and endotherapy–how far have we come? The role of endoscopic treatment for acute recurrent pancreatitis (ARP) with sphincter of Oddi dysfunction (SOD). Endoscopy 2011;43(3):230–2.

150. Mark DH, Lefevre F, Flamm CR, et al. Evidence-based assessment of ERCP in the treatment of pancreatitis. Gastrointest Endosc 2002;56(Suppl 6):S249–54.

151. Coté GA, Imperiale TF, Schmidt SE, et al. Similar efficacies of biliary, with or without pancreatic, sphincterotomy in treatment of idiopathic recurrent acute pancreatitis. Gastroenterology 2012;143(6):1502–9.

152. Botoman VA, Kozarek RA, Novell LA, et al. Long term outcome after endoscopic sphincterotomy in patients with biliary colic and suspected sphincter of Oddi dysfunction. Gastrointest Endosc 1994;40:165–70.

153. Bozkurt T, Orth KH, Butsch B, et al. Long-term clinical outcome of post-cholecystectomy patients with biliary-type pain: Results of manometry, non-invasive techniques and endoscopic sphincterotomy. Eur J Gastroenterol Hepatol 1996;8:245–9.

154. Wehrmann T, Wiemer K, Lembcke B, et al. Do patients with sphincter of Oddi dysfunction benefit from endoscopic sphincterotomy? A 5-year prospective trial. Eur J Gastroenterol Hepatol 1996;8:251–6.

Endoscopic Ultrasonographic Access and Drainage of the Common Bile Duct

Savreet Sarkaria, MD, Subha Sundararajan, MD, Michel Kahaleh, MD*

KEYWORDS

- Endoscopic ultrasonography • Endoscopic retrograde cholangiopancreatography
- Rendezvous • Biliary drainage • Biliary obstruction • EUS-guided cholangiography
- EUS-guided biliary drainage • EUS-guided choledochoduodenostomy

KEY POINTS

- When conventional endoscopic retrograde cholangiopancreatography for biliary drainage is not possible, endoscopic ultrasound-guided biliary drainage (EUS-BD) should be considered as an alternative to percutaneous biliary drainage or surgical options.
- EUS-BD can be performed either via a transhepatic approach or an extrahepatic approach, with or without rendezvous.
- This article discusses the evolving role of EUS-BD and reviews the published data that support EUS-BD as an effective and attractive option for biliary drainage when performed in centers with expertise.

INTRODUCTION

Endoscopic retrograde cholangiography (ERCP) is the current standard of care for biliary drainage. When an initial ERCP attempt is unsuccessful, the recommended next step is referral to an expert endoscopist. In expert hands, ERCP is successful in 90% to 98% of patients, with complication rates of less than 10%.[1,2]

Traditionally, patients with failed conventional ERCP were referred for either percutaneous transhepatic biliary drainage (PTBD) or surgical intervention. However, PTBD can be difficult to perform or even contraindicated in patients with obesity, ascites, or intervening structures, such as vasculature or lungs. Complication rates of PTBD range from 10% to 20%, and common complications include cholangitis, bile leak, bleeding, fistula formation, peritonitis, empyema, pneumothorax, and stent occlusion.[3–5] The mortality rate associated with PTBD has been reported to be as high as 6%,[6] and

Division of Gastroenterology & Hepatology, Weill Cornell Medical College, 1305 York Avenue, New York, NY 10021, USA
* Corresponding author. Division of Gastroenterology & Hepatology, Department of Medicine, Weill Cornell Medical College, New York, NY 10021.
E-mail address: mkahaleh@gmail.com

Gastrointest Endoscopy Clin N Am 23 (2013) 435–452
http://dx.doi.org/10.1016/j.giec.2012.12.013
1052-5157/13/$ – see front matter © 2013 Elsevier Inc. All rights reserved.

long-term efficacy was recently questioned. In addition, the external drainage associated with PTBD can lead to significant patient dissatisfaction and a decrease in quality of life; this can be secondary to pain from the external biliary drain, difficulty taking care of the drain, or complications related to infection or leakage.[3–5]

Endoscopic ultrasound-guided biliary drainage (EUS-BD) is a novel and attractive alternative after failed ERCP. Artifon and colleagues[7] found EUS-BD and PTBD to have similar efficacy, complication rates, and costs. EUS-BD has the additional advantage that it can be performed while under the same sedation as attempted ERCP.

Although surgical drainage is reasonably effective, it is associated with 2% to 5% mortality and 17% to 37% morbidity.[8] Moreover, surgery requires a longer recovery time. In patients with malignant biliary obstruction who already have a poor prognosis and short life expectancy, the invasive nature, longer recovery, and delay in chemotherapy make surgery a less attractive option.

The development of therapeutic linear-array echoendoscopes and the evolution of endoscopic ultrasonography (EUS) from a diagnostic to a therapeutic modality has made EUS an attractive tool in our armamentarium to provide biliary drainage. EUS has been a widely accepted modality for diagnosing and treating many pancreatobiliary diseases for years. The proximity of the stomach and duodenum to the pancreatobiliary tree has allowed high-frequency transducers to provide high-resolution images of the pancreas, pancreatic ducts, bile ducts, and gallbladder.

Contrast injection through the fine-needle aspiration (FNA) needle allows for EUS-guided cholangiography (ESC). Once the cholangiogram has been obtained, ERCP accessories are then used through the working channel of the echoendoscope to complete the procedure and accomplish biliary drainage. ESC therefore represents a hybrid technique that combines EUS-guided FNA and ERCP.

This article discusses the evolving role of EUS-BD and reviews data that support EUS-BD as an effective and attractive option when conventional ERCP for biliary drainage is not possible.

INDICATIONS FOR EUS-GUIDED BILIARY DRAINAGE

Guidelines have not yet been established as to when EUS-BD should be performed. EUS-BD, however, should be considered any time that successful cannulation of the bile duct cannot be achieved via ERCP in the hands of an expert endoscopist. This situation can arise in patients with surgically altered anatomy such as those with Roux-en-Y anatomy, Billroth II anatomy, or postbariatric biliopancreatic diversion. Inability to cannulate the biliary system can also be encountered in patients with gastric-outlet obstruction, tumor infiltration at the level of the duodenum, periampullary diverticula, tortuous bile ducts, impacted stones, or malignancy with bile-duct infiltration.[9–11]

EUS-GUIDED BILIARY DRAINAGE: PROCEDURAL CONSIDERATIONS
Patient Selection and Evaluation

Consent for EUS-BD should be incorporated into the consent for ERCP any time when failed ERCP may be anticipated.

The preprocedure evaluation is similar to that of a standard ERCP, and should include evaluation for cardiopulmonary risk and the use of anticoagulants for coagulation disorders. In addition, the use of general anesthesia should be strongly considered. If the patient is not already on antibiotics to cover biliary pathogens, the authors routinely administer antibiotics both during the procedure and for 7 to 14 days after the procedure, depending on the clinical scenario, adequacy of drainage, and patient course.

Materials and Instruments

It is important to ensure that all required equipment is readily available before puncturing the bile ducts. Once the bile duct has been accessed via EUS, it is crucial to proceed in an expeditious manner without any additional or unnecessary manipulation to reduce the chances of losing access and minimize complications. It is also imperative that the team in the room is familiar with the techniques and instruments used during these procedures so that wires and instruments are successfully exchanged.

1. *Fluoroscopy.* Fluoroscopy equipment should be set up before starting the procedure. Fluoroscopy is needed to evaluate the angle of bile-duct puncture. The fluoroscopy image should be centered with the tip of the scope, bile ducts, and duodenum all in view.
2. *Contrast.* Contrast to perform cholangiography should be available and prefilled in labeled syringes.
3. *Water.* Plenty of water to flush catheters and hydrophilic wires should be in easily accessible containers and syringes. Water is much more effective than saline; saline is sticky because of its salt content.
4. *Echoendoscope.* Echoendoscopes with a 3.8-mm working channel (therapeutic echoendoscope) will permit a variety of catheters and stent diameters to be used. In addition, a duodenoscope should be available if there is the possibility of rendezvous technique and conversion to retrograde procedure.
5. CO_2 should be used for insufflation to decrease barotrauma.
6. *FNA needles.* 19-gauge FNA needles are preferred over 22-gauge needles because they allow manipulation of 0.035-in guide wires.
7. *Guide wires.* Hydrophilic 0.035-in guide wires are preferred because of their ease of manipulation and ability to support a variety of catheters and stents. In addition, it is important to use uncoated wires, when possible, because of the "shearing" effect that the FNA needle can have on the coating of the guide wire.
8. *Dilation.* It is preferable to have both 4 - to 6-mm wire-guided dilating balloons and 6F to 7F dilating bougie catheters.
9. *Sphincterotome.* A rotatable sphincterotome or bending catheter should be available if the wire needs to be redirected to facilitate transpapillary passage of wire.
10. *Stents.* Appropriate stent selection is crucial for adequate biliary drainage and fewer complications. Refer to the later discussion regarding placement of plastic versus self-expanding metal stents (SEMS).

Techniques

Choice of approach

EUS-BD is typically performed using either the EUS-guided rendezvous technique followed by conversion to ERCP, with placement of transpapillary stent in retrograde fashion, or by creating a tract from either the stomach or the duodenum into the bile ducts and placing a stent in an antegrade fashion. When the duodenoscope can be advanced to the ampulla, it is preferable to attempt an EUS-guided rendezvous procedure.

EUS-guided rendezvous

This approach can only be used when a duodenoscope can be advanced to the second portion of the duodenum. It may be appropriately used after failed ERCP attributable to periampullary diverticula, tortuous bile ducts, impacted stones, or malignancy with bile-duct infiltration. Transpapillary drainage via EUS-BD can be attempted using classic rendezvous, parallel rendezvous,[9] or standard cannulation, without rendezvous, after cholangiography by contrast injection through an EUS needle.[10,11]

In this procedure, under EUS and Doppler guidance a needle is inserted into either the left hepatic or common bile duct. The authors find it helpful to have the echoendoscope in the stomach or duodenal bulb; under fluoroscopic guidance one is then able to visualize the FNA needle pointing caudad before accessing the duct with the FNA needle (**Fig. 1**). This caudad position of the FNA needle facilitates advancing the guide wire distally into the duodenum (**Figs. 2** and **3**).

Once EUS imaging shows insertion into the duct, a syringe is attached to the FNA needle and bile aspiration is performed to confirm position. Contrast injection through the FNA needle provides a cholangiogram. The needle is then flushed with water and the guide wire is inserted through the FNA needle, advanced beyond the ampulla, and into the duodenum. Conventional ERCP in a retrograde fashion is then completed.

The limiting step for any method of transpapillary drainage is guide-wire manipulation. Because the FNA needle is rigid and has a sharp cutting edge, to and fro movements of the needle over the wire may bend or shear the guide wire, which in turn can lead to an inability to further manipulate the wire or thread catheters over the wire. If this happens, both the wire and the needle need to be removed, resulting in loss of access. Furthermore, shearing of the wire can potentially result in parts of the wire and coating becoming displaced and left behind in the equipment or the patient's bile duct.

Hence, it is crucial to flush both the FNA needle and the guide wire with copious amounts of water before inserting the guide wire. In addition, avoiding unnecessary friction between the guide wire and the FNA needle is of paramount importance. When the wire is being advanced, it should be done with enough speed to maximize likelihood of crossing the stricture. If the wire must be pulled back, this should be done cautiously and aborted at the moment any resistance is met.

To facilitate passing the guide wire into the duodenum, EUS and fluoroscopy should be used to select a site and position as distal as possible in the bile duct with a tangential needle orientation to the duct before the actual puncture. Transpapillary wire advancement is much more difficult from an intrahepatic puncture, as the wire may

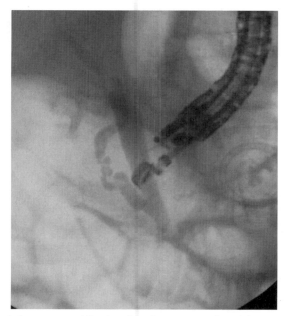

Fig. 1. Puncture of the common bile duct by ultrasonography with contrast injection.

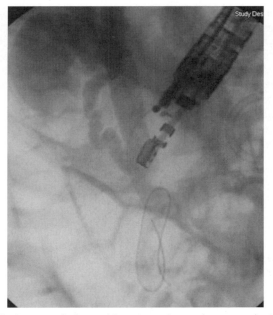

Fig. 2. Fluoroscopic image of the guide wire advanced antegrade into the common bile duct.

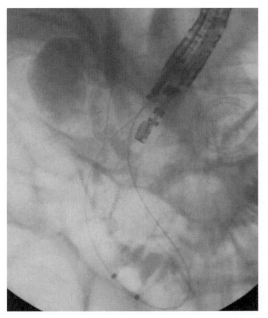

Fig. 3. Fluoroscopic image of a retrieval balloon advanced across the distal biliary stricture in the duodenum.

go peripherally into another branch of the left intrahepatic ducts or into the right-lobe ducts. With intrahepatic duct puncture, passage of the transpapillary guide wire often requires dilation of the puncture tract to allow intraductal passage of catheters or sphincterotomes. Once the wire is in the bile duct, if transpapillary passage is not achieved, the FNA needle should be exchanged for a sphincterotome or dilating bougie. At this point, the wire can be manipulated back and forth safely to facilitate passage beyond the ampulla.

In this rendezvous technique the echoendoscope is removed, with the FNA needle, still attached to the biopsy channel and guide wire, left in place (**Fig. 4**). The assistant feeds the wire into the needle at the same rate that the endoscopist removes the scope and needle assembly. The position of the guide wire is monitored fluoroscopically to prevent both looping in the stomach and dislodgment of the transpapillary looped wire. It is helpful to have at least 3 to 5 large loops of guide wire in the small bowel to ensure that transpapillary access is maintained.

After the echoendoscope is removed, a duodenoscope is advanced side by side with the guide wire while the assistant holds the wire under gentle traction from the patient's mouth to prevent looping. In the classic rendezvous technique, once the papilla is reached with the duodenoscope (or a longer endoscope in patients with altered anatomy), the transpapillary guide wire can be grasped with a polypectomy snare and retrieved through the working channel for subsequent over-the-wire cannulation. Standard ERCP catheters can then be threaded over the wire once it has exited from the endoscope channel. The procedure can then be converted and completed by conventional ERCP with stent placement in a retrograde manner (**Fig. 5**).

Alternatively, the guide wire can be left in place, the echoendoscope can be removed, and a duodenoscope can be used to cannulate next to the previously placed guide wire, in a parallel rendezvous technique. In the parallel rendezvous technique, once the duodenoscope reaches the papilla, a sphincterotome is used to cannulate the bile duct alongside the ESC-placed wire.

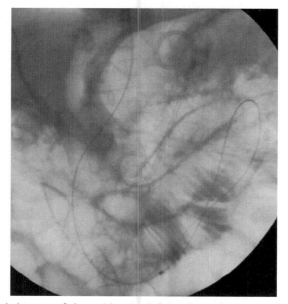

Fig. 4. Fluoroscopic images of the guide wire left in place after removal of the echoendoscope, to permit a rendezvous.

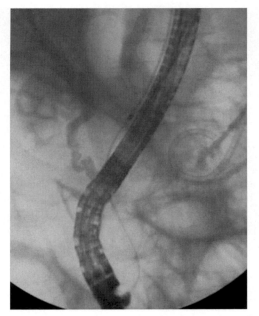

Fig. 5. Fluoroscopic images of the guide wire pulled in the working channel of the duode-noscope advanced into the duodenum.

If the guide wire cannot be advanced beyond the ampulla and into the duodenum, a transenteric tract must be created into the bile duct. This action can be accomplished by dilating over the guide wire with a 4- to 6-mm wire-guided balloon catheter or a 6F to 7F dilating bougie followed by stent placement in an anterograde manner.

A third approach, which is less commonly performed, is contrast injection via EUS followed by standard cannulation ERCP. This method obtains a cholangiogram, via the EUS FNA needle, that provides a road map for cannulation. In addition, the injection of contrast either may make a patulous papilla more evident (eg, an intradiverticular papilla) or the pressure created by the flow of contrast may open the biliary orifice. Furthermore, as has been described for minor papilla cannulation, combining contrast with methylene blue may be of additional benefit with bile-duct cannulation.[12]

Transmural drainage: EUS-guided choledochoduodenostomy and hepaticogastrostomy

When the transpapillary approach cannot be accomplished with the EUS-guided rendezvous, either the transgastric-transhepatic (intrahepatic) or transenteric-transcholedochal (extrahepatic) approach must be used. In these cases, a tract between the digestive tract and bile ducts is created by performing either an EUS-guided choledochoduodenostomy (EUS-CDS) or an EUS-guided hepaticogastrostomy (EUS-HGS).

The intrahepatic approach is performed via the neighboring gastrointestinal tract (usually the cardia or in the lesser curvature of the stomach) to allow visualization of the left intrahepatic bile ducts. After checking local vasculature with color flow Doppler (**Fig. 6**), the EUS needle is then advanced into an intrahepatic duct (**Fig. 7**). This maneuver is followed once again by bile aspiration, cholangiogram, and advancement of the guide wire with fluoroscopic guidance across the ampulla and into the duodenum (**Figs. 8–10**). Then, in an antegrade manner, a 6F or 7F bougie or dilating

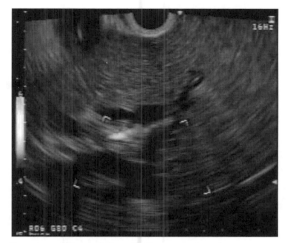

Fig. 6. Color flow Doppler of the left liver before puncture.

catheter is inserted over the guide wire to dilate the tract (**Fig. 11**) followed by antegrade stent deployment with drainage into the stomach (**Figs. 12** and **13**).

In the extrahepatic approach, the echoendoscope is typically advanced into the duodenum and the EUS needle is inserted directly into the common bile duct (see **Fig. 1**). The guide wire is then advanced in an antegrade fashion across the ampulla and into the duodenum (see **Figs. 2** and **3**). From this point, the remainder of the procedure is performed in the same way as the intrahepatic approach, with deployment of the stent in the duodenum.

Choice of plastic versus metal stent

Both plastic and metal stents have been used during EUS-BD. Initially plastic stents were primarily used,[11,13–26] but more recently reported cases have been published using SEMS.[7,11,13,16,18–20,22,24,27–31] These studies have included placement of uncovered, partially covered, and fully covered SEMS, as well as plastic stents within SEMS and fully covered SEMS within uncovered SEMS.[32]

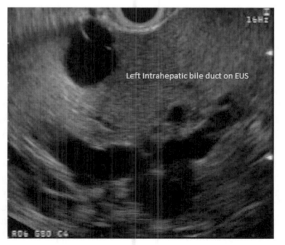

Fig. 7. Endoscopic ultrasonogram of the left hepatic duct before puncture.

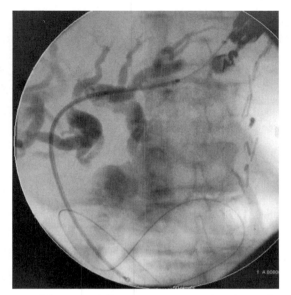

Fig. 12. Advancement of the stent delivery system across the obstruction.

complications with precut papillotomy.[33] Complications that are more specific or more likely to occur with EUS-BD include pneumoperitoneum with or without bile peritonitis, and possibly bleeding from creation or dilation of the biliary enteric tract. Overall complication rates for EUS-BD in the literature range from 10% to 36%.[11–43] Major complications requiring surgery, however, are far less common.

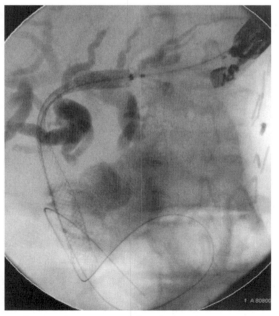

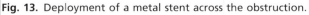

Fig. 13. Deployment of a metal stent across the obstruction.

Table 1
Published data on EUS-BD with extrahepatic approach

Authors,[Ref.] Year	No./ Total Sample	Method	Disease	Approach	Initial Stent	Success Rate (%)	Complication
Giovannini et al,[21] 2001	1	Direct (1)	Malig. (1)	Duodenum	PS (1)	100	None
Burmester et al,[15] 2003	3	Direct (3)	Malig. (3)	Duodenum (2), Jejunum (1)	PS (3)	66.6	Bile leak (1)
Mallery et al,[30] 2004	2	Rendezvous (2)	Malig. (2)	Duodenum (2)	SEMS (2)	100	None
Lai and Freeman,[31] 2005	1	Rendezvous (1)	Malig. (1)	Duodenum (1)	SEMS (1)	100	None
Puspok et al,[16] 2005	6	Direct (6)	Malig. (5), Benign (1)	Duodenum (5), Jejunum (1)	PS (5), SEMS (1)	83	Subacute phlegmonous cholecystitis (1)
Kahaleh et al,[19] 2006	10	Direct (2), rendezvous (7)	Malig. (8), Benign (2)	Duodenum (5), Jejunum (5)	PS (4), SEMS (5)	90	Bile leak (1), pneumoperitoneum (2)
Will et al,[18] 2007	8	Direct (8)	Malig. (7), Benign (1)	Stomach (4), Jejunum (3), Esophagus (1)	PS (2), SEMS (5)	88	Slight pain (2), cholangitis (1)
Tarantino et al,[17] 2008	8	Direct (4), rendezvous (4)	Malig. (7), Benign (1)	Duodenal (8)	PS (8)	100	None
Yamao et al,[14] 2008	5	Direct (5)	Malig. (5)	Duodenal (5)	PS (5)	100	Pneumoperitoneum (1)
Brauer et al,[11] 2009	12	Direct (4), rendezvous (7)	Malig. (8), Benign (4)	N/A	PS (5), SEMS (5)	92	Pneumoperitoneum (1), respiratory failure (1)
Hanada et al,[23] 2009	4	Direct (4)	Malig. (4)	Duodenal (4)	PS (4)	100	None
Horaguchi et al,[22] 2009	9	N/A	Malig. (9)	Duodenal (8), Stomach (1)	PS (15), Nasobiliary tube (1)	100	Peritonitis (1)

Study	N	Approach	Type	Location	Stent	Success (%)	Complications
Maranki et al,[39] 2009	14	Direct (6), rendezvous (8)	Malig. (9), Benign (5)	N/A	N/A	86	Biliary peritonitis (1), abdominal pain and pneumoperitoneum (1)
Kim et al,[24] 2010	15	Rendezvous (15)	Malig. (10), Benign (5)	Duodenum (15)	PS (4), SEMS (8)	80	Pancreatitis (1)
Nguyen-Tang et al,[27] 2010	1	Rendezvous (1)	Malig. (1)	N/A	SEMS (1)	100	None
Park et al,[20,a] 2011	26	Direct (26)	Malig. (51), Benign (6)[b]	Duodenum (26)	PS (12), SEMS (12)	92	Pneumoperitoneum (6), mild bleeding (2)
Fabbri et al,[28] 2011	16	Direct (13), rendezvous (3)	Malig. (16)	Duodenum (15), Stomach (1)	SEMS (12)	75	Pneumoperitoneum (1)
Hara et al,[25,a] 2011	18	Direct (18)	Malig. (18)	N/A	PS (17)	94	Peritonitis (2), bleeding (1)
Ramirez-Luna et al,[26] 2011	9	Direct (9)	Malig. (9)	Duodenum (9)	PS (9)	89	Biloma (1)
Kim et al,[29] 2012	9	Direct (9)	Malig. (9)	Duodenum (9)	SEMS (9)	100	Pneumoperitoneum (1), migration (1), mild peritonitis (1)
Dhir et al,[43] 2012	58	Rendezvous (58)	Malig. (43), Benign (15)		SEMS (13)	98.3	Pericholedochal contrast medium leak (2)
Artifon et al,[7] 2012	13	Direct (13)	Malig. (13)	Duodenum (13)	SEMS (13)	100	Mild bleeding (1), bile leak (1)

Abbreviations: Malig, malignant; N/A, no data available; PS, plastic stents; SEMS, self-expanding metal stents.

[a] Prospective study.

[b] Malig. and Benign in Park and colleagues[20] reflect total numbers for intrahepatic and extrahepatic approach.

EUS-BD requires manipulation of the gastrointestinal tract wall integrity and the creation of a tract to directly gain access to the hepatobiliary system. This procedure can result in pneumoperitoneum and leakage of bile. Less commonly, biloma, pneumoperitoneum, or bile peritonitis can occur, although they are usually asymptomatic. Theoretically, placing a stent should help minimize this risk by sealing the tract. Although there are some data in the literature to support this proposal, further studies evaluating the different types of stents and their success are still needed. Pneumoperitoneum can usually be managed conservatively if the patient has no signs of peritonitis. Similar to treatment of pneumoperitoneum seen after percutaneous endoscopic gastrostomy (PEG) tube placement and laparoscopy, the authors use CO_2 insufflation during ERCP to minimize the effects of pneumoperitoneum.

As with conventional ERCP, bleeding can be related to sphincterotomy, but specifically with EUS-BD bleeding can also arise from transmural FNA needle instrumentation. In addition, the use of cautery can increase the risk of bleeding and formation of fistulous tracts. Using a needle-knife during ESC has been suggested in one series to be the most significant predictor of complications during EUS-BD.[33]

The results of published data are summarized in **Tables 1** and **2**.[11–43]

DISCUSSION

The first case of EUS-BD was reported by Wiersema and colleagues[38] in 1996 among 11 patients in whom conventional ERCP failed. Giovannini and colleagues[21] subsequently described the first case of choledochoduodenal fistula with stent placement for biliary decompression in 2003. Since that time, EUS-BD has been shown to be a technically feasible procedure, with approximately 400 cases reported in the literature.[11–43] The overall success rate for EUS-BD in the literature is reported to be approximately 90% (range 75%–100%).[11–43]

As this technique is still evolving, several issues need to be established. At present, it remains uncertain whether the intrahepatic approach or extrahepatic approach is preferable. In clinical practice, because of anatomic constraints and the level of obstruction, typically only a single EUS access site is possible in approximately 80% of biliary cases, allowing a choice between intrahepatic and extrahepatic bileduct puncture only in about 20% or fewer of cases. The choice between an intrahepatic or extrahepatic approach is based on multiple factors including: access to the duodenum, degree of dilation of the left intrahepatic bile ducts, presence of ascites, and level of the obstruction based on preprocedure cross-sectional imaging. Patient anatomy and operator preference and skill are also important when considering the drainage approach.

The authors' group demonstrated that the extrahepatic approach carried a greater risk of complications compared with the intrahepatic approach, mainly in terms of bile leakage. The results in **Tables 1** and **2**, however, suggest that the extrahepatic approach has higher success rates without additional risk. The authors believe that the duodenal (transbulbar) route is easier and safer because the distance between the duodenum and the bile duct is short, the duodenal wall is thin and without any major intervening vascular structures, and the direction of the puncture is caudad. Recently Kim and colleagues[24] also found the transduodenal approach to be safer and more effective. It is clear that more studies are needed to evaluate this further.

Itoi and colleagues[35] reported that the limitations of the intrahepatic approach technique included: (1) nonapposed gastric wall and left liver lobe, resulting in the possibility of procedure failure; (2) risk of mediastinitis with a transesophageal

Table 2
Published data on EUS-BD with intrahepatic approach

Authors,[Ref.] Year	No./Total Sample	Method	Disease	Approach	Initial Stent	Success Rate (%)	Complication
Burmester et al,[15] 2003	1	Direct (1)	Malig. (1)	Stomach (1)	PS (1)	100	Bile leak (1)
Kahaleh et al,[19] 2006	13	Direct (1), rendezvous (12)	Malig. (9), Benign (4)	Stomach (13)	PS (6), SEMS (6)	92	Minor bleeding (1)
Bories et al,[13] 2007	11	Direct (9), Transpapillary (2)	Malig. (3), Benign (8)	Stomach (3), Duodenal (3), Stenosis (5)	PS (7), SFMS (3)	91	Transient ilcus (1), biloma (1), cholangitis (1)
Horaguchi et al,[22] 2009	7	N/A	Malig. (7)	Stomach (5), esophagus (2)	PS (2), SEMS (5)	100	None
Maranki et al,[39] 2009	35	Direct (9), Transpapillary (24)	Malig. (26), Benign (9)	N/A	N/A	83	Self-resolving bleeding (1), pneumoperitoneum (3), aspiration pneumonia (1)
Nguyen-Tang et al,[27] 2010	4	Rendezvous (4)	Malig. (3), Benign (1)	Duodenum (1), Stomach (3)	SEMS (5)	100	None
Park et al,[20,a] 2011	31	Direct (31)	Malig. (51), Benign (6)[b]	Stomach (31)	PS (6), SEMS (25)	100	Pneumoperitoneum (1), Bile peritonitis (2)
Ramirez-Luna et al,[26] 2011	2	Direct (2)	Malig. (2)	Stomach (2)	PS (2)	100	Stent migration (1)
Kim et al,[29] 2012	4	Direct (4)	Malig. (4)	Stomach (4)	SEMS (4)	75	Mild peritonitis (1), stent migration (1)

Abbreviations: Malig, malignant; PS, plastic stents; SEMS, self-expanding metal stents.
[a] Prospective study.
[b] Malig. and Benign in Park and colleagues[20] 2011 reflect total numbers for intrahepatic and extrahepatic approach.

approach; (3) difficulty of puncture in the case of liver cirrhosis; and (4) risk of injuring the portal vein with use of small-caliber stents or SEMS with a small-diameter delivery.

The appropriate indications for EUS-BD require evaluation. At present, most literature supports considering EUS-BD when conventional ERCP methods fail. The aspects of what falls under conventional ERCP are being evaluated, including the issue of precut papillotomy, as this technique is associated with a risk of post-ERCP pancreatitis. Dhir and colleagues[43] published a retrospective series of cases in which EUS-guided rendezvous was performed in patients who failed selective cannulation (ie, with wire and sphincterotome only, and no precut technique) in comparison with patients who had precut papillotomy performed. EUS-guided rendezvous access in patients with distal biliary obstruction was found to have a higher success rate than precut papillotomy for single-session biliary access (98% vs 90.3%; $P = .03$), with no significant difference in terms of complications. More prospective studies are needed to evaluate the role of EUS-BD.

Consensus agreements to define the role and indications for ESC and EUS-BD techniques are also needed. Meetings were held for the first time during Digestive Disorders Week in Chicago in 2011 and again in San Diego in 2012.

SUMMARY

The high success rates reported in the literature would indicate that EUS-BD is a technically feasible and effective procedure when performed by endoscopists highly skilled in both EUS and ERCP at tertiary care and expert centers. This technique offers a clear alternative to both the percutaneous and surgical approaches in patients in whom conventional ERCP is unsuccessful or not possible. ESC holds promise as a technique for gaining access and draining the bile ducts when conventional ERCP has failed.

Further clinical trials are needed to more comprehensively evaluate the techniques used during EUS-BD, including which types of stents should be placed, and to evaluate complications associated with EUS-BD. In addition, consensus regarding the following questions is also needed: what nomenclature to use, how training should be offered, how to capture all cases performed, how to grant privileges, and how to secure reimbursement.

REFERENCES

1. Huibregtse KM. Endoscopic retrograde cholangiopancreatography, endoscopic sphincterotomy and endoscopic biliary and pancreatic drainage. In: Yamada T, editor. Textbook of gastroenterology. Philadelphia: J.B. Lippincott; 1995. p. 2590–617.
2. Baron TH, Petersen BT, Mergener K, et al. Quality indicators for endoscopic retrograde cholangiopancreatography. Gastrointest Endosc 2006;63:S29–34.
3. Lameris JS, Stoker J, Nijs HG, et al. Malignant biliary obstruction: percutaneous use of self-expandable stents. Radiology 1991;179(3):703–7.
4. Beissert M, Wittenberg G, Sandstede J, et al. Metallic stents and plastic endoprostheses in percutaneous treatment of biliary obstruction. Z Gastroenterol 2002;40(7):503–10.
5. Yee AC, Ho CS. Complications of percutaneous biliary drainage: benign vs malignant diseases. AJR Am J Roentgenol 1987;148:1207–9.
6. van Delden OM, Lameris JS. Percutaneous drainage and stenting for palliation of malignant bile duct obstruction. Eur Radiol 2008;18:448–56.

7. Artifon E, Aparicio D, Paione JB, et al. Biliary drainage in patients with unresectable, malignant obstruction where ERCP fails: endoscopic ultrasonography-guided choledochoduodenostomy versus percutaneous drainage. J Clin Gastroenterol 2012;46:763–74.

8. Sohn TA, Lillemoe KD, Cameron JL, et al. Surgical Palliation of unresecatable periampullary adenocarcinoma in the 1990's. J Am Coll Surg 1999;188:658–66.

9. Dickey W. Paralleled cannulation technique at ERCP rendezvous. Gastrointest Endosc 2006;63:686–7.

10. Kahaleh M, Yoshida C, Kare L, et al. Interventional EUS cholangiography: a report of five cases. Gastrointest Endosc 2004;60:138–42.

11. Brauer BC, Chen YK, Fukami N, et al. Single-operator EUS-guided cholangiopancreatography for difficult pancreatobiliary access (with video). Gastrointest Endosc 2009;70:471–9.

12. Dewitt J, McHenry L, Fogel E, et al. EUS-guided methylene blue pancreatography for minor papilla localization after unsuccessful ERCP. Gastrointest Endosc 2004;59:133–6.

13. Bories E, Pseenti C, Caillol F, et al. Transgastric endoscopic ultrasonography-guided biliary drainage: results of a pilot study. Endoscopy 2007;39:287–91.

14. Yamao K, Bhatia V, Mizuno N, et al. EUS-guided choledochoduodenostomy for palliative biliary drainage in patients with malignant biliary obstruction: results of long term follow up. Endoscopy 2008;40:340–2.

15. Burmester E, Niehaus J, Leineweber T, et al. EUS-cholangio-drainage of the bile duct: report of 4 cases. Gastrointest Endosc 2003;57:246–51.

16. Puspok A, Lomoschitz F, Dejaco C, et al. Endoscopic ultrasound guided therapy of benign and malignant biliary obstruction: a case series. Am J Gastroenterol 2005;100:1743–7.

17. Tarantino I, Barresi L, Repici A, et al. EUS-guided biliary drainage: a case series. Endoscopy 2008;40:336–9

18. Will U, Thieme A, Fueldner F, et al. Treatment of biliary obstruction in selected patients by endoscopic ultrasonography (EUS)-guided transluminal biliary drainage. Endoscopy 2007;39:292–5.

19. Kahaleh M, Hernandez AJ, Tokar J, et al. Interventional EUS-guided cholangiography: evaluation of a technique in evolution. Gastrointest Endosc 2006;64:52–9.

20. Park do H, Jang JW, Lee SS, et al. EUS-guided biliary drainage with transluminal stenting after failed ERCP: predictors of adverse events and long-term results. Gastrointest Endosc 2011;74:1276–84.

21. Giovannini M, Mourardier V, Pesenti C, et al. Endoscopic ultrasound-guided bilioduodenal anastomosis: a new technique for biliary drainage. Endoscopy 2001; 33:898–900.

22. Horaguchi J, Fujita N, Noda Y, et al. Endosonography-guided biliary drainage in cases with difficult transpapillary endoscopic biliary drainage. Dig Endosc 2009; 21:239–44.

23. Hanada K, Iiboshi T, Ishii Y. Endoscopic ultrasound-guided choledochoduodenostomy for palliative biliary drainage in cases with inoperable pancreas head carcinoma. Dig Endosc 2009;21(Suppl 1):S75–8.

24. Kim YS, Gupta K, Mallery S, et al. Endoscopic ultrasound rendezvous for bile duct access using a transduodenal approach: cumulative experience at a single center. A case series. Endoscopy 2010;42:496–502.

25. Hara K, Yamao K, Niwa Y, et al. Prospective clinical study of EUS-guided choledochoduodenostomy for malignant lower biliary tract obstruction. Am J Gastroenterol 2011;106:1239–45.

26. Ramirez-Luna MA, Tellez-Avila FI, Giovannini M, et al. Endoscopic ultrasound-guided biliodigestive drainage is a good alternative in patients with unresectable cancer. Endoscopy 2011;43(9):826–30.

27. Nguyen-Tang T, Binmoeller KF, Sanchez-Yague A, et al. Endoscopic Ultrasound (EUS)-guided transhepatic anterograde SEMS placement across malignant biliary obstruction. Endoscopy 2012;42:232–6.

28. Fabbri C, Luigiano C, Fuccio L, et al. EUS-guided biliary drainage with placement of a new partially covered biliary stent for palliation of malignant biliary obstruction: a case series. Endoscopy 2011;43:438–41.

29. Kim TH, Kim SH, Oh HJ, et al. Endoscopic ultrasound-guided biliary drainage with placement of a fully covered metal stent for malignant biliary obstruction. World J Gastroenterol 2012;18(20):2526–32.

30. Mallery S, Matlock J, Freeman ML. EUS-guided rendezvous drainage of obstructed biliary and pancreatic ducts: report of 6 cases. Gastrointest Endosc 2004;59:100–7.

31. Lai R, Freeman ML. Endoscopic ultrasound-guided bile duct access for rendezvous ERCP drainage in the setting of intradiverticular papilla. Endoscopy 2005; 37:487–9.

32. Giovannini M, Bories E. EUS-guided biliary drainage. Gastroenterol Res Pract 2012;2012:348719.

33. Yamao K, Hara K, Mizuno N, et al. EUS- guided biliary drainage. Gut Liver 2010; 4:S67–75.

34. Yamao K, Sawaki A, Takahashi K, et al. EUS-guided choledocholduodenostomy for palliative biliary drainage in case of papillary obstruction: report of 2 cases. Gastrointest Endosc 2006;64:663–7.

35. Itoi T, Itokawa F, Sofuni A, et al. Endoscopic ultrasound-guided choledochoduodenostomy in patients with failed endoscopic retrograde cholangiopancreatography. World J Gastroenterol 2008;14:6078–82.

36. Park do H, Koo JE, Oh J, et al. EUS-guided biliary drainage with one-step placement of a fully covered metal stent for malignant biliary obstruction: a prospective feasibility study. Am J Gastroenterol 2009;104:2168–74.

37. Perez-Miranda M, de la Sema C, Diez-Redondo P, et al. Endosonography-guided cholangiopancreatography as a salvage drainage procedure for obstructed biliary and pancreatic ducts. World J Gastrointest Endosc 2010;2:212–22.

38. Wiersema MJ, Sandusky D, Carr R, et al. Endosonography-guided cholangiopancreatography. Gastrointest Endosc 1996;43:102–6.

39. Maranki J, Hernandez AJ, Arslan B, et al. Interventional endoscopic ultrasound-guided cholangiography: long-term experience of an emerging alternative to percutaneous transhepatic cholangiography. Endoscopy 2009;41:532–8.

40. Fujita N, Noda Y, Kobayashi G, et al. Temporary endosonography-guided biliary drainage for transgastrointestinal deployment of a self-expandable metallic stent. J Gastroenterol 2008;43:637–40.

41. Fujita N, Sugawara T, Noda Y, et al. Snare-over-the-wire technique for safe exchange of a stent following endosonography-guided biliary drainage. Dig Endosc 2009;21:48–52.

42. Itoi T, Sofuni A, Itokawa F, et al. Endoscopic ultrasonography-guided biliary drainage. J Hepatobiliary Pancreat Sci 2010;17:611–6.

43. Dhir V, Bhandari S, Bapat M, et al. Comparison of EUS-guided rendezvous and precut papillotomy techniques for biliary access (with videos). Gastrointest Endosc 2012;75:354–9.

Endoscopic Management of Acute Cholecystitis

Muhammad K. Hasan, MD[a], Takao Itoi, MD[b],
Shyam Varadarajulu, MD[a],*

KEYWORDS

- Endoscopy • Acute cholecystitis • Gallbladder drainage
- Endoscopic ultrasonography • Endoscopic ultrasound guided gallbladder drainage

KEY POINTS

- In high-risk surgical patients with acute cholecystitis, alternative treatment modalities are required for gallbladder decompression.
- For patients in whom temporary decompression is preferred, nasocystic drainage guided by endoscopic retrograde cholangiopancreatography is an effective treatment option.
- For patients who require permanent decompression, transluminal drainage guided by endoscopic ultrasonography is an alternative treatment option.

Cholecystectomy, performed either laparoscopically or through open surgery, is the mainstay of the treatment of acute cholecystitis, which affects nearly 20 million Americans annually.[1] Although the laparoscopic approach is less invasive and is the treatment of choice for a majority of patients, some critically or terminally ill patients may not be able to withstand the morbidity of surgery.[2] Therefore a less invasive procedure, such as percutaneous gallbladder drainage, could be a life-saving treatment option or serve as bridge to elective surgery.[3–7] Percutaneous drainage is technically easy to perform; however, the physical discomfort from the catheter renders this a less desirable option for patients with limited life expectancy from terminal cancer or those patients with contraindications to the procedure.

This article reviews the 2 endoscopic treatment approaches that are feasible for patients with acute cholecystitis, particularly for high-risk surgical candidates who require gallbladder decompression: (1) transpapillary drainage of the gallbladder at endoscopic retrograde cholangiopancreatography (ERCP) by nasocystic catheter or stent placement; and (2) endoscopic ultrasonography (EUS)-guided gallbladder drainage via the transluminal route.

a Center for Interventional Endoscopy, Florida Hospital, 601 East Rollins Street, Orlando, FL 32803, USA; b Department of Gastroenterology and Hepatology, Tokyo Medical University, 6-7-1 Nishishinjuku, Shinjuku-ku, Tokyo 160-0023, Japan
* Corresponding author.
E-mail address: svaradarajulu@yahoo.com

Gastrointest Endoscopy Clin N Am 23 (2013) 453–459
http://dx.doi.org/10.1016/j.giec.2012.12.010

PROCEDURAL INDICATIONS AND CHOICE OF TECHNIQUE

Endoscopic decompression of the gallbladder is usually attempted only when standard treatment options fail or are contraindicated. Specifically, endoscopic decompression is considered in patients with acute or acalculous cholecystitis who (1) are critically ill or have severe comorbidity that precludes a surgical cholecystectomy and/or (2) have contraindications for placement of a percutaneous cholecystostomy tube, such as the presence of large amounts of ascites, hypercoagulopathy, or an intervening loop of bowel between the diaphragm and the liver that precludes percutaneous access. Endoscopic management is contraindicated, however, in patients (1) with perforated gallbladder, (2) who are too unstable to undergo endoscopy or sedation, or (3) who are pregnant, because of the risks of radiation exposure from a prolonged procedure.

For patients who require only temporary gallbladder decompression as a bridge to elective surgery, transpapillary drainage by means of stenting or nasocystic catheter placement are effective options.[8–10] The advantage of nasocystic catheters over stents is that they can be flushed periodically, whereas stents tend to clog easily. On the other hand, nasocystic catheters, unlike stents, are prone to dislodgment and can be a source of physical discomfort to patients. Some experts advocate the deployment of nasocystic catheters as a temporizing measure followed by placement of transpapillary internal stents as a bridge to elective surgery.[8] For patients who require a more definitive treatment, such as high-risk surgical candidates, EUS-guided transluminal drainage of the gallbladder by means of internal stenting could offer permanent palliation.[11]

Transpapillary Gallbladder Drainage

ERCP can aid in gallbladder decompression by facilitating access to the cystic duct.[8–10] After successful cannulation of the common bile duct using an ERCP catheter, a 0.035-inch (0.889 mm) guide wire (stiff or hydrophilic) is advanced into the cystic duct and then the gallbladder (**Fig. 1**). In patients with a difficult cystic duct configuration, the choice of a biliary catheter may vary: for a left-side cystic duct takeoff, a flexible-tip catheter (Swing-tip; Olympus Medical Systems, Tokyo, Japan) or a rotatable sphincterotome may be used; for a right-sided takeoff, a standard sphincterotome may be used because it usually bows toward the cystic duct when it takes off on the right side. Alternatively, the sphincterotome may be advanced deep into the bile duct, bowed, and then withdrawn slowly, so that the tip may position itself into the cystic duct opening on pull-down. When the gallbladder or the cystic duct cannot be opacified because of cholecystitis, a balloon is inflated below the expected takeoff of the cystic duct, and an occlusion cholangiogram obtained to allow cystic duct visualization. Alternatively, the cystic duct can be identified by mere manipulation of the guide wire. In some patients, SpyGlass-assisted cystic duct cannulation has been performed successfully, with good technical outcomes.[12,13] Once the guide wire is advanced and coiled within the gallbladder lumen, the catheter is exchanged for a 5F to 7F pigtail nasocystic drainage tube or a 7F to 10F double-pigtail transpapillary stent. The length of the stent depends on lengths of the cystic duct and gallbladder lumen from the major duodenal papilla. When large-caliber (10F) stents are placed, a biliary sphincterotomy should be performed to minimize the chances of post-ERCP pancreatitis caused by the fulcrum effect.

EUS-Guided Transluminal Gallbladder Drainage

The therapeutic linear-array echoendoscope is used for EUS-guided transgastric/transduodenal gallbladder drainage. The drainage access point chosen is based on

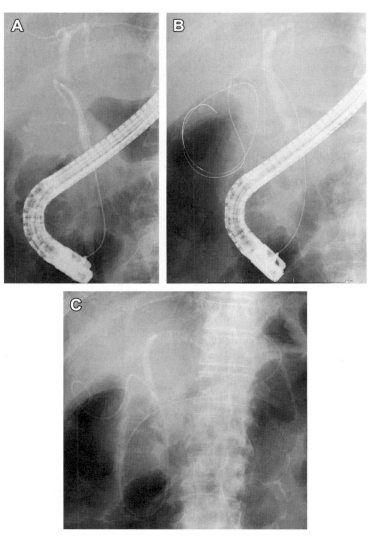

Fig. 1. (*A*) Cholangiogram revealing the cystic duct takeoff and the gallbladder being opacified. (*B*) A 0.035-inch (0.889-mm) stiff guide wire is advanced into the gallbladder lumen. (*C*) A transpapillary nasobiliary drain is deployed within the gallbladder lumen to facilitate drainage.

the smallest distance between the gallbladder and the enteral lumen (gastric antrum or the duodenal bulb). Theoretically, the risk of leakage into the peritoneum can be minimized if inflammatory adhesion exists between the gallbladder and enteral lumen. A 19-gauge needle punctures the gastric or the duodenal wall to access the gallbladder (**Fig. 2**). A 0.035-inch guide wire is then passed through the needle and coiled within the gallbladder lumen. The fine-needle aspiration needle is then exchanged for a needle knife or stiff catheter, which is then advanced over the guide wire into the gallbladder lumen to create a fistula. The transmural tract is then sequentially dilated using a graded dilation catheter or a dilating balloon. To minimize the chances of bile leak, the balloon should not be inflated more than 6 mm. Following dilation,

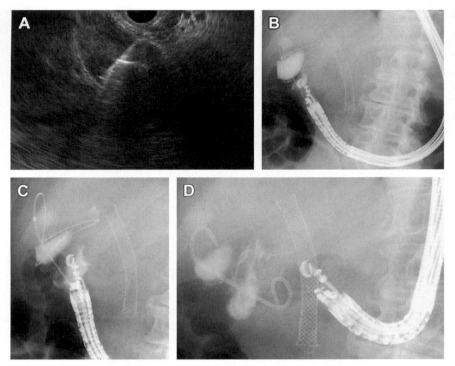

Fig. 2. (*A*) Under EUS guidance, the gallbladder is accessed via the transduodenal route using a 19-gauge fine-needle aspiration needle. (*B*) A 0.035-inch guide wire is coiled within the gallbladder lumen. (*C*) The transluminal tract is sequentially dilated with a catheter to create a fistula. (*D*) A transduodenal double-pigtail stent is deployed within the gallbladder lumen.

a nasocystic catheter, double-pigtail plastic stent, or self-expandable metal stent (SEMS) is deployed to facilitate biliary drainage within the enteral lumen.

A prototype novel lumen-apposing stent (AXIOS; Xlumena Inc, Mountain View, CA) that appears to minimize the risk of bile leakage and SEMS migration has been recently developed.[14] The lumen-apposing stent is a fully covered, 10-mm diameter, nitinol, braided stent with bilateral anchor flanges. The diameter of the flanges, when fully expanded, is twice that of the "saddle" section and is designed to hold the tissue layers in apposition. The stent is delivered constrained through a 10.5F catheter and the delivery system is Luer locked to the proximal end of the biopsy port of the endoscope, which gives the endoscopist control of stent deployment. The handle enables a 2-step release of each flange. The distal flange is first deployed under EUS guidance, followed by proximal traction of the distal flange to place the target lumen in firm apposition to the duodenal or gastric walls. The proximal flange is then deployed under endoscopic guidance. The length of the stent (6 or 10 mm) is determined by the combined thickness of the interposed tissue.

TREATMENT OUTCOMES
ERCP-Assisted Transpapillary Drainage

The pooled technical success rate for the nasocystic drainage-catheter placement technique in 194 patients has been reported to be 80.9%, with a clinical response rate of 75.3%.[10] The pooled technical success rate for the transpapillary gallbladder stenting technique in 127 patients has been reported to be 96%, with a clinical response rate of 88%.[10] In one study, the mean duration to symptom relief after successful endoscopic transpapillary drainage was 5.5 days.[15] The rate of pooled adverse events for both techniques is reported at 4.7% with the incidence varying between 0% and 16%.[10] In a study of 51 patients who underwent endoscopic transpapillary gallbladder drainage (both stenting and drainage-catheter placement), at a mean follow-up of 10 ± 13 months, septic shock was reported in 14% of cases when the stents were left in place as long-term strategy.[16] Although 56% of patients had no recurrence of cholecystitis, 10% of the patients were readmitted for recurrent cholangitis or ongoing symptoms. Other procedure-related adverse events include post-ERCP pancreatitis, perforation of the cystic duct or gallbladder, and sepsis.

EUS-Guided Transluminal Drainage

Reports of studies using plastic stents, nasocystic drainage catheters, SEMS, and prototype lumen-apposing stents for EUS-guided transluminal drainage of the gallbladder have been published. In a study of 8 patients in whom 7F double-pigtail plastic stents were deployed, the treatment was successful in all patients.[17] Two of 8 patients developed complications of bile leak and pneumoperitoneum, which were managed conservatively. Two studies evaluated the use of nasocystic drainage catheters in a total of 38 patients.[10,18] Although the technical and clinical success was reported to be 100%, pneumoperitoneum was observed in 3 patients (10.3%), who were treated conservatively.

A recent study evaluated the technical feasibility and safety of EUS-guided transgastric/transduodenal gallbladder drainage with single-step placement of a modified covered SEMS in 15 patients who were unsuitable for cholecystectomy.[19] The stents were deployed via the transgastric route in 10 patients and via the duodenum in 5. Although the treatment success was 100%, pneumoperitoneum occurred in 2 patients who were treated conservatively. During a median follow-up of 145 days, no patient experienced recurrent cholecystitis.

In another case series of 5 patients with acute cholecystitis, EUS-guided gallbladder drainage was undertaken using the novel tissue-apposing fully covered SEMS that is designed with bilateral anchor flanges.[14] Four patients underwent cholecystoduodenostomy and 1 underwent cholecystogastrostomy. Resolution of acute cholecystitis was observed immediately after stent deployment in all patients, and there was no recurrence of symptoms during a median follow-up period of 9 months.

CONSENSUS APPROACH TO ENDOSCOPIC MANAGEMENT OF ACUTE CHOLECYSTITIS

Endoscopic treatment of acute cholecystitis is a viable and relatively safe option for a select group of patients who are not candidates for surgery or percutaneous drainage. The transpapillary approach is usually a temporizing measure that provides short-term to medium-term palliation or serves as a bridge to surgery. On the other hand, the transluminal drainage technique offers long-term palliation for patients who, because of other comorbidities, may not be surgical candidates. In a recent randomized trial that compared EUS-guided transluminal gallbladder drainage with percutaneous cholecystostomy, both techniques were found to be equivalent in terms of clinical efficacy and safety profile.[11] Patients who underwent EUS-guided transluminal drainage reported significantly less postprocedure pain. Moreover, the intervention did not impede subsequent cholecystectomy in any patient. Despite these recent advances, pneumoperitoneum has been reported in almost every series on transluminal gallbladder drainage. More data are needed to confirm whether the tissue-apposing metal stent will eliminate the risk of pneumoperitoneum in these patients.

REFERENCES

1. Everhart JE, Khare M, Hill M, et al. Prevalence and ethnic differences in gallbladder disease in the United States. Gastroenterology 1999;117:632–9.
2. Csikesz NG, Tseng JF, Shah SA. Trends in surgical management for acute cholecystitis. Surgery 2008;144:283–9.
3. Bakkaloglu H, Yanar H, Guloglu R, et al. Ultrasound guided percutaneous cholecystostomy in high-risk patients for surgical intervention. World J Gastroenterol 2006;12:7179–82.
4. Patterson EJ, McLoughlin RF, Mathieson JR, et al. An alternative approach to acute cholecystitis: percutaneous cholecystostomy and interval laparoscopic cholecystectomy. Surg Endosc 1996;10:1185–8.
5. Chopra S, Dodd GD III, Mumbower AL, et al. Treatment of acute cholecystitis in non-critically ill patients at high surgical risk: comparison of clinical outcomes after gallbladder aspiration and after percutaneous cholecystostomy. AJR Am J Roentgenol 2001;176:1025–31.
6. Ito K, Fujita N, Noda Y, et al. Percutaneous cholecystostomy versus gallbladder aspiration for acute cholecystitis: a prospective randomized controlled trial. AJR Am J Roentgenol 2004;183:193–6.
7. Cherng N, Witkowski ET, Sneider EB. Use of cholecystostomy tubes in the management of patients with primary diagnosis of acute cholecystitis. J Am Coll Surg 2012;214:196–201.
8. Itoi T, Sofuni A, Itokawa F, et al. Endoscopic transpapillary gallbladder drainage in patients with acute cholecystitis in whom percutaneous transhepatic approach is contraindicated or anatomically impossible (with video). Gastrointest Endosc 2008;68:455–60.
9. Feretis C, Apostolidis N, Mallas E, et al. Endoscopic drainage of acute obstructive cholecystitis in patients with increased operative risk. Endoscopy 1993;25:392–5.
10. Itoi T, Coelho-Prabhu N, Baron TH. Endoscopic gallbladder drainage for management of acute cholecystitis. Gastrointest Endosc 2010;71:1038–45.
11. Jang JW, Lee SS, Song TJ, et al. Endoscopic ultrasound-guided transmural and percutaneous transhepatic gallbladder drainage are comparable for acute cholecystitis. Gastroenterology 2012;142:805–11.
12. Barkay O, Bucksot L, Sherman S. Endoscopic transpapillary gallbladder drainage with the SpyGlass cholangiopancreatoscopy system. Gastrointest Endosc 2009;70:1039–40.
13. Chen YK, Pleskow DK. SpyGlass single-operator peroral cholangiopancreatoscopy system for the diagnosis and therapy of bile-duct disorders: a clinical feasibility study (with video). Gastrointest Endosc 2007;65:832–41.
14. Itoi T, Binmoeller KF, Shah J, et al. Clinical evaluation of a novel lumen-apposing metal stent for endosonography-guided pancreatic pseudocyst and gallbladder drainage (with videos). Gastrointest Endosc 2012;75:870–6.
15. Kjaer DW, Kruse A, Funch-Jensen P. Endoscopic gallbladder drainage of patients with acute cholecystitis. Endoscopy 2007;39:304–8.
16. Pannala R, Petersen BT, Gostout CJ, et al. Endoscopic transpapillary gallbladder drainage: 10-year single center experience. Minnerva Gastroenterol Dietol 2008;54:107–13.

17. Song TJ, Park do H, Eum JB, et al. EUS-guided cholecystoenterostomy with single-step placement of a 7F double-pigtail plastic stent in patients who are unsuitable for cholecystectomy: a pilot study (with video). Gastrointest Endosc 2010;71:634–40.
18. Lee SS, Park DH, Hwang CY, et al. EUS-guided transmural cholecystostomy as rescue management for acute cholecystitis in elderly or high-risk patients: a prospective feasibility study. Gastrointest Endosc 2007;66:1008–12.
19. Jang JW, Lee SS, Park do H, et al. Feasibility and safety of EUS-guided transgastric/transduodenal gallbladder drainage with single-step placement of a modified covered self-expandable metal stent in patients unsuitable for cholecystectomy. Gastrointest Endosc 2011;74:176–81.

Endoscopic Approach to the Patient with Bile Duct Injury

John Baillie, MB, ChB, FRCP

KEYWORDS

- Laparoscopic cholecystectomy • Biliary injury • Bile duct leak
- Endoscopic retrograde cholangiopancreatography
- Percutaneous transhepatic cholangiography
- Magnetic resonance cholangiopancreatography • Bismuth classification
- Strasberg classification

KEY POINTS

- The majority of bile duct injuries are iatrogenic, and most commonly follow laparoscopic cholecystectomy (LC).
- Less than one-third of LC-related injuries are identified at the time of surgery.
- If an injury is observed during LC, a drain should be left and the patient urgently referred to a specialist hepatobiliary surgeon for management.
- Patients who develop symptoms suggestive of a bile leak following LC should undergo cross-sectional imaging to check for a contained or free bile collection (which should be drained).
- Complete transection of the bile duct at LC cannot be managed solely by endoscopy; surgical reconstruction after percutaneous drain placement is almost always necessary.

INTRODUCTION

A variety of insults can result in injury to the biliary tree, including blunt and penetrating trauma, radiation, chronic pancreatitis, choledocholithiasis, autoimmune disorders (eg, cholangiopathy, primary sclerosing cholangitis, pancreatitis), interventional radiology, and surgery. This review focuses principally on by far the most common cause, gallbladder surgery (cholecystectomy), the vast majority of which are performed laparoscopically. Data from large population studies indicate that injuries to the biliary tree occur in 0.1% to 0.3% of open and 0.3% to 0.6% of laparoscopic cholecystectomies.[1,2] Bile duct injuries can be classified according to mechanism and type of injury, location, effect on biliary continuity, and the timing of identification. Identification of the location of bile duct injury is critical to successful management. A length of healthy bile duct without ischemia, tension, or loss of length is necessary to ensure

Department of Medical Gastroenterology, Carteret General Hospital, Arendell Street, Morehead City, NC 28557, USA
E-mail address: jbaillie@ccgh.org

Gastrointest Endoscopy Clin N Am 23 (2013) 461–472
http://dx.doi.org/10.1016/j.giec.2013.01.002
1052-5157/13/$ – see front matter © 2013 Elsevier Inc. All rights reserved.

successful repair. Starting in 1982, Bismuth and colleagues[3] classified biliary strictures based on their proximity to the biliary confluence (**Fig. 1** and **Table 1**). In 1995, Strasberg and colleagues[4] expanded on this classification (**Table 2**): they classified injuries by location, mechanism, and results, and separated leaks from strictures (**Fig. 2**). The clinical presentation of bile duct injury is determined by its type and timing. Depending on the nature of the injury, endoscopic therapy alone, principally the placement of plastic biliary stents, may correct the problem. However, complex ductal injuries, especially duct clippings and transections causing vascular injury and arterial ischemia, almost always require surgery, usually after percutaneous drain placement.

Although this review concerns the endoscopic approach to bile duct injury, the endoscopist does not work in isolation when managing these problems: a multidisciplinary approach and a solid understanding of the biliary anatomy and surgical principles involved in managing bile leaks and strictures is essential to their successful resolution.

RECOGNITION OF POSTOPERATIVE BILIARY INJURIES

Less than one-third of iatrogenic biliary injuries are detected at the time of LC.[5] When a bile duct injury is identified at the time of the initial surgery, measures should be taken to try to define its extent. If the level of the injury is clearly defined and the surgeon is comfortable undertaking biliary reconstruction, immediate repair can be performed. However, if there is any question that the anatomy of the injury is unclear, the patient should have a drain placed in the gallbladder fossa and then be referred without delay to a center with an experienced hepatobiliary surgeon. Careful evaluation of the extent of the injury before attempted reconstruction optimizes the chances for favorable outcome. An obvious intraoperative sign of bile duct injury is sudden, unexpected leakage of bile from the liver or soft tissue adjacent to the porta hepatis. Encountering a second duct during cholecystectomy may lure the unsuspecting surgeon into clipping a right posterior duct, which has been wrongly assumed to be a benign accessory duct. If there is any question about the biliary anatomy, an intraoperative cholangiogram should be performed, although this does not always prevent injury. If an immediate repair is not going to be performed for a bile duct injury, immediate conversion to open laparotomy is not indicated; placement of a drain and immediate referral to an experienced hepatobiliary surgeon is appropriate, and may reduce liability.[6]

An important part of the evaluation of any bile duct injury is the identifying the patency of vascular structures. Intraoperative Doppler ultrasonography should be performed to evaluate vascular integrity, because up to one-third of patients who have LC-associated bile duct injury have a concomitant arterial injury. Vascular injury significantly increases morbidity and mortality, and increases the likelihood of later stricture formation.

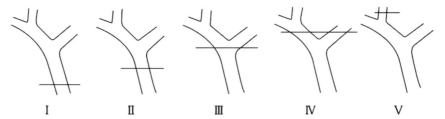

I   II   III   IV   V

Fig. 1. Bismuth classification of biliary strictures. (*From* Jabłońska B, Lampe P. Iatrogenic bile duct injuries: etiology, diagnosis and management. World J Gastroenterol 2009;15(33):4097-104)

Table 1
Bismuth classification of biliary stricture

Type	Criteria
1	Low common hepatic duct stricture with a length of common hepatic duct stump of >2 cm
2	Proximal common hepatic duct stricture with hepatic duct stump <2 cm
3	Hilar stricture, no residual common hepatic duct, but the hepatic ductal confluence is preserved
4	Hilar stricture with involvement of confluence and loss of communication between right and left hepatic duct
5	Involvement of an aberrant right sectoral duct alone or with concomitant stricture of the common hepatic duct

Adapted from Jarnagin WR, Blumgart LH. Benign biliary strictures. In: Blumgart LH, editor. Surgery of the liver, biliary tract, and pancreas. 4th edition. Philadelphia: Saunders; 2007. p. 634; with permission.

There is usually a delay in diagnosing biliary injuries that occur during LC. Affected patients often present with nonspecific symptoms, such as vague abdominal pain and low-grade fever, resulting from uncontrolled bile leakage into the peritoneal cavity. Some patients may present with established sepsis from severe bile peritonitis. Patients who have suffered bile duct ligation or stricture formation may present with jaundice with or without cholangitis. Patients with a significant postoperative bile duct leak may be recognized by bilious drainage from a drain placed during surgery. Leaking bile may form a walled-off collection (a biloma) (**Fig. 3**) or bilious ascites, resulting in bile peritonitis.

ROLE OF VASCULAR INJURY

The outcome of iatrogenic biliary injury is worsened by concomitant arterial injury. The right hepatic artery lies behind the common hepatic duct at the usual level of injury, and is often caught up in it (**Fig. 4**). Injury to the right hepatic artery increases morbidity, and is more commonly seen in Bismuth class III and IV biliary injuries. When nonspecialist primary surgeons attempt repair of damaged right hepatic

Table 2
Strasberg classification of laparoscopic bile duct injury

Type	Criteria
A	Cystic duct leak or leak from small ducts in the liver bed
B	Occlusion of an aberrant right hepatic duct
C	Transection without ligation of an aberrant right hepatic duct
D	Lateral injury to a major bile duct
E1	Transection >2 cm from the hilum
E2	Transection <2 cm from the hilum
E3	Transection in the hilum
E4	Separation of major ducts in the hilum
E5	Type C injury plus injury in the hilum

Modified from Strasberg SM, Hertl M, Soper NJ. An analysis of the problem of biliary injury during laparoscopic cholecystectomy. J Am Coll Surg 1995;180:101–25; with permission.

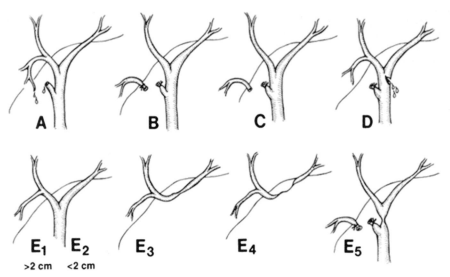

Fig. 2. Strasberg classification of biliary injuries. (*Adapted from* Strasberg SM, Hertl M, Soper NJ. An analysis of the problem of biliary injury during laparoscopic cholecystectomy. J Am Coll Surg 1995;180:101–25; with permission.)

arteries, there is a greater chance of abscess, bleeding (including hemobilia), liver ischemia, and the need for hepatic resection. These repairs should be left to experienced hepatobiliary surgeons.

TRIAGE OF A PATIENT REFERRED TO A SPECIALIST CENTER WITH SUSPECTED BILE DUCT INJURY

Imaging techniques, especially transabdominal ultrasonography and computed tomography (CT), are valuable during the initial evaluation of a patient suspected of

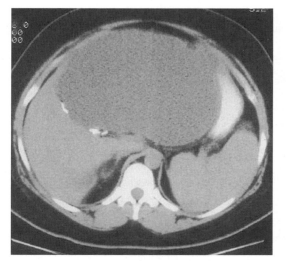

Fig. 3. Abdominal computed tomography scan showing a large, homogeneous fluid collection overlying the liver in a patient with a bile leak, commonly referred to as a biloma.

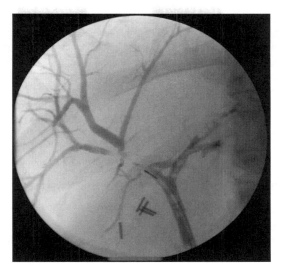

Fig. 4. Endoscopic retrograde cholangiopancreatography (ERCP) showing right-sided intra-hepatic stricturing proximal to the biliary confluence from a surgical injury. This injury is likely to be associated with right hepatic artery damage.

having a biliary injury. The presence of localized fluid collections, or ascites in the peritoneal cavity, suggests the presence of a bile leak. Percutaneous drainage confirms the presence of bile in the fluid, and is a vital part of the initial treatment. It has been the author's personal observation over many years that patients transferred to tertiary centers for urgent endoscopic retrograde cholangiopancreatography (ERCP) to define suspected biliary injuries frequently have not had cross-sectional imaging. Often these patients are no longer under the care of the surgeon who performed their LC; instead, they have returned to an emergency room (sometimes in a different hospital) and have been admitted under a hospitalist on a Medicine service. A surgical consultation may or may not have been obtained, but even if one has, the usual recommendation is to transfer the patient out as soon as possible if iatrogenic biliary injury is suspected. Along the way, cross-sectional imaging of the abdomen is often overlooked. Especially if transfer to a surgical center of excellence involves transportation over a long distance, or other delays supervene, the patient may become septic and be very unwell by the time his or her destination is reached. For this reason, the first question to referring physicians who call requesting transfer of such patients is "What did the abdominal CT scan show?" If the answer is, "We haven't done one," the author insists that transfer is postponed until an urgent CT scan has been performed and any significant intra-abdominal fluid collection drained percutaneously. Ideally such patients should be transferred directly to a Surgery service, but as the calls rarely come from surgeons these patients typically get admitted to Medicine services where hospitalists look after patients admitted for ERCP. Having a patient with a surgical complication admitted to a medical ward is suboptimal management, in the author's opinion, but unfortunately it is the reality faced on a daily basis by those who practice therapeutic endoscopy. It is essential in these circumstances to obtain an early surgical consultation from a hepatobiliary surgeon and not just the duty surgical resident-on-call. The rigid surgical chain of command in large centers can be another obstacle to timely and effective management. If you are the gastroenterologist consulting on the case, you are probably going to have to be "calling the shots" (directing management) until the appropriate surgical specialist gets involved. Ensuring that bile collections are being drained adequately is a priority: a drain that stops draining may be kinked or have become dislodged. Do not assume that the bile leak has sealed off until this is confirmed by further imaging. Patients with suspected bile leaks should be started on broad-spectrum intravenous antibiotics, even if they do not appear septic when they arrive. Daily liver-function tests should be performed to look for evidence of progressive biliary obstruction, coagulation status should be checked and corrected, and volume depletion aggressively managed. If the patients are elderly, their existing comorbidities often add to their morbidity and mortality: loss of diabetic control, worsening renal function, hypoxemia, the onset of heart failure, and confusion all predict poor outcome.

WHAT IMAGING BEYOND ULTRASONOGRAPHY AND CT SCANNING IS HELPFUL?

Hepatobiliary iminodiacetic acid (HIDA) scanning can be helpful in the diagnosis of bile leakage[7]; however, this nuclear medicine study lacks specificity to accurately define biliary anatomy or the level of the leak. HIDA scanning can be useful in the investigation of the symptomatic post-LC patient in whom ultrasonography and/or CT imaging fails to demonstrate an abdominal fluid collection that would typically accompany a bile leak. In such patients the HIDA scan can confirm the presence of a leak, and prompt further evaluation and treatment with ERCP. ERCP can confirm the presence of a biliary injury and provides a way to definitively manage many injuries using temporary internal stents. If complete disruption or occlusion of the bile duct is identified by ERCP, prompt evaluation with percutaneous transhepatic cholangiography (PTC) is necessary to define the proximal biliary anatomy and decompress the biliary system (by percutaneous drain placement) (**Fig. 5**).

Occlusion or transection of an aberrant right hepatic duct (Strasberg injury types B and C) may be especially difficult to diagnose, as ERCP may fail to identify the obstruction or leak and be interpreted as "normal."[8] Careful examination of the ERCP films is required to look for a subtle "missing" duct appearance that results

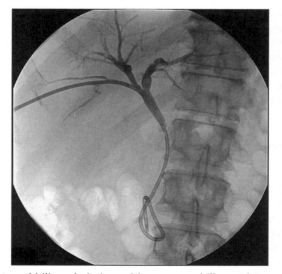

Fig. 5. Internal-external biliary drain in position across a biliary stricture, with its distal tip coiled in the duodenum.

from failure to opacify the posterior segments of the right liver lobe. In the case of a bile leak from an aberrant right hepatic duct not in communication with the common duct (Strasberg type C), a retrograde contrast study by way of a percutaneously placed drain may reveal the injured duct. When these injuries are identified, reconstruction of the isolated segment can be performed with Roux-en-Y hepaticojejunostomy. Noninvasive imaging techniques, such as magnetic resonance cholangiopancreatography (MRCP), can be used to evaluate bile duct injuries. Several small clinical studies have indicated that MRCP can be used postoperatively to classify bile duct injuries, potentially obviating invasive procedures such as ERCP or PTC. CT cholangiography has also been shown to be an effective means of imaging the biliary tree, but its specific role in evaluating bile duct injury needs further study.

CAUSES OF BILE DUCT INJURY

The majority of bile duct injuries are iatrogenic and associated with cholecystectomy, which nowadays is almost always performed laparoscopically. In the early postsurgical patient, the cause of the bile leak or stricture is rarely in doubt. However, the bile duct can also be injured by blunt or penetrating trauma, including iatrogenic causes, such as percutaneous liver biopsy and guide-wire/catheter trauma during ERCP. In patients undergoing laparotomy for stab wounds of the abdomen, 40% will be found to have an injury to the liver (approximately 30% in patients with gunshots).[9] Rarely, the bile duct may develop a stricture following irradiation for cancer therapy. Bile duct stones can cause strictures, a unique variety of which is seen in Mirizzi syndrome. Intrahepatic stones can embed (epithelialize) into the bile duct wall, giving the appearance of a malignant or benign stricture. Stones embedded at the biliary confluence may present a radiologic appearance indistinguishable from hilar cholangiocarcinoma (Klatskin tumor). The bile duct is frequently caught up in the inflammatory process of chronic pancreatitis: as the common bile duct (CBD) runs through the "head" of the pancreas, it may develop an extrinsic stricture. These strictures may become tight enough the obstruct bile flow and cause elevations of the patient's liver-function tests. Surgical drainage of biliary strictures in chronic pancreatitis is often necessary (by choledochoduodenoscopy vs hepaticojejunostomy), but short-term palliation is usually achieved by endoscopic stenting.[10] If portal hypertension and/or coagulopathy render surgery "high risk" in these patients, prolonged stenting with large-bore plastic stents is an option. Large-bore (caliber) plastic stents (ie, 10F, 11.5F) are preferred because they last longer than 7F stents. Experience has shown that uncovered self-expanding metallic stents (SEMS) are unsuitable for long-term palliation of benign biliary strictures because of their permanence (they embed in the bile duct wall) and inevitable occlusion. However, partially and wholly covered SEMS, which are usually removable, may prove suitable for managing these strictures in patients considered poor operative candidates.[11] The multiple stent placement and serial dilation approach pioneered by Costamagna and colleagues[12] works well in chronic pancreatitis, as in other kinds of benign biliary stricture.

If stricturing resulting from any disease process that damages the bile duct can be considered "injury," then postsurgical anastomotic strictures and those seen in primary sclerosing cholangitis (PSC), autoimmune cholangiopathy, and pancreatitis should also be included in this discussion. Most post–liver transplant strictures occur at duct-to-duct (**Fig. 6**) or biliary-enteric anastomoses. There is great variation in the reported success rates of endotherapy for these strictures, ranging from 27% to 91%.[13] Dilation of these strictures alone is rarely sufficient, unlike those of PSC, which tend to open, and stay open, after treatment using small-caliber biliary balloons. In

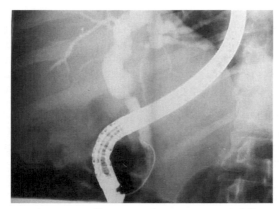

Fig. 6. ERCP demonstrating a post–liver transplant anastomotic biliary stricture: Note the mismatch in proximal (donor) and distal (recipient) bile duct segments.

PSC, exclusion of malignancy is an important goal, but often a difficult one to achieve. Injury to the bile duct from catheters and guide wires is a particular risk of endotherapy for PSC, and infection is an omnipresent problem that should be addressed with prophylactic broad-spectrum antibiotics.

TYPES OF INJURY RESULTING IN BILIARY LEAKS
Cystic Duct Stump Leak

This leak may result from dislodgment of clips from the cystic duct remnant or avulsion of the stump from the CBD caused by excessive traction on it. At ERCP, an early "blush" of contrast material is seen in the vicinity of the cystic duct stump during cholangiography. Cystic duct leaks typically can be treated with a short transpapillary stent (ie, the fistula itself does not have to be occluded by the stent). Generally, 10F stents are favored over 7F stents, as the small increase in internal diameter greatly increases the potential flow rate through a cylinder (from Pouseuille's equation). Biliary sphincterotomy is usually not performed because this encourages stent migration, but may be appropriate to reduce post-ERCP pancreatitis if the "fit" feels tight. Biliary sphincterotomy alone may be used as an alternative to stent placement, with roughly equivalent results. However, this exposes the patient to the potential complications of biliary sphincterotomy. Nasobiliary (NB) drainage is also an effective way to deal with biliary leaks, but NB drains are technically more difficult to place than stents and are poorly tolerated by many patients. It is also difficult to send patients with NB drains home with the drains in place. Rarely, these leaks fail to resolve with endoscopic therapy. Surgical resolution may be achieved by primary repair or a local diverting procedure.

Transected Duct of Luschka Leak

The so-called duct of Luschka was once considered to be a communication between the right intrahepatic ductal system and the gallbladder bed. However, most of these aberrant ducts drain into the common hepatic duct or cystic duct within 30 mm of the hepatocystic angle. The aberrant right hepatic duct serves as the only route of bile drainage for the portion of the right hepatic lobe that it serves. Severed aberrant ducts should be suspected when a bile leak persists despite cholangiography interpreted as normal, when there is failure of a bile leak to close after stenting, or when a surgeon reports ligation of an injured aberrant bile duct during cholecystectomy. MRCP and helical CT scanning have been recommended to identify severed aberrant ducts. Although some duct of Luschka leaks seal with endoscopic stenting, noncommunicating leaks can only be fixed by surgery (eg, Roux-en-Y hepaticojejunostomy). In a study from Duke University Medical Center (Durham, NC) that the author participated in, 86 postcholecystectomy leaks were reviewed,[14] of which 15 (17%) were found to be from accessory ducts: 11 were diagnosed by ERCP, 2 required percutaneous fistulography, and 2 others required percutaneous cholangiography to confirm the diagnosis. Two of these leaks required surgery and the remainder resolved with endotherapy.

Inadvertent Clipping of the Common Bile Duct

Clips placed close to the bile duct may interrupt its fragile vasculature, resulting in early or late ischemic structuring. Transection is a devascularizing injury, the fragile blood supply of the duct having been acutely interrupted. The two ends of the disrupted duct tend to drift apart in a mush of ischemic necrosis. A clip placed entirely across the duct will result in biliary obstruction, with progressive jaundice. A concomitant bile leak is typical after transection. The diagnosis is usually obvious from the cholangiogram at ERCP; endotherapy is rarely an option, especially not if the transection is complete.[15]

Partial or Complete Resection of the Extrahepatic Bile Duct

This potentially catastrophic injury results from misidentification of the ducts in and around the liver. There is no endoscopic remedy for this; a major surgical reconstruction is required.

MANAGEMENT OF POSTSURGICAL BILIARY INJURIES

Bile duct injury following cholecystectomy is associated with perioperative morbidity and mortality, reduced long-term survival and quality of life, and high rates of litigation. The management of these injuries depends significantly on when the injury is recognized (ie, at the time or later), the severity of the injury, the patient's comorbidities, and the availability of experienced hepatobiliary surgeons to effect the repair. Immediate detection and repair are typically associated with better outcome. The current standard of care for the management of a bile duct injury is urgent referral to a surgeon with experience in the repair of such injuries. The goal of the repair is restoration of the biliary ductal system and prevention of complications such as biliary fistula, intraabdominal abscess, bile duct stricture, recurrent cholangitis, and (secondary) biliary cirrhosis. Strictures involving the CBD or distal common hepatic duct (CHD) are more easily repaired than more proximal strictures. As a rule, the higher the location of the injury, the more difficult the repair and the more likely it is to recur.

The Bismuth classification of postoperative biliary strictures, first promulgated in 1982 (during the era of open cholecystectomy), is based on the most distal site proximal to the site of injury at which healthy biliary mucosa is available for anastomosis (see **Fig. 1**).[1] This classification has proved useful for indicating the most appropriate technique for repair, and has been shown to correlate well with the final outcome. For example, Type 1 Bismuth strictures can be repaired without opening the left main hepatic duct or lowering the hilar plate, whereas Type 2 strictures do require one to open the left duct to create the anastomosis. In Bismuth Type 4 lesions, the biliary confluence is interrupted and surgical reconstruction is needed (or 2 or more anastomoses). There have been numerous modifications of the Bismuth classification, such as that proposed by McMahon and colleagues[16] in 1995, which addresses laceration versus transection or excision of the bile duct, and provides weightings for minor versus major ductal injury. The Bismuth classification does not address every possible variant of biliary injury.

A different classification is appropriate for injuries following LC, which are often more severe than those seen after open cholecystectomy. The classic LC injury follows misidentification of the CBD for the cystic duct, resulting in resection of part of the CBD and CHD; it is usually associated with injury to the right hepatic artery. Clip ligation of the CBD with proximal ligation and division of the cystic duct results in biliary obstruction and leakage. Another injury results from "tenting": the cystic duct is correctly identified and grasped, with a portion of the CBD removed between the clips by traction. Strasberg and colleagues[4] extended the Bismuth classification by including a variety of laparoscopic injuries to the extrahepatic biliary tree. The classification ranges from Type A to Type E, with subdivision of the latter into E1 to E5 (see **Fig. 2**). Other investigators, including Neuhaus and colleagues,[17] Csendes and colleagues,[18] and Stewart and colleagues,[19] have proposed additional classification systems. Finally, the so-called Amsterdam classification[20] of bile duct injuries provides yet another perspective on the benefits of endotherapy versus surgery:

Type A: leakage from cystic duct or peripheral radicals (Strasberg type A). Treatment of choice is endoscopic sphincterotomy, biliary stenting and, if necessary, percutaneous drainage. Success rate approaches 100%.

Type B: major bile duct injury with leakage (Strasberg types C and D). The size of leak determines success of endoscopic therapy. If leakage can be adequately controlled by percutaneous drainage, endoscopic sphincterotomy, and biliary stenting, repeat procedures later prove effective in managing strictures without surgery.

Type C: bile duct stricture without leakage (Strasberg types E). This type has only about 40% success rate with endotherapy. Rendezvous procedures may improve this.

Most patients with Type B and C injuries can be treated nonoperatively.

Type D: complete transection or excision (Strasberg types E with long strictures or defects). The role of endoscopy is diagnostic only, and patients need to be managed operatively.

Postoperative strictures arising from the ligation or clipping of the bile duct present early and usually require definitive surgical management (**Box 1**). Ischemic injuries resulting from excessive cautery or dissection along the duct present after weeks to years. Most strictures occurring after LC occur at or above the level of the cystic duct. Endoscopic therapy for postoperative strictures using dilation and multiple stents results in 74% to 89% "good to excellent" results 3 to 5 years after stent removal, and at least 80% "good to excellent" results at 9 to 10 years.[21]

ENDOSCOPIC THERAPY FOR BILE DUCT LEAKS

An interesting perspective on endotherapy for bile leaks is available from a recent retrospective study[22] using a new classification: "low-grade" leaks are only visible after intrahepatic opacification at ERCP; "high-grade" leaks are visible on initial contrast injection, before intrahepatic opacification. In a study of 207 patients with bile leaks after cholecystectomies, 134 of the cholecystectomies were laparoscopic and 72 were open. These patients presented at a median of 9 days (range 1–50 days). Their predominant sign or symptom was pain in 56%, jaundice in 16%, fever in 11%, and

---

Box 1
Surgical management of bile duct injury

Avulsion of the Cystic Duct or Laceration

Primary repair

Local diversion procedure

Transection of the Bile Duct Without Loss of Tissue

End-to-end anastomosis

Choledochoduodenostomy

Roux-en-Y choledochojejunostomy

Segmental Loss of Ductal Tissue

Roux-en-Y choledochojejunostomy

Cholecystojejunostomy

Choledochoduodenostomy

Roux-en-Y hepatoportal enterostomy

Combined Injury

Hepatic resection (proximal injury)

Ligation of right or left main hepatic duct

Whipple procedure (distal injury)

---

abdominal distention in 7%. Persistent percutaneous bile drainage was present in 48% of cases. ERCP identified the leak site in 204 of 207 patients: cystic duct stump in 159 (78%), duct of Luschka in 26 (13%), and "other" in 19 (9%). Of 104 patients with low-grade leaks, 75 had biliary sphincterotomy alone, of whom 68 (91%) improved. The remainder needed stent placement (6) or surgery (1). Of 100 patients with high-grade leaks, 97 had stents placed. Bile duct stones were found and removed in 41 cases (28 in the low-grade group, 13 in the high-grade group). Three complications occurred: 2 cases of pancreatitis and 1 perforation (all 3 were managed conservatively, with no mortality). The investigators preferred biliary sphincterotomy over stenting for low-grade leaks, and used it with a high success rate and few complications. Many contemporary ERCP endoscopists would start with stenting and reserve sphincterotomy for cases in which stents failed to resolve the leak. Stenting was used in almost all cases of high-grade leaks, with obvious success. Surgery was needed to fix a persistent leak in only 1 case (0.5%). As the majority of post-LC bile leaks arise from the cystic duct stump and are immediately apparent on contrast injection, stenting is the treatment of first choice. It is the author's preference not to use sphincterotomy routinely in such cases because it adds some risk, increases stent migration, and permanently destroys the biliary sphincter mechanism.

REFERENCES

1. Flenn DR, Cheadle A, Prela C, et al. Bile duct injury during cholecystectomy and survival in Medicare beneficiaries. JAMA 2003;290:2168–73.
2. Krohenbuhl L, Sclobos C, Wente MN, et al. Incidence, risk factors and prevention of bile duct injuries during laparoscopic cholecystectomy in Switzerland. World J Surg 2001;25:1325–30.

3. Bismuth H, Majno PE. Biliary strictures: classification based on the principles of surgical treatment. World J Surg 2001;25:1241–4.
4. Strasberg SM, Hentl M, Soper NJ. An analysis of the problem of biliary injury during laparoscopic cholecystectomy. J Am Coll Surg 1995;180:101–25.
5. Haney JC, Pappas TN. Management of common bile duct injuries. Operative techniques in general surgery 2007;9(4):175–84.
6. Nordin A, Gronroos JM, Makisalo H. Treatment of biliary complications after laparoscopic cholecystectomy. Scand J Surg 2011;100:42–8.
7. Shinhar S, Nobel M, Shimonov M, et al. Tc99m-HIDA scintigraphy versus endoscopic retrograde cholangiopancreatography in demonstrating bile leaks after laparoscopic cholecystectomy. J Nucl Med 1998;39:1802–4.
8. Mutignani M, Shah SK, Trignali A, et al. Endoscopic therapy for biliary leaks from aberrant right hepatic ducts severed during cholecystectomy. Gastrointest Endosc 2002;55:932–6.
9. Felciano DV, Rozycki GS. Hepatic trauma. Scand J Surg 2002;91:72–9.
10. Isayama H, Nakai Y, Togawa O, et al. Covered metallic stents in the management of malignant and benign pancreatobiliary strictures. J Hepatobiliary Pancreat Surg 2009;16(5):624–7.
11. Akbar A, Irani S, Baron TH, et al. Use of covered self-expandable metal stents for endoscopic management of benign biliary disease not related to stricture. Gastrointest Endosc 2012;76:196–201.
12. Costamagna G, Pandolfi M, Mutignani M, et al. Long term results of endoscopic management of postoperative bile duct strictures with increasing numbers of stents. Gastrointest Endosc 2001;54:162–8.
13. Judah JR, Draganov PV. Endoscopic therapy of benign biliary strictures. World J Gastroenterol 2007;13:3531–9.
14. Mergener K, Stobel JC, Suhocki P, et al. The role of ERCP in diagnosis and management of accessory bile duct leaks after cholecystectomy. Gastrointest Endosc 1999;50:527–31.
15. Fiocca F, Salvatori FM, Fanelli F, et al. Complete transaction of the main bile duct: minimally invasive treatment with an endoscopic-radiologic rendezvous. Gastrointest Endosc 2011;74:1393–8.
16. McMahon AJ, Fullarton G, Baxter JN, et al. Bile duct injury and bile leakage in laparoscopic cholecystectomy. Br J Surg 1995;82:307–13.
17. Neuhaus P, Schmidt SC, Huntze RE, et al. Classification and treatment of bile duct injuries after laparoscopic cholecystectomy. Chirurg 2000;71:166–73.
18. Csendes A, Navarrete C, Burdiles P, et al. Treatment of common bile duct injuries during laparoscopic cholecystectomy: endoscopic and surgical management. World J Surg 2001;25:1346–51.
19. Stewart L, Robinson TN, Lee CM, et al. Right hepatic artery injury associated with laparoscopic bile duct injury: incidence, mechanism and consequences. J Gastrointest Surg 2004;8:523–31.
20. Bergman JJ, van den Brink GR, Rauws EA, et al. Treatment of bile duct lesions after laparoscopic cholecystectomy. Gut 1996;38:141–7.
21. Vitale GC, Tran TC, Davis BR, et al. Endoscopic management of post-cholecystectomy bile duct strictures. J Am Coll Surg 2008;206:918–23.
22. Sandha GS, Bourke MJ, Haber GB, et al. Endoscopic therapy for bile leak based on a new classification: results in 207 patients. Gastrointest Endosc 2004;60:567–74.

Endoscopic Approach to the Post Liver Transplant Patient

John Y. Nasr, MD, Adam Slivka, MD, PhD*

KEYWORDS

- Endoscopic Retrograde Cholangiography (ERCP) • Liver transplant
- Biliary complications • Bile Leak • Choledocholithiasis

KEY POINTS

- Management of biliary complications following liver transplant.
- Methods of stone extraction following liver transplant.
- Management of bile leak following liver transplant.

INTRODUCTION

Liver transplant has evolved as the treatment of choice for selected patients with end-stage liver disease, fulminant hepatic failure, and early stage hepatoma.

As the number of liver transplants has increased, so has the number of postoperative biliary complications requiring endoscopic treatment and management using endoscopic retrograde cholangiopancreatography (ERCP).

Biliary complications occur in up to 5%–25% of patients after liver transplant and can be categorized based on time of onset as early, occurring within 30 days of transplant, or late, occurring more than 30 days after transplant.[1–4]

Although some postoperative biliary complications require surgical reintervention or percutaneous transhepatic cholangiography, the advancement of endoscopic techniques has made endoscopic therapy a safe and effective first approach to managing postoperative biliary complications in most patients.

This review focuses on the endoscopic diagnosis and treatment of post-liver transplant complications.

TYPES OF BILIARY COMPLICATIONS AFTER TRANSPLANT

Biliary complications after liver transplant commonly include biliary strictures, biliary leaks, choledocholithiasis, ischemic biliary injury, biliary cast syndrome, and sphincter

Division of Gastroenterology, Hepatology, and Nutrition, University of Pittsburgh Medical Center, 200 Lothrop street, Pittsburgh, PA 15213, USA
* Corresponding author.
E-mail address: slivax@upmc.edu

Gastrointest Endoscopy Clin N Am 23 (2013) 473–481
http://dx.doi.org/10.1016/j.giec.2012.12.014
1052-5157/13/$ – see front matter © 2013 Elsevier Inc. All rights reserved.

of Oddi dysfunction (SOD). Hemobilia, mucocele formation, and bactobilia are less commonly seen.

LIVER TRANSPLANT ANATOMY

Liver transplant success and graft survival are highly dependent on adequate blood flow through both the hepatic artery and the portal vein. Any injury to the vasculature will result in ischemic injury and potential graft failure.

Knowledge of the biliary reconstruction after transplant is critical when considering posttransplant endoscopic therapy. Around 75%–88% of transplants are performed using a choledochocholedochostomy. The remaining 12%–25% of reconstructions are performed using a Roux-en-Y choledochojejunostomy.[5–8] The benefits of creating a choledochocholedochostomy may include shorter operating times, use of a T-tube for access, maintenance of intestinal integrity and continuity, sterility of the biliary tract, and ease of access for ERCP.[5,9–14] As recipient sphincter of Oddi function is preserved, the incidence of reflux-associated biliary injury and disease are less compared with Roux-en-Y choledochojejunostomy reconstruction.[12] In cases in which the donor bile duct is inadequate to perform a choledochocholedochostomy, or when the native common bile duct is diseased or absent (eg, primary sclerosing cholangitis, biliary atresia), a Roux-en-Y choledochojejunostomy is performed.

Biliary tract complications after liver transplant depend on the type of biliary reconstruction, injury during donor harvesting, cold ischemic time, surgical technique, and the integrity of the portal vein and hepatic artery anastomosis.

BILIARY STRICTURES

One of the most common complications is a biliary stricture (**Fig. 1**). Biliary strictures constitute around 40%–45% of posttransplant biliary complications.[12,15] Strictures occur in around 5%–15% of deceased donor liver transplants[16–19] and have been reported in up to 32% of live-donor–related transplants.[18] Biliary strictures are divided into early biliary strictures, which are usually secondary to technical surgical complications, and late biliary strictures, which are usually secondary to ischemic injury.

Posttransplant biliary strictures can occur at the anastomotic site or at nonanastomotic regions. Anastomotic strictures are defined as strictures that occur at the site of the anastomosis between the donor and recipient bile duct. Anastomotic strictures

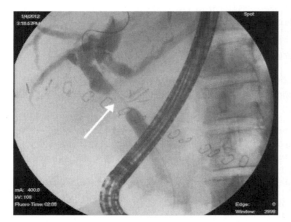

Fig. 1. Post duct to duct liver transplant, anastomotic stricture (*arrow* points to stricture).

usually develop within 1 year after transplant.[18] These strictures appear as a narrowing at the area of the surgical choledochal anastomosis. Dilation of the donor ducts can be seen. The anastomotic narrowing can be related to postsurgical edema, usually seen in the first few weeks after transplant, or to fibrotic or ischemic injury at the anastomosis, which are persistent or delayed in onset. Care should be taken to avoid incorrectly diagnosing anastomotic strictures in patients who have mismatch in size between the donor and the recipient duct (**Fig. 2**). In these cases, the donor or recipient duct is usually larger in size, but no narrowing or stricture is seen at the anastomosis.

Patients who present with anastomotic strictures usually require balloon dilation and biliary stent placement across the stricture. Conventionally, plastic biliary stents have been used with great success. Preliminary studies have reported on the effectiveness of off-label covered metal stents in managing anastomotic biliary strictures.[20,21] A recent prospective study, including 54 patients, concluded that covered metal stents should not be used as a primary treatment modality for post–liver transplant biliary complications, although they may be effective in three-quarters of patients who do not respond to standard therapy.[22] The authors concluded that stent migration remains a major complication.

For early strictures, which may be caused by postoperative edema, placing a single plastic stent without balloon dilation is preferred to avoid both injury to the anastomosis and unnecessary therapy in patients who might have a resolution to their obstruction in several weeks. For strictures that persist beyond the first month, the authors' practice is to place a guide wire across the stricture and to dilate the stricture with a biliary balloon. The balloon diameter is sized to the smallest duct on either side of the stricture to prevent perforation. We then place plastic biliary stents, preferably of 10F. The number of stents placed usually depends on the size of the ducts, the diameter of the stricture, and the number of sessions the patient has undergone for stricture treatment. We tend to exchange the stents every 3 months, because these stents tend to occlude, and repeat procedures will allow assessment of response to stenting.

Treatment for most patients with biliary anastomotic strictures will require more than one endoscopic procedure over a period of 9–12 months. Fluoroscopic resolution of the stricture indicates successful therapy, but recurrences have been reported. The long-term success of biliary stenting has been reported at 65%–100%.[16,18,23–26]

Patients who received a choledochojejunostomy also have strictures at the anastomosis between the donor bile duct and the recipient jejunum. These are usually

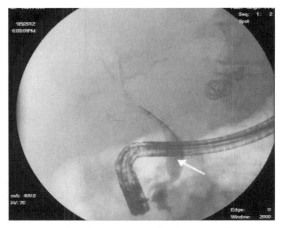

Fig. 2. Donor-recipient duct mismatch (*arrow* at recipient duct).

treated with balloon dilation and placement of plastic biliary stents across the anastomosis. Endoscopic access to the anastomosis can be attempted but may be difficult and usually requires longer front-viewing instruments. Percutaneous approaches represent an acceptable alternative for these patients. Follow-up interval blood work is mandatory for all patients who have had endotherapy for anastomotic strictures to monitor for recurrence.

Patients may also have nonanastomotic strictures after liver transplant. These are usually related to hepatic ischemia from vascular injury or thrombosis or from recurrence of primary liver disease, as in primary sclerosing cholangitis. The incidence of nonanastomotic strictures has been reported to be as high as 25%.[27]

Ischemic strictures tend to be diffuse, multiple, and intrahepatic (**Fig. 3**). Nonanastomotic strictures are usually more difficult to treat, with studies reporting 50%–75% rate of response to biliary stenting.[3,19,23,26,28] These strictures are usually treated with a combination of endoscopic dilation and stenting, in addition to percutaneous biliary stenting and draining of any fluid collections or abscesses that may form secondary to biliary obstruction. Ultimately, patients with severe ischemic strictures will require retransplantation.

BILE DUCT STONES

Biliary lithiasis is common after liver transplant, and the stones are typically of the pigmented or mixed type (**Fig. 4**). Bile duct stones develop in around 4%–30% of patients after transplant.[26,29,30]

Stones can develop early or late. In one study, the stones developed at a mean of 19 months after transplant and, in most patients, were cleared in a single endoscopic session.[26] Biliary stones are usually treated with biliary sphincterotomy and balloon or basket extraction. Lithotripsy may be required for large stones or donor duct stones above an anastomotic narrowing. Stones that occur in setting of biliary strictures may require stricture dilation and stent placement. These patients usually require multiple endoscopic sessions for stone extraction and stricture resolution.

BILE DUCT CASTS

Biliary casts are filling defects seen in the biliary tree after liver transplant. They are commonly brown and conform to the shape the biliary duct (**Fig. 5**). Casts usually

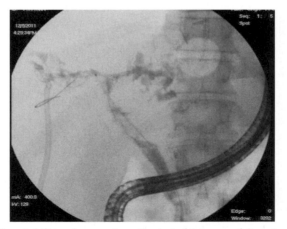

Fig. 3. Diffuse ischemic biliary damage in patient s/p (status post) liver transplant.

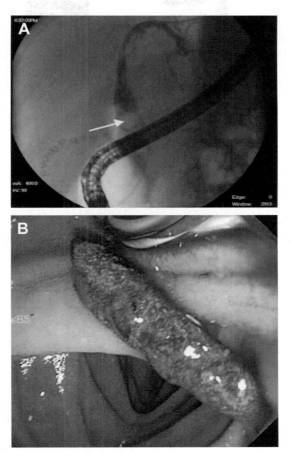

Fig. 4. (*A*) Choledocholithiasis (*arrow* points to CBD stone) in transplant patient. (*B*) Choledocholithiasis extraction.

form in the setting of hepatic ischemic injury, and patients who are found to have casts during ERCP should undergo Doppler testing of the hepatic vasculature to ensure adequate arterial perfusion.

Biliary cast syndrome is described as biliary obstruction secondary to presence of biliary casts and debris. Biliary cast syndrome in present in 2.5%–18% of posttransplant patients.[31,32] Endoscopic treatment of biliary cast syndrome is similar in approach to treatment of isolated biliary casts but is associated with worse outcome compared with patients without casts.[31] A combination of percutaneous and endoscopic treatment approaches have been reported to clear the biliary tree in 60% of cases.[32]

SPHINCTER OF ODDI DYSFUNCTION

SOD has been described de novo in patients after liver transplantation. In one series, SOD was reported in 7% of patients after liver transplant.[26] The cause of SOD after transplant is unclear, but is thought to be secondary to denervation of the biliary sphincter after surgical intervention. Patients with SOD usually present with cholestasis, with imaging studies showing diffuse biliary dilation of either or both the donor

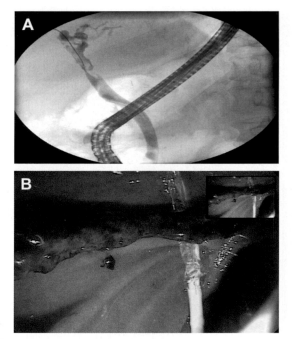

Fig. 5. (*A, B*) Biliary cast.

and recipient segment, with no evidence of filling defects or biliary strictures. Pain is not a common presentation. Treatment of patients with SOD is with biliary endoscopic sphincterotomy, which allows drainage and decompression of the biliary tree.

BILE LEAK

Bile leaks have been reported in around 10%–15% of patients after liver transplant.[33] They usually occur early in the posttransplant course and may cause significant morbidity. Posttransplant bile leaks are treated either surgically or endoscopically. Endoscopic treatment consists of biliary endoscopic sphincterotomy to decrease the transpapillary pressure gradient or placement of a transpapillary plastic stent, allowing preferential drainage of bile into the intestine. Often, both endoscopic sphincterotomy and stent placement are performed, but, occasionally, either one could be performed independently. Endoscopic therapy has been found to be effective in around 95% of posttransplant bile leaks.[3,19]

Recently, covered self-expandable metal stents were evaluated in treatment of postoperative biliary leaks.[34] Although these stents were clinically effective for managing posttransplant bile leaks, a significant number of biliary strictures were observed after stent removal; therefore, these stents were not recommended in the posttransplant setting.

The authors treat patients who have postoperative bile leaks with biliary endoscopic sphincterotomy and placement of plastic biliary stents, usually by placing a single 10F stent. The authors also recommend percutaneous drainage of any significant residual bilomas to prevent abscess formation in these immune-suppressed patients. If the bile leak does not respond to initial biliary stent placement, ERCP is repeated with an attempt at placing additional stent(s), to increase diameter of the drainage channel, and to further decrease the pressure gradient across the papilla. The number of stents placed depends on the size of both the donor and recipient bile ducts and the presence of a concomitant biliary stricture. Any leak above a stricture mandates crossing the stricture with the stent to relieve the pressure gradient.

OTHER POSTTRANSPLANT BILIARY COMPLICATIONS

Other complications after liver transplant include mucoceles, hemobilia, and infections.

Mucoceles have been described after liver transplant.[35,36] These are usually related to collection of mucus in the donor cystic duct. This leads to mass formation and extrinsic compression of the biliary tree. Management of mucoceles is usually surgical, requiring excision of the cystic duct remnant.

Hemobilia also can develop in patients after liver transplant. This is usually related to percutaneous transhepatic catheter drain placement or liver biopsy, although spontaneous bleeding can occur. Management of active hemobilia is usually through angiography and arterial embolization, although patients with intraductal blood clots, causing biliary obstruction, usually require endoscopic removal, similar to stone extraction.

BILIARY COMPLICATIONS AFTER LIVING DONOR LIVER TRANSPLANTATION

Biliary complications occur after living donor liver transplantation at an incidence higher than those seen in orthotopic transplants.[37] A recent systematic review, published in 2011, compared biliary complications in patients who underwent orthotopic liver transplantation with those of patients with living donor liver transplant.[8] The incidence of biliary strictures was higher in the living donor liver transplant group, whereas no significant difference was seen in the incidence of biliary leaks between the 2 groups. The difference in biliary stricture incidence was thought to be related to smaller ductal size, technically challenging reconstruction, and ductal devascularization at time of harvesting.

COMPLICATIONS OF ENDOSCOPIC THERAPY

Complications of endoscopic therapy in patients after liver transplant are similar to complications in nontransplant patients. Complications include pancreatitis, bleeding, perforation, infection, and sedation-related complications. Other potential complications include bile leak and damage of surgical anastomosis.

The incidence of post-ERCP complications has been reported to be around 5% in nontransplant patients.[38] This is compared with around 9% in posttransplant patients in a recent retrospective review,[39] although a more recent study reported no statistical difference in post-ERCP complications when comparing liver transplant patients with nontransplant patients.[40]

SUMMARY

Biliary complications occur after liver transplantation. These complications can be effectively and safely managed using endoscopic approaches and can prevent unnecessary and potentially morbid surgery.

REFERENCES

1. Stratta RJ, Wood RP, Langnas AN, et al. Diagnosis and treatment of biliary tract complications after orthotopic liver transplantation. Surgery 1989;106(4):675–83 [discussion: 683–4].

2. Thethy S, Thomson B, Pleass H, et al. Management of biliary tract complications after orthotopic liver transplantation. Clin Transplant 2004;18(6):647–53.
3. Pfau PR, Kochman ML, Lewis JD, et al. Endoscopic management of postoperative biliary complications in orthotopic liver transplantation. Gastrointest Endosc 2000;52(1):55–63.
4. Krok KL, Cardenas A, Thuluvath PJ. Endoscopic management of biliary complications after liver transplantation. Clin Liver Dis 2010;14(2):359–71.
5. Friend PJ. Overview: biliary reconstruction after liver transplantation. Liver Transpl Surg 1995;1(3):153–5.
6. Starzl TE, Demetris AJ, Van Thiel D. Liver transplantation (2). N Engl J Med 1989; 321(16):1092–9.
7. Starzl TE, Demetris AJ, Van Thiel D. Liver transplantation (1). N Engl J Med 1989; 321(15):1014–22.
8. Akamatsu N, Sugawara Y, Hashimoto D. Biliary reconstruction, its complications and management of biliary complications after adult liver transplantation: a systematic review of the incidence, risk factors and outcome. Transpl Int 2011;24(4): 379–92.
9. Porayko MK, Kondo M, Steers JL. Liver transplantation: late complications of the biliary tract and their management. Semin Liver Dis 1995;15(2):139–55.
10. Vallera RA, Cotton PB, Clavien PA. Biliary reconstruction for liver transplantation and management of biliary complications: overview and survey of current practices in the United States. Liver Transpl Surg 1995;1(3):143–52.
11. Gholson CF, Zibari G, McDonald JC. Endoscopic diagnosis and management of biliary complications following orthotopic liver transplantation. Dig Dis Sci 1996; 41(6):1045–53.
12. Pascher A, Neuhaus P. Biliary complications after deceased-donor orthotopic liver transplantation. J Hepatobiliary Pancreat Surg 2006;13(6):487–96.
13. Hwang S, Lee SG, Sung KB, et al. Long-term incidence, risk factors, and management of biliary complications after adult living donor liver transplantation. Liver Transpl 2006;12(5):831–8.
14. Marubashi S, Dono K, Nagano H, et al. Biliary reconstruction in living donor liver transplantation: technical invention and risk factor analysis for anastomotic stricture. Transplantation 2009;88(9):1123–30.
15. Sossenheimer M, Slivka A, Carr-Locke D. Management of extrahepatic biliary disease after orthotopic liver transplantation: review of the literature and results of a multicenter survey. Endoscopy 1996;28(7):565–71.
16. Verdonk RC, Buis CI, Porte RJ, et al. Anastomotic biliary strictures after liver transplantation: causes and consequences. Liver Transpl 2006;12(5):726–35.
17. Verdonk RC, Buis CI, Porte RJ, et al. Biliary complications after liver transplantation: a review. Scand J Gastroenterol Suppl 2006;(243):89–101.
18. Sharma S, Gurakar A, Jabbour N. Biliary strictures following liver transplantation: past, present and preventive strategies. Liver Transpl 2008;14(6):759–69.
19. Thuluvath PJ, Pfau PR, Kimmey MB, et al. Biliary complications after liver transplantation: the role of endoscopy. Endoscopy 2005;37(9):857–63.
20. Mahajan A, Ho H, Sauer B, et al. Temporary placement of fully covered self-expandable metal stents in benign biliary strictures: midterm evaluation (with video). Gastrointest Endosc 2009;70(2):303–9.
21. Marin-Gomez LM, Sobrino-Rodriguez S, Alamo-Martinez JM, et al. Use of fully covered self-expandable stent in biliary complications after liver transplantation: a case series. Transplant Proc 2010;42(8):2975–7.

22. Tarantino I, Traina M, Mocciaro F, et al. Fully covered metallic stents in biliary stenosis after orthotopic liver transplantation. Endoscopy 2012;44(3):246–50.
23. Graziadei IW, Schwaighofer H, Koch R, et al. Long-term outcome of endoscopic treatment of biliary strictures after liver transplantation. Liver Transpl 2006;12(5): 718–25.
24. Pasha SF, Harrison ME, Das A, et al. Endoscopic treatment of anastomotic biliary strictures after deceased donor liver transplantation: outcomes after maximal stent therapy. Gastrointes Endosc 2007;66(1):44–51.
25. Seo JK, Ryu JK, Lee SH, et al. Endoscopic treatment for biliary stricture after adult living donor liver transplantation. Liver Transpl 2009;15(4):369–80.
26. Rerknimitr R, Sherman S, Fogel EL, et al. Biliary tract complications after orthotopic liver transplantation with choledochocholedochostomy anastomosis: endoscopic findings and results of therapy. Gastrointest Endosc 2002;55(2):224–31.
27. Dacha S, Barad A, Martin J, et al. Association of hepatic artery stenosis and biliary strictures in liver transplant recipients. Liver Transpl 2011;17(7):849–54.
28. Rizk RS, McVicar JP, Emond MJ, et al. Endoscopic management of biliary strictures in liver transplant recipients: effect on patient and graft survival. Gastrointest Endosc 1998;47(2):128–35.
29. Spier BJ, Pfau PR, Lorenze KR, et al. Risk factors and outcomes in post-liver transplantation bile duct stones and casts: a case-control study. Liver Transpl 2008;14(10):1461–5.
30. Sheng R, Ramirez CB, Zajko AB, et al. Biliary stones and sludge in liver transplant patients: a 13-year experience. Radiology 1996;198(1):243–7.
31. Gor NV, Levy RM, Ahn J, et al. Biliary cast syndrome following liver transplantation: predictive factors and clinical outcomes. Liver Transpl 2008;14(10):1466–72.
32. Shah JN, Haigh WG, Lee SP, et al. Biliary casts after orthotopic liver transplantation: clinical factors, treatment, biochemical analysis. Am J Gastroenterol 2003; 98(8):1861–7.
33. Shah JN, Ahmad NA, Shetty K, et al. Endoscopic management of biliary complications after adult living donor liver transplantation. Am J Gastroenterol 2004; 99(7):1291–5.
34. Martins FP, Phillips M, Gaidhane MR, et al. Biliary leak in post-liver-transplant patients: is there any place for metal stent? HPB Surg 2012;2012:684172.
35. Zajko AB, Bennett MJ, Campbell WL, et al. Mucocele of the cystic duct remnant in eight liver transplant recipients: findings at cholangiography, CT, and US. Radiology 1990;177(3):691–3.
36. Chatterjee S, Das D, Hudson M, et al. Mucocele of the cystic duct remnant after orthotopic liver transplant a problem revisited. Exp Clin Transplant 2011;9(3): 214–6.
37. Wang SF, Huang ZY, Chen XP. Biliary complications after living donor liver transplantation. Liver Transpl 2011;17(10):1127–36.
38. Williams EJ, Taylor S, Fairclough P, et al. Risk factors for complication following ERCP; results of a large-scale, prospective multicenter study. Endoscopy 2007; 39(9):793–801.
39. Balderramo D, Bordas JM, Sendino O, et al. Complications after ERCP in liver transplant recipients. Gastrointest Endosc 2011;74(2):285–94.
40. Sanna C, Giordanino C, Giono I, et al. Safety and efficacy of endoscopic retrograde cholangiopancreatography in patients with post-liver transplant biliary complications: results of a cohort study with long-term follow-up. Gut Liver 2011;5(3):328–34.

Endoscopic Approach to the Bile Duct in the Patient with Surgically Altered Anatomy

Alexander Lee, MD[a], Janak N. Shah, MD[b],*

KEYWORDS

- Endoscopic retrograde cholangiopancreatography • Billroth II
- Roux-en-Y anastomosis • Gastric bypass • Double-balloon enteroscopy
- Push and pull enteroscopy

KEY POINTS

- Endoscopic retrograde cholangiopancreatography (ERCP) in patients with surgically altered anatomy can be technically challenging because of the difficulty in traversing altered anatomy, cannulation from an altered position, and the lack of standard ERCP accessories for use with longer-length endoscopes.
- For ERCP in most patients with Billroth II anatomy, standard duodenoscopes or gastroscopes (with or without caps) can be used with high success rates.
- For ERCP in patients post Roux-en-Y, longer-length endoscopes or deep enteroscopy techniques are usually necessary. After the biliary orifice is reached, success rates for ERCP are reasonably high. Percutaneous or laparoscopic-assisted access for ERCP may be preferred in patients with long-limb Roux-en-Y gastric bypass.
- An endoscopist's thorough understanding of the postsurgical anatomy, along with careful preparation and availability of all potentially needed accessories, maximizes the chances of successful ERCP in the patient with surgically altered anatomy.

INTRODUCTION

Endoscopic retrograde cholangiopancreatography (ERCP) in surgically altered anatomy can be technically challenging, because of three main problems that must be overcome: (1) endoscopically traversing the altered luminal anatomy, (2) cannulating the biliary orifice from an altered position, and (3) performing biliary interventions with available ERCP instruments. This article addresses the most common and

Financial Disclosures: None.
[a] Division of Gastroenterology, University of California, San Francisco, 513 Parnassus Avenue, Room S-357, San Francisco, CA 94143, USA; [b] Paul May and Frank Stein Interventional Endoscopy Center, California Pacific Medical Center, University of California, San Francisco, 2351 Clay Street, 6th Floor, IES Lab, San Francisco, CA 94109, USA
* Corresponding author.
E-mail address: shahj@sutterhealth.org

Gastrointest Endoscopy Clin N Am 23 (2013) 483–504
http://dx.doi.org/10.1016/j.giec.2012.12.005
giendo.theclinics.com

most challenging variations in anatomy encountered by a gastroenterologist performing ERCP. It also highlights the innovations and progress that have been made in coping with these anatomic variations, with special attention paid to altered anatomy from bariatric surgery.

POSTSURGICAL ANATOMY WITH CONVENTIONALLY ACCESSIBLE BILIARY SYSTEM

Certain types of postsurgical anatomy feature a conventionally accessible biliary system, so ERCP can be performed with a standard duodenoscope and from the usual ERCP position. This offers two important advantages: endoscopist familiarity with standard ERCP techniques, and complete compatibility with standard ERCP tools.

There are several common operations that do not affect access to the patient's biliary systems: (1) sleeve gastrectomy, in which the greater curvature of the stomach is resected, and the remnant stomach is kept in continuity with the small bowel; (2) laparoscopic adjustable gastric band, in which a band-like device is placed around the stomach immediately beneath the gastroesophageal junction, with the inner portion of the band consisting of a saline-filled silicon balloon that can be inflated or deflated by a subcutaneous access port; and (3) Billroth I distal gastrectomy, in which antrectomy is performed and an end-to-end anastomosis is created between the remnant stomach and the duodenum.[1]

Advancement of the duodenoscope is usually relatively straightforward in these cases. The anatomic variations may be apparent as the stomach is traversed, and there may be variations in endoscope looping and position. However, with the duodenum remaining in continuity, establishing a good position for cannulation of the major papilla is generally not difficult, and the usual ERCP accessories are used for cannulation and therapy.

POSTSURGICAL ANATOMY WITH DIFFICULT-TO-ACCESS BILIARY SYSTEM

Many surgical procedures create variations in gastrointestinal anatomy, making ERCP challenging or even impossible. The difficulty arises because the gastric outlet is no longer contiguous with the duodenum. Altered anatomy leads to a longer gastrointestinal tract length to traverse to reach the biliary tree and to an unusual cannulation approach from a caudal angle. Duodenoscopes may be of insufficient length to reach the papilla, and ERCP in altered anatomy often requires the use of longer endoscopes, deep enteroscopy techniques, surgically assisted approaches, or additional supporting instruments. Common operations that result in difficult-to-access biliary systems are described next.

Gastrojejunostomy (Including Billroth II)

An anastomosis is created between the stomach and a loop of the jejunum. Typical procedures that use this type of anastomosis include gastrojejunostomy after partial gastrectomy or gastrojejunostomy without gastric resection for treatment of gastric outlet obstruction. The Billroth II distal gastrectomy uses a gastrojejunostomy (**Fig. 1**). Although this type of operation is performed infrequently in the current era of proton pump inhibitors, it is still encountered by biliary endoscopists, because it was popular in the past for complicated peptic ulcer disease.[2] During the procedure, the distal stomach is resected and an end-to-side gastrojejunostomy is created. From the anastomosis, an afferent limb leads to the more proximal small bowel and duodenum, and an efferent limb leads to the distal small bowel. Approach to the

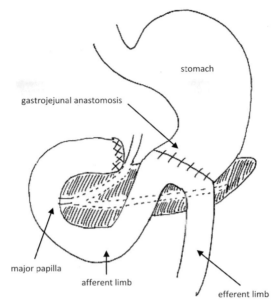

Fig. 1. Schematic of anatomy after Billroth II.

bile duct involves identifying the afferent limb and subsequently advancing the endoscope up the afferent limb and to the papilla.

Roux-en-Y Reconstruction

Roux-en-Y reconstruction adds a level of complexity for the biliary endoscopist. In this operation, the small bowel is divided, usually in the jejunum. The small bowel proximal to the division, which contains the biliary orifice, is anastomosed to a point distal to the location of the division, forming a jejunojejunostomy, and is termed the "biliopancreatic limb." The portion of small bowel distal to the division is anastomosed to the stomach and is termed the "Roux limb." Thus, the two upper limbs of the "Y" are the biliopancreatic and Roux limbs. This type of anastomosis is used in several procedures, such as pancreaticoduodenectomy (Whipple operation) (**Fig. 2**); bariatric surgery; and Roux-en-Y reconstructions after gastric resection, liver transplant, and certain biliary tract operations. ERCP in patients with Roux-en-Y anatomy can be difficult because of the length of bowel that must be traversed. The length varies depending on the type of surgery performed, with bariatric operations, such as Roux-en-Y with gastric bypass (RYGB), often resulting in the longest limbs (**Fig. 3**). Additionally, some types of Roux-en-Y reconstructions (eg, bariatric surgery or gastric resections) do not alter the native papilla but add an additional challenge of successful cannulation because the endoscopist must approach the papilla from the reverse position.[3–5]

APPROACH TO THE BILE DUCT IN GASTROJEJUNOSTOMY AND BILLROTH II

The most commonly used endoscopes to perform ERCP in patients with gastrojejunostomy (short-limb) or Billroth II anatomy are duodenoscopes and gastroscopes. Obstacles to success include difficulties in identifying the afferent limb, advancing the endoscope through the afferent limb to the papilla, and cannulating from an inverted or caudal angle. Techniques and instruments that facilitate successful biliary

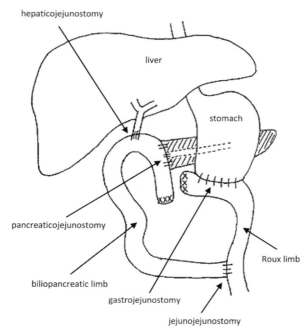

Fig. 2. Schematic of anatomy after pancreaticoduodenectomy (Whipple operation) with Roux-en-Y anastomosis anatomy.

access in these patients are discussed next. Performing biliary interventions can also be challenging, and are discussed in a subsequent section.

Duodenoscope

The duodenoscope remains a popular choice among biliary endoscopists for patients with Billroth II or similar anatomy. Obviously, the afferent limb must be of limited length to allow the duodenoscope to reach the papilla. Because of the side-view optics, identifying the afferent limb and negotiating the duodenoscope to the correct position can be difficult. Several techniques may help facilitate successful insertion of the duodenoscope. Use of fluoroscopy during insertion may confirm that the endoscope is heading toward the expected location of the papilla. Changing patient position or applying external compression may help advance duodenoscopes across acute angulations at the gastrojejunal anastomosis. Using a gastroscope before duodenoscopy may also allow the endoscopist to confirm the correct limb and evaluate for any unexpected anatomic angulations or variations. The correct limb can be marked with submucosal ink tattoo, or a guidewire can be left in place to facilitate immediate duodenoscope insertion.[6]

After the duodenoscope is advanced to the second portion of the duodenum, the papilla is usually readily visible. The presence of an elevator allows for additional fine control during cannulation attempts and subsequent instrumentation. When seeing the papilla "head-on" from the second portion of the duodenum, the reverse angle of approach for biliary cannulation toward the 5-o'clock position compared with the usual 11- to 12-o'clock position for standard ERCP should be recognized (**Fig. 4**). The authors recommend using standard, straight cannulas with or without guidewires for selective biliary access. These cannulas can also be "pushed" against

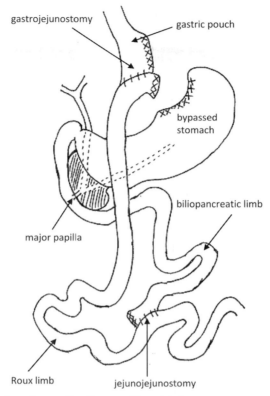

Fig. 3. Schematic of anatomy after Roux-en-Y gastric bypass.

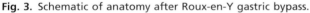

the duodenal wall to create a reverse angulation (from the usual angulation produced by the elevator), which improves the trajectory toward the biliary orifice.

The largest published experience of ERCP in Billroth II anatomy is in association with duodenoscopes. In larger series (each including 45–110 patients with Billroth II distal gastrectomies), success rates using duodenoscopes for reaching the papilla and for selective biliary cannulation are 70% to 97% and 60% to 91%, respectively.[2,7,8]

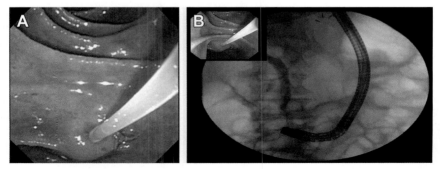

Fig. 4. Endoscopic (A) and fluoroscopic (B) images after successful biliary cannulation in a patient with Billroth II anatomy using a duodenoscope. The cannula extends toward the 5-o'clock position with respect to the papilla.

Gastroscope Versus Duodenoscope

Some experts advocate using gastroscopes over duodenoscopes in Billroth II anatomy. The main advantage of this instrument is the ease of recognizing and nego-tiating the afferent limb. The front-view optics facilitates advancing the endoscope through the afferent limb and into the second portion of the duodenum. However, can-nulation can be difficult, because the papilla may not be located in a favorable position with respect to the instrument channel. Lack of an elevator also compromises fine control of cannulation tools and accessories. That said, a few centers have reported high cannulation rates, ranging from 81% to 87%, using front-view endoscopes in ERCP in Billroth II.[7,9]

One prospective, randomized trial directly compared gastroscopes with duodeno-scopes in a group of 45 patients with Billroth II in need of ERCP.[9] Cannulation rates trended higher (87% vs 68%) in patients undergoing ERCP using gastroscopes. However, these results should be interpreted with caution because all cannulation "failures" in the duodenoscope group (total of 7) occurred in settings where the papilla was not reached. These were attributed to perforations during endoscope insertion (N = 4); difficulty in entering or negotiating the afferent limb (N = 2); or abdominal pain during insertion (N = 1). Other centers have reported high cannulation rates with duodenoscopes when the papilla is reached.[2] The cannulation failures in the gastroscope group were related to long afferent limbs (N = 2) or failed cannulation despite reaching the papilla (N = 1).

When using a gastroscope, one method to facilitate successful ERCP is the use of a transparent cap on the tip of the endoscope (**Fig. 5**). This allows the operator to better visualize the papilla by displacing any adjacent folds, stabilizing the endoscope during attempted cannulation, and optimizing the angle of approach. It also may assist the endoscopist in negotiating any acute angles in the afferent limb during intubation. In a case series from Korea, cap-assisted ERCP with a gastroscope allowed for successful cannulation and biliary therapy in 10 (100%) of 10 patients.[10]

An oblique-viewing gastroscope may combine the relative benefits of gastroscopes and duodenoscopes for Billroth II ERCP. Use of this instrument was first reported by Law and Freeman in 2004,[11] in which it was successfully used to perform therapeutic

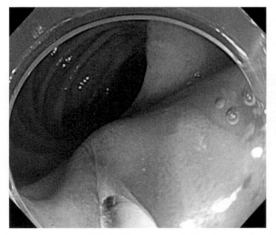

Fig. 5. Endoscopic image of cap-assisted biliary cannulation in a patient with prior gastro-jejunostomy. The transparent cap at the tip of the gastroscope helps the endoscopist locate the papilla and stabilize the endoscope during cannulation attempts.

ERCP in a single patient. Subsequently, a larger case series reported use of this endo-scope with a high success rate of reaching the papilla (88%) and high cannulation success (95%) in patients with Billroth II anatomy.[12] Unfortunately, these instruments were prototype models that are not currently available commercially for widespread use.

Complications

Performing ERCP in Billroth II anatomy increases the risk of complications. In addition to the usual complications that are associated with ERCP, there is the added concern for perforation while attempting to traverse the afferent limb, because perforations can occur near the gastrojejunal anastomosis. This may occur with use of either gastro-scopes or duodenoscopes. Perforations can also occur within the afferent limb itself, and these are usually related to passage of side-viewing duodenoscopes under limited visibility.

The previously mentioned randomized trial comparing gastroscopes with duodeno-scopes in patients with Billroth II did reveal a higher perforation rate with the duodeno-scope (4 of 22) compared with the gastroscope (0 of 23).[9] However, other series with larger numbers of patients (100+) have suggested more modest perforation rates ranging from 2% to 6%.[8,13,14]

Ultimately, the decision of whether to use a duodenoscope or gastroscope is likely best guided by personal experience and operator success rates. However, one should be prepared to switch to the alternative technique based on intraprocedural findings. Some studies have shown success even when the initial method fails.[7] In patients with long afferent limbs in which there is difficulty reaching the papilla, techniques used to perform ERCP in patients with Roux-en-Y anatomy should be considered, as dis-cussed next.

APPROACH TO THE BILE DUCT IN ROUX-EN-Y RECONSTRUCTION

Performing ERCP in patients with Roux-en-Y anatomy was once thought to be virtually impossible because of the long length of interposed bowel. This is of special concern in bariatric operations with long Roux limbs. Endoscopic techniques and tips to facil-itate successful biliary access in patients with Roux-en-Y anatomy are discussed next **(Table 1)**.

General Considerations

Earlier reports of attempting ERCP using duodenoscopes in patients with Roux-en-Y anatomy revealed poor success rates (33%), essentially caused by inability to reach the biliary orifice.[15] Push enteroscopy (using enteroscope or pediatric colonoscope) and deep enteroscopy technology (eg, balloon or spiral enteroscopy [SE]) may allow the endoscopist to overcome the technical limitations of insufficient length. However, there remain several challenges to successful ERCP when using either of these platforms:

1. Maneuverability and reaching the biliary orifice: Although the enteroscope may be of sufficient length, distal advancement down the Roux limb and up the biliopancre-atic limb may still be difficult because of angulations, adhesions, and looping in the small bowel. Deep enteroscopy technology confers some advantage over standard push enteroscopy with regards to this issue. Additionally, fluoroscopy to aid in identifying and eliminating loops and to verify appropriate advancement toward the right upper quadrant may be of benefit.

Table 1
Approaches and success rates for biliary ERCP in patients with postsurgical anatomy

Technique	Success in Reaching Biliary Orifice[a]	Success in Cannulation, if Biliary Orifice Reached[a]	Success in Therapy After Cannulation, if Indicated[a]	Comments
Push enteroscopy or colonoscopy[17,18]	67%–84%	95%–100%	86%–100%	Widely available Reasonable first choice in short-limb Roux-en-Y Use of colonoscope allows wider array of ERCP accessories
Deep enteroscopy: DBE[26–29,34] SBE[30–34,40] Short DBE[35–37] Spiral[34,40,41]	74%–100% 55%–92% 86%–97% 64%–77%	85%–100% 83%–100% 90%–98% 63%–90%	92%–100% 77%–100% 100% 88%–100%	No major differences among technologies Limited ERCP accessories through enteroscopes Various methods to advance "shorter" endoscopes may improve cannulation and therapy
ERCP by gastrostomy[48,49] or laparoscopic-assisted[50–52]	100%	100%	100%	More invasive and resource intensive than purely endoscopic methods Highest success rates Best option for patients requiring multiple ERCPs Better than deep enteroscopy–assisted ERCP for long-limb Roux-en-Y

Percentages derived from 21 studies with a total of 632 patients (95% Roux-en-Y, 5% Billroth II).
   [a] When possible, success rates were calculated using the actual number of ERCPs as denominator; in some studies, limitations in the reported data required using the number of patients as denominator.

2. Limited ERCP accessories: There are limited ERCP tools that are compatible with longer-length endoscopes and their smaller-size accessory channels. The authors recommend preparing a special "ERCP tool kit" that matches appropriate length and size ERCP instruments to the type of endoscope used. Tools that may be needed for biliary access or therapy should be anticipated.
3. Cannulation difficulty: As discussed with regards to cannulation difficulty when using gastroscopes in Billroth II anatomy, attempting cannulation with a front-view pediatric colonoscope or enteroscope from a caudal angle can also be a challenge in Roux-en-Y reconstruction. In patients with bilioenteric anastomoses (eg, post–Whipple surgery), this is not an issue. However, in patients with a native papilla (eg, post-RYGB), the papilla may be at an unfavorable angle with respect to the instrument channel. Lack of an elevator may also limit the fine control that is often needed during cannulation.

Push Enteroscopy

Colonoscopes and push enteroscopes are available in most endoscopy units, and may be a reasonable first choice, especially in patients with relatively short Roux limbs. The first report of a pediatric colonoscope used to perform ERCP on a patient with Roux-en-Y reconstruction was published in 1988.[16] A subsequent case series of 18 patients with Roux-en-Y reconstruction (including three with gastric bypass) revealed high success rates for reaching the papilla or ductal anastomosis (86% for enteroscope, 82% for pediatric colonoscope). Cannulation rates in this series were also high (94%), and included five of six procedures in patients with native papilla.[17]

Given the larger experience with duodenoscopes in ERCP in Billroth II, some experts have developed methods to introduce duodenoscopes to the papilla in Roux-en-Y anatomy. One technique involves advancing a colonoscope to the papilla, followed by placing a guidewire in the biliopancreatic limb. A duodenoscope can then be advanced over the wire or can be pulled into the biliopancreatic limb using an inflated wire-guided balloon as an anchor. A case series highlighting this technique showed successful insertion of duodenoscopes to the papilla in 10 (67%) of 15 with long-limb Roux-en-Y anatomy, with subsequent diagnostic or therapeutic ERCP success in all 10 of these patients.[18]

Deep Enteroscopy

Deep enteroscopy platforms were developed to help endoscopists evaluate and reach the distal small bowel. Double-balloon enteroscopy (DBE) was first reported in 2001.[19] Single-balloon enteroscopy (SBE) and SE were developed by other manufacturers and became available in the United States about 6 to 7 years later. All of these technologies are similar in that they are designed to allow deeper endoscope insertion into the small bowel, and therefore all of these may facilitate reaching the biliary orifice after Roux-en-Y reconstruction.

Balloon enteroscopy

DBE involves two separate inflatable balloons at the tip of the enteroscope and overtube. By alternating inflation-deflation and reduction-advancement on both the enteroscope and overtube, the endoscope tip can be advanced to the further depths of the small bowel (**Fig. 6**). Use of DBE to reach the bypassed stomach in a small series of patients with RYGB was first described in 2005.[20]

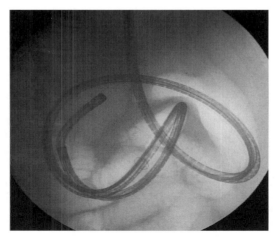

Fig. 6. Fluoroscopic image during ERCP using double-balloon enteroscopy in a patient with a Roux-en-Y hepaticojejunostomy. Alternating inflations-deflations on the endoscope and overtube anchoring balloons, along with push-pull maneuvers, has allowed the endoscope to reach the area of the biliary anastomosis in a tortuous position.

Since then, numerous case reports have emerged using DBE for ERCP in Roux-en-Y anatomy.[21–25] Larger series with 13 to 31 patients have published success rates of reaching the biliary orifice and subsequently achieving successful cannulation in 74% to 100% and 85% to 100%, respectively; in the subset of patients requiring interventions, therapeutic success was reported in 92% to 100% after successful cannulation.[26–29] As might be expected, cannulation and endobiliary therapy are more difficult in Roux-en-Y patients with native papilla (eg, post–gastric bypass) compared with Roux-en-Y patients with bilioenteric anastomoses.[26,28]

SBE uses only one balloon at the tip of the overtube, but essentially similar types of maneuvers are performed to help advance the enteroscope distally. Five large case series involving 13 to 50 patients have reported successful reaching of the biliary orifice in 55% to 92%, subsequent successful cannulation in 83% to 100%, and successful therapy in 83% to 100% among those needing interventions based on diagnostic ERCP findings.[30–34]

"Short" endoscope – balloon enteroscopy

The longer length of the standard enteroscope used for balloon enteroscopy limits the types of ERCP accessories that may be used. For DBE and SBE, techniques have been developed to allow use of shorter-length endoscopes that can accommodate a larger array of standard ERCP catheters. Manufacturers of the DBE platform have developed a shorter system that uses an enteroscope with a 152-cm working length. In three of the largest case series reporting outcomes of a "short" DBE system for Roux-en-Y ERCP involving 20, 68, and 79 patients with altered anatomy, diagnostic cholangiography was successfully obtained in 81% to 95%, with treatment success in almost all cases requiring therapy.[35–37]

Another technique that has been used with SBE involves modifying the overtube. After the papilla is reached, the longer enteroscope can be removed while maintaining overtube position near the biliary orifice. A shorter-length gastroscope can then be inserted to the area of the papilla (or bilioenteric anastomosis) by a slot created in the side of the overtube at a distance that allows the instrument to extend past the tip of the overtube. Itoi and colleagues[32] described this technique and managed successful therapeutic ERCP in 10 (77%) of 13 patients with altered anatomy, including 8 (72%) of 11 with intact papilla. The main benefit of allowing the endoscopist to reach the biliary orifice with a short length endoscope is the availability of a wider spectrum of ERCP accessories that maximize the chances for successful cannulation and therapy.

Spiral enteroscopy

SE uses an endoscope in conjunction with a rotational overtube with a spiral design on the exterior surface. By using clockwise rotational movements the endoscopist can "engage" the small intestinal mucosa and pleat the folds, allowing for deeper access (**Fig. 7**). In studies focusing on evaluation of small bowel disorders, SE offers shorter examination time compared with DBE but at the cost of less depth of insertion.[38,39] With respect to using this platform for ERCP in altered anatomy, it is not known whether a decreased insertion depth would be relevant; reaching the biliary orifice is all that is needed. However, a potentially decreased time to reach the biliary orifice would certainly be beneficial, because the time required to perform the ERCP portion of the procedure can be substantial.

Large recent retrospective series have demonstrated modest rates of reaching the biliary orifice (64%–72%).[34,40] Wagh and Draganov[41] recently published the first prospective series on SE-assisted ERCP in surgically altered anatomy and described

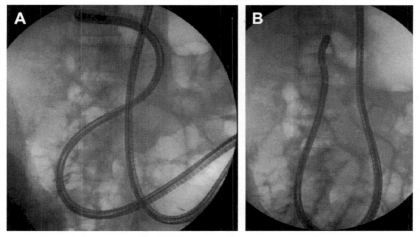

Fig. 7. Fluoroscopic images during ERCP using spiral overtube enteroscopy after the biliary orifice was reached in a patient with Roux-en-Y hepaticojejunostomy. The endoscope was initially in a tortuous position (A), but rotational movements on the overtube allowed for reduction of loops and a straighter and more stable endoscope position (B) for biliary interventions.

outcomes among seven patients undergoing 13 attempted ERCPs. The papilla-bilioenteric anastomosis was reached in 77%. In cases when the biliary orifice was reached, deep cannulation was successful in 89% and therapy was successful in 90%.

Comparative studies: deep enteroscopy technologies

There are few studies directly comparing the various deep enteroscopy technologies with respect to their use in ERCP in altered anatomy. The largest series was a multi-center US study reporting outcomes from 129 patients with long-limb Roux-en-Y anatomy.[34] The deep enteroscopy method allowed successful access to the papilla or bilioenteric anastomosis using SBE in 69% (31 of 45); DBE in 74% (20 of 27); and SE in 72% (41 of 57). ERCP was successful in 60% (27 of 45) of the SBE; 63% (17 of 27) of the DBE; and 65% (37 of 57) of the SE groups. As expected, these procedures required extended time compared with standard ERCP. The mean procedural duration was 110 minutes. There were no significant differences among the three deep enteroscopy technologies. Although overall ERCP success was 63% (81 of 129), ERCP success among patients in whom the biliary orifice could be accessed was 88% (81 of 92), suggesting that the most important issue in these patients was getting the endoscope to the right location. On reaching the area of the papilla or bil-ioenteric anastomosis, cannulation failures occurred in only 11 patients (12%). Other published studies with smaller cohorts have compared ERCP using DBE versus SBE and SBE versus SE, and such studies have also shown no significant differences between these technologies.[40,42]

Complications

Performing ERCP in patients with Roux-en-Y reconstruction may be associated with an increased risk of complications. In addition to the usual inherent risks associated with ERCP and deep enteroscopy, there may be added risks related to endoscope insertion across multiple anastomoses. In a large multicenter retrospective study collating complications after 2478 DBE procedures at nine US centers, the overall major complication rate was 0.9%, which included a 0.4% perforation rate. However, in the subset of patients with altered anatomy, the perforation rate was higher at 3%.[43] In a large series of 86 DBE-ERCPs, Raithel and colleagues[27] reported 2.3% pancreatitis rate and 2.3% perforation rate.

Studies on other deep enteroscopy-ERCP platforms (SBE, short-DBE, SE) involving at least 50 cases have reported similar pancreatitis and perforation rates as have been seen with DBE.[33,37,40] The aforementioned multicenter study comparing DBE, SBE, and SE-ERCPs in 129 patients with long-limb Roux-en-Y reported overall complications in 16 patients (12.4%). These included pancreatitis (3%); bleeding (0.8%); and perforation (1.6%). Distribution of complications by modality was not reported.[34]

Special Considerations for RYGB

The increasing prevalence of obesity is well known.[44] Bariatric surgery is now the second most common abdominal procedure in the United States, amounting to more than 150,000 cases annually, and more than 60% of these are the RYGB.[45] Moreover, there is a high prevalence of gallstone formation associated with weight loss after RYGB.[46] ERCP is becoming an increasingly requested procedure in post-RYGB patients.

ERCP in RYGB can be particularly challenging compared with other types of Roux-en-Y reconstructions because of the relatively longer Roux and biliopancreatic limbs that must be traversed. Additionally, cannulation of native papilla after RYGB can be more difficult than accessing bilioenteric anastomoses. However, one advantage that patients with RYGB have is the presence of a remnant stomach that can be accessed either percutaneously or laparoscopically, allowing for a route to the papilla using a duodenoscope. Either percutaneous access or laparoscopic-assisted ERCP allows a duodenoscope to approach the papilla in a standard position and allows for full use of all ERCP accessories.

Percutaneous access

This technique was first reported in 1998 in a post-RYGB patient with recurrent pancreatitis.[47] A surgical gastrostomy was created first, for the sole purpose of facilitating subsequent ERCP. Gastrostomy patency was maintained with a large-diameter tube. After a 2-week period for tract maturation, a duodenoscope was inserted after tract dilation, and successful ERCP was performed. Multiple studies have shown this technique to be efficacious, with all patients undergoing successful therapeutic ERCP where indicated.[48,49]

The gastrostomy can be created either surgically or by percutaneous puncture (by interventional radiology), but does require delay for tract maturity before ERCP. Thus, this approach is not useful in cases requiring urgent ERCP. The need for this intermediate step and second procedure is the main drawback of this technique compared with deep enteroscopy ERCP. However, one main advantage is that the gastrostomy tract can be maintained for quick access in patients in need of additional ERCPs to complete therapy.

Laparoscopy-assisted ERCP

Laparoscopy can also be used to create a point of access to the gastric remnant in patients with RYGB. As opposed to the two-stage procedure by gastrostomy, laparoscopic-assisted ERCP is performed during one session in the operating room. The duodenoscope can be advanced into the peritoneal cavity by a large-diameter trocar. The surgeon then inserts the duodenoscope directly into the gastric lumen through a laparoscopic gastrostomy. The entire procedure is performed under sterile conditions in the operating room.

This technique seems to be gaining popularity, as evidenced by increasing case reports and small series in recent years. Two of the largest series involving 15 and 23 patients with RYGB reported 100% success with ERCP.[50,51] In a recent single-center retrospective comparison of 24 laparoscopy-assisted ERCPs versus 32 DBE/ SBE-ERCPs in patients with prior RYGB, the former was significantly superior in reaching the papilla (100% vs 72%), cannulating (100% vs 59%), and performing therapy (100% vs 59%).[52] However, overall procedure times were shorter, but with increased endoscopist time, in the DBE-SBE cohort. There were no differences in hospital stay or complications rates between groups. Interestingly, an overall limb length (including Roux and biliopancreatic) of less than 150 cm was associated with procedural success and cost-savings in the deep enteroscopy ERCP group, suggesting that laparoscopy-assisted ERCP may be a better first choice in patients with long-limb RYGB.

Advantages of laparoscopy-assisted ERCP over deep enteroscopy–ERCP include use of the duodenoscope in a standard position for cannulation and therapy; availability of the complete array of ERCP tools; ability to perform other laparoscopic procedures if needed (eg, cholecystectomy, internal hernia repair, lysis of adhesions, and so forth); and the option to create a percutaneous gastrostomy if repeated ERCPs are anticipated. However, the main disadvantages are the increased invasiveness of this technique with the associated risks of anesthesia and surgery, and the logistical difficulties of coordinating with surgeon and operating room schedules.

BILIARY INTERVENTIONS IN SURGICALLY ALTERED ANATOMY

Most biliary interventions, such as stone removal, stricture dilation, or stent placement, require widening the biliary orifice in some manner (eg, sphincterotomy or dilation). However, even after cannulation is achieved, performing these maneuvers in patients with altered anatomy can still remain a challenge. Tips and techniques to facilitate interventions are discussed in this section.

General Considerations

Because most ERCPs are performed for therapeutic indications, it is imperative for the endoscopist to be prepared for any possible interventions that may be required. There is no point in pursuing a difficult procedure in a patient with altered anatomy without having the appropriate tools ready. Thus, the endoscopist should have available the appropriate sphincterotome, stone extraction device, dilation device, or stent relevant for a particular procedure. The size and length of the instrument channel should be taken into account. Thorough lists of ERCP accessories with details on their lengths and sizes are available through various gastrointestinal professional society publications.[53–57] Local representatives of ERCP device manufacturers are also excellent resources in this regard.

Sphincterotomy

Sphincterotomy is one of the basic techniques required for most biliary interventions. Several methods can be used to perform a biliary sphincterotomy in altered anatomy. When a duodenoscope can be used to reach the papilla, sphincterotomy can be performed using specially modified sphincterotomes in which the electrosurgical cutting wire extends in an arc shape or retracts leading to an S-shaped catheter curvature (thereby exposing the cutting wire in correct angle).[58] Care must be taken that this instrument exits and the cutting wire extends in the correct orientation with respect to the biliary orifice. With a duodenoscope positioned en face with the papilla, the cut should extend toward the 5-o'clock position. High rates of successful sphincterotomy (>92%) and low complication rates (<5%) using modified sphincterotomes through duodenoscopes in patients with Billroth II have been described.[15,59]

However, the modified sphincterotomes ("Billroth II sphincterotomes") do not always exit the papilla at the correct angle. This is even more of an issue when using these devices through a forward-view endoscope. Rotatable sphincterotomes are available and may allow for an appropriate cutting orientation.[57] Use of this type of device was safe and associated with a high success rate for sphincterotomy (89%) in a small series of patients with Billroth II.[60]

A third method to perform sphincterotomy involves placing a biliary stent and then using a needle-knife to incise the overlying tissue (**Fig. 8**). One benefit of this technique over the others is that proper cutting orientation is verified during stepwise incisions over the biliary stent. This technique was associated with high success (95%) and a low complication rate (5%) in one series,[61] and is the preferred method for sphincterotomy in altered anatomy at the authors' center.

Balloon Dilation or Sphincteroplasty

Balloon dilation of an intact papilla is another method to facilitate biliary interventions (**Fig. 9**). The pros and cons of this technique in patients with normal anatomy undergoing standard ERCP have been hotly debated. The main controversy has been a perceived higher risk of postdilation pancreatitis. Two recent meta-analyses of trials comparing ERCP with papillary balloon dilation versus biliary sphincterotomy have had varied results. One revealed no difference in postprocedure pancreatitis,[62] whereas the other revealed a significantly higher rate of pancreatitis (9% vs 3%) in the papillary dilation group.[63] However, they both revealed a higher rate of postprocedure hemorrhage in patients treated with sphincterotomy.

Several issues make balloon dilation an attractive or only option compared with sphincterotomy in the setting of altered anatomy. (1) After wire access has been achieved, balloon dilation catheters can be easily advanced into position without consideration of the angle of approach to the papilla. (2) Balloon dilation catheters

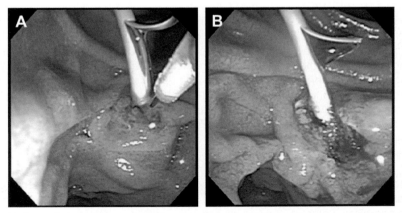

Fig. 8. Endoscopic images demonstrating needle-knife sphincterotomy over a biliary stent in a patient with Billroth II anatomy (duodenoscope used). (*A*) The proper angle for incision should be toward the 5-o'clock position. (*B*) Sphincterotomy is performed by incising the tissue overlying the biliary stent.

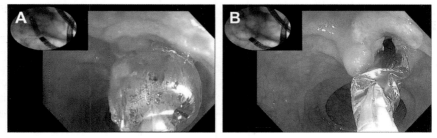

Fig. 9. Endoscopic images (with fluoroscopic insets) of balloon sphincteroplasty in a patient with Roux-en-Y gastric bypass. (*A*) After successful wire access into the biliary system, an over-the-wire balloon dilator is advanced across the papilla and inflated to 10 mm. (*B*) Post-dilation the biliary orifice is widely patent to allow subsequent stone removal (not shown).

of a sufficient length for use with enteroscopes are more widely available and stocked in most endoscopy units. (3) In a patient at risk for postprocedure hemorrhage or with a difficult-to-reach papilla, balloon dilation may be preferred because of its decreased risk of bleeding. (4) Balloon dilation is the safest option to widen the orifice and perform biliary interventions in patients with bilioenteric anastomoses.

In a recent Korean series of 13 patients with Billroth II anatomy and choledocholi-thiasis, transpapillary balloon dilation (using a cap-fitted gastroscope) was performed without preceding sphincterotomy. Selective biliary cannulation was achieved in 92%, and duct clearance was successful in each of these.[64] Depending on the endoscope used, balloon dilation can also be performed after a partial or small sphincterotomy. Theoretically, this might combine advantages of both techniques, and minimize the perforation and bleeding risk while widening the orifice to fit the desired intervention. Several groups have reported high success rates (89%–100%) without complications for stone removal in small series of up to 26 patients with Billroth II using this technique.[60,65,66]

Ultimately, deciding whether to pursue sphincterotomy or balloon dilation to facili-tate a biliary intervention in a particular case depends on several factors, including (1) presence or absence of a bilioenteric anastomosis; (2) type of endoscope used to reach the biliary orifice; (3) type of therapy required; (4) angle of access to the biliary orifice; (5) types, sizes, and lengths of ERCP tools available; and (6) underlying patient factors (eg, bleeding diathesis, need for antiplatelet medications, and so forth). One randomized trial comparing sphincterotomy with dilation for facilitating stone removal in 34 patients with Billroth II revealed similar success rates (78% for sphincterotomy, 88% for dilation) and a similar overall complication rate.[67]

NOVEL TECHNIQUES AND TECHNOLOGIES

Several new technologies have emerged, and novel techniques have been described, to facilitate bile duct access and therapy in patients with surgically altered anatomy. These are discussed next.

Multibending Gastroscope

Koo and colleagues[68] used a novel gastroscope (called an M-scope) to improve orien-tation and biliary access in 14 patients with Billroth II anatomy. Attempts at selective cannulation using standard gastroscopes had failed in all patients. The M-scope is unique in that its distal end can bend in two discrete points, with separate control dials for each. Selective bile duct cannulation was successful in 13 (92.9%) cases using this prototype. All attempted therapeutic maneuvers were also successful, including sphincterotomy, papillary balloon dilation, and stone removal.

EUS-guided Access and Therapy

A recent report demonstrated a novel technique involving therapeutic endoscopic ultrasound (EUS) to access the biliary tree and treat biliary stones in patients with RYGB. This involved the following steps: (1) EUS fine-needle aspiration puncture into an intrahepatic bile duct, (2) EUS-guided cholangiography, (3) guidewire advancement across the ampulla, (4) catheter dilation of the transhepatic-transgastric access tract, (5) anterograde balloon sphincteroplasty, and (6) anterograde advancement of stones across the ampulla using an extraction balloon. Six patients with past RYGB and symptomatic choledocholithiasis underwent the procedure. EUS-guided transhepatic puncture and cholangiography was successful in 100%; tract dilation, anterograde balloon sphincteroplasty, and stone extraction were successful in four (67%). In the remaining two patients, successful retrograde stone extraction was accomplished with ease after advancing a wire into the afferent limb and then performing rendezvous DBE-ERCP.[69]

Direct Cholangioscopy

A Japanese group recently demonstrated successful direct cholangioscopy in three patients with altered anatomy (one with Roux-en-Y gastrojeunostomy, two with Billroth II). Initially, the papilla was reached using DBE. After biliary access and sphincterotomy, an ultraslim endoscope was placed through an incision in the overtube and advanced to the biliary orifice. Direct cholangioscopy was performed, facilitating stone removal in two and confirming stone clearance in one patient.[70] Depending on the size of the biliary orifice, it may not be necessary to switch to an ultraslim endoscope, and a larger-diameter enteroscope could be immediately advanced into the bile duct for direct evaluation and therapy (**Fig. 10**).

Motorized Spiral Enteroscope

In 2011, Akerman and colleagues[71] described a modification of the SE system with the addition of an integrated motor device. A more recent study published in abstract form reported outcomes using this technology in 27 patients. An average anterograde

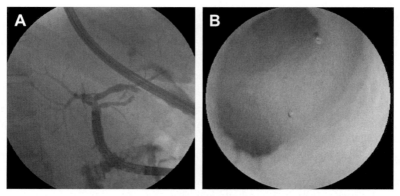

Fig. 10. Fluoroscopic (A) and endoscopic (B) images during direct cholangioscopy in a patient with Roux-en-Y hepaticojejunostomy. Double-balloon enteroscopy was used to reach the biliary anastomosis. After balloon dilation, the tip of the endoscope was directly advanced into the biliary tree.

insertion depth of 530 cm (range, 350–700 cm) was reached in an average of just 36 minutes (range, 24–46), and included three peroral cecal intubations.[72] Use of the motorized spiral enteroscope to perform ERCP has not yet been reported, but given the apparent quicker procedure times with consistent deep advancement into the small bowel, this technology may have potential use for ERCP in the postsurgical population.

Percutaneous Stent-assisted ERCP

To improve methods for ERCP in RYGB, one group investigated the feasibility of immediate ERCP after creation of a percutaneous-transgastric conduit using large-diameter self-expandable metal stents (SEMS). Duodenoscopes were successfully inserted directly into the stomach and advanced to the papilla immediately after transgastric SEMS access in all nine animals. Cholangiography was successful in all attempted cases. This series also included one human case, in which initial ERCP and follow-up duodenoscopy for pancreatic stent removal were successfully performed by the transgastric SEMS.[73] This technique offers the advantage of allowing repeated access for ERCP while obviating the need to wait for tract maturity; a laparoscopic approach also allows immediate access but requires collaboration with a second physician (surgeon) and use of the operating room.

SUMMARY AND TIPS FOR SUCCESS

Accessing the bile duct and performing biliary interventions in patients with altered anatomy is challenging. The authors recommend the following measures to maximize success:

1. Understand the anatomy: Familiarize oneself with the exact anatomy, lengths of surgical limbs, and presence or absence of a native major papilla. This impacts the choice of endoscope and devices needed for the procedure. The operative report should be reviewed in detail. Discussing the particulars with the surgeon who performed the procedure is even better.
2. Prepare an "ERCP toolkit": Have available ERCP cannulation instruments, wires, and therapeutic accessories that are appropriate for the instrument channel size and length of the endoscope used for the procedure. All possible access and therapeutic maneuvers that may be required should be anticipated, and the corresponding ERCP instruments should be at-hand for the procedure.

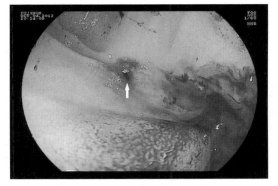

Fig. 11. Endoscopic image after placement of submucosal tattoo near the biliary anastomosis in a patient with Roux-en-Y hepaticojejunostomy. Ink marking facilitates identification of the biliary orifice (*arrow*) during future ERCPs, if needed.

3. Facilitate future ERCP procedures: A few measures can be taken to maximize success for future procedures, if needed. Submucosal ink tattoos can provide a useful roadmap. It is recommended to place a submucosal tattoo near the entrance of the correct limb (eg, afferent limb in Billroth II or biliopancreatic limb in Roux-en-Y), and near the bilioenteric anastomosis (when appropriate) to facilitate future procedures (**Fig. 11**). Additionally, a detailed procedure note is quite helpful. Specifics as to what maneuvers were helpful (eg, position change, external pressure, endoscope and accessories used) and what methods failed are equally important in saving the endoscopist valuable time and effort during a repeat procedure.

Postsurgical anatomy presents significant challenges to the pancreaticobiliary endoscopist. Selection of the appropriate technique should be determined on a case-by-case basis, and above all, the endoscopist's experience and technical familiarity with a particular method should dictate which modality is used for ERCP. Advances are ongoing and should facilitate increasingly effective and efficient ways to perform ERCP in this unique patient population.

REFERENCES

1. Herron DM, Roohipour R. Bariatric surgical anatomy and mechanisms of action. Gastrointest Endosc Clin N Am 2011;21:213–8.
2. Cicek B, Parlak E, Disibeyaz S, et al. Endoscopic retrograde cholangiopancreatography in patients with Billroth II gastroenterostomy. J Gastroenterol Hepatol 2007;22(8):1210–3.
3. Lopes TL, Wilcox CM. Endoscopic retrograde cholangiopancreatography in patients with Roux-en-Y anatomy. Gastroenterol Clin North Am 2010;39:99–107.
4. Khashab MA, Okolo PI. Accessing the pancreatobiliary limb and ERCP in the bariatric patient. Gastrointest Endosc Clin N Am 2011;21:305–13.
5. Lopes TL, Baron TH. Endoscopic retrograde cholangiopancreatography in patients with Roux-en-Y anatomy. J Hepatobiliary Pancreat Sci 2011;18:332–8.
6. Garcia-Cano J. A simple technique to aid intubation of the duodenoscope in the afferent limb of Billroth II gastrectomies for endoscopic retrograde cholangiopancreatography. Endoscopy 2008;40:E21–2.
7. Lin LF, Siauw CP, Ho KS, et al. ERCP in post-Billroth II gastrectomy patients: emphasis on technique. Am J Gastroenterol 1999;94(1):144–8.
8. Faylona JM, Qadir A, Chan AC, et al. Small-bowel perforations related to endoscopic retrograde cholangiopancreatography (ERCP) in patients with Billroth II gastrectomy. Endoscopy 1999;31:546–9.
9. Kim MH, Lee SK, Lee MH, et al. Endoscopic retrograde cholangiopancreatography and needle-knife sphincterotomy in patients with Billroth II gastrectomy: a comparative study of the forward-viewing endoscope and the side-viewing duodenoscope. Endoscopy 1997;29:82–5.
10. Park CH, Lee WS, Joo YE, et al. Cap-assisted ERCP in patients with a Billroth II gastrectomy. Gastrointest Endosc 2007;66(3):612–5.
11. Law N, Freeman ML. ERCP by using a prototype oblique-viewing endoscope in patients with surgically altered anatomy. Gastrointest Endosc 2004;59(6):724–8.
12. Nakahara K, Horaguchi J, Fujita N, et al. Therapeutic endoscope retrograde cholangiopancreatography using an anterior oblique-viewing endoscope for bile duct stones in patients with Billroth II gastrectomy. J Gastroenterol 2009;44:212–7.
13. Demarquay JF, Dumas R, Buckley MJ, et al. Endoscopic retrograde cholangiopancreatography in patients with Billroth II gastrectomy. Ital J Gastroenterol Hepatol 1998;30(3):297–300.

14. Aabakken L, Holthe B, Sandstad O, et al. Endoscopic pancreaticobiliary procedures in patients with a Billroth II resection: a 10-year follow up study. Ital J Gastroenterol Hepatol 1998;30(3):301–5.
15. Hintze RE, Adler A, Veltzke W, et al. Endoscopic access to the papilla of Vater for endoscopic retrograde cholangiopancreatography in patients with Billroth II or Roux-en-Y gastrojejunostomy. Endoscopy 1997;29(2):69–73.
16. Gostout CJ, Bender CE. Cholangiopancreatography, sphincterotomy, and common duct stone removal via Roux-en-Y limb enteroscopy. Gastroenterology 1988;95:156–63.
17. Elton E, Hanson BL, Qaseem T, et al. Diagnostic and therapeutic ERCP using an enteroscope and a pediatric colonoscope in long-limb surgical bypass patients. Gastrointest Endosc 1998;47:62–7.
18. Wright BE, Cass OW, Freeman ML. ERCP in patients with long-limb Roux-en-Y gastrojejunostomy and intact papilla. Gastrointest Endosc 2002;56(2):225–32.
19. Yamamoto H, Sekine Y, Sato Y, et al. Total enteroscopy with a nonsurgical steerable double-balloon method. Gastrointest Endosc 2001;53(2):216–20.
20. Sakai P, Kuga R, Safatle-Ribeiro AV, et al. Is it feasible to reach the bypassed stomach after Roux-en-Y gastric bypass for morbid obesity? The use of the double-balloon enteroscope. Endoscopy 2005;37(6):566–9.
21. Iwamoto S, Ryozawa S, Yamamoto H, et al. Double balloon endoscope facilitates endoscopic retrograde cholangiopancreatography in Roux-en-Y anastomosis patients. Dig Endosc 2010;22(1):64–8.
22. Kuga R, Furuya CK Jr, Hondo FY, et al. ERCP using double-balloon enteroscopy in patients with Roux-en-Y anatomy. Dig Dis 2008;26(4):330–5.
23. Monkemuller K, Fry LC, Bellutti M, et al. ERCP with the double balloon enteroscope in patients with Roux-en-Y anastomosis. Surg Endosc 2009;23(9):1961–7.
24. Ryozawa S, Iwamoto S, Iwano H, et al. ERCP using double-balloon endoscope in patients with Roux-en-Y anastomosis. J Hepatobiliary Pancreat Surg 2006;16: 613–7.
25. Haber GB. Double balloon endoscopy for pancreatic and biliary access in altered anatomy (with videos). Gastrointest Endosc 2007;66(3):S47–50.
26. Aabakken L, Bretthauer M, Line PD. Double-balloon enteroscopy for endoscopic retrograde cholangiography in patients with a Roux-en-Y anastomosis. Endoscopy 2007;39(12):1068–71.
27. Raithel M, Dormann H, Naegel A, et al. Double-balloon-enteroscopy-based endoscopic retrograde cholangiopancreatography in post-surgical patients. World J Gastroenterol 2011;17(18):2302–14.
28. Emmett DS, Mallat DB. Double-balloon ERCP in patients who have undergone Roux-en-Y surgery: a case series. Gastrointest Endosc 2007;66(5):1038–41.
29. Parlak E, Cicek B, Disibeyaz S, et al. Endoscopic retrograde cholangiography by double balloon enteroscopy in patients with Roux-en-Y hepaticojejunostomy. Surg Endosc 2010;24(2):466–70.
30. Neumann H, Fry LC, Meyer F, et al. Endoscopic retrograde cholangiopancreatography using the single balloon enteroscope technique in patients with Roux-en-anastomosis. Digestion 2009;80(1):52–7.
31. Wang AY, Sauer BG, Behm BW, et al. Single-balloon enteroscopy effectively enables diagnostic and therapeutic retrograde cholangiography in patients with surgically altered anatomy. Gastrointest Endosc 2010;71(3):641–9.
32. Itoi T, Ishii K, Sofuni A, et al. Single-balloon enteroscopy-assisted ERCP in patients with Billroth II gastrectomy or Roux-en-Y anastomosis (with video). Am J Gastroenterol 2010;105(1):93–9.

33. Saleem A, Baron TH, Gostout CJ, et al. Endoscopic retrograde cholangiopancreatography using a single-balloon enteroscope in patients with altered Roux-en-Y anatomy. Endoscopy 2010;42(8):656–60.

34. Shah RJ, Smolkin M, Ross AS, et al. A multi-center, U.S. experience of single balloon, double balloon, and rotational overtube enteroscopy-assisted ERCP in long limb surgical bypass patients. Gastrointest Endosc 2010;71:AB134.

35. Shimatani M, Matsushita M, Takaoka M, et al. Effective "short" double-balloon enteroscope for diagnostic and therapeutic ERCP in patients with altered gastrointestinal anatomy: a large case series. Endoscopy 2009;41(10):849–54.

36. Cho S, Kamalaporn P, Kandel G, et al. Short double-balloon enteroscope endoscopic retrograde cholangiopancreatography in patients with a surgically altered upper gastrointestinal tract. Can J Gastroenterol 2011;25(11):615–9.

37. Siddiqui AA, Chaaya A, Shelton C, et al. Utility of the short double-balloon enteroscope to perform pancreaticobiliary interventions in patients with surgically altered anatomy in a US multicenter study. Dig Dis Sci 2012. [Epub ahead of print].

38. May A, Manner H, Aschmoneit I, et al. Prospective, cross-over, single-center trial comparing oral double-balloon enteroscopy and oral spiral enteroscopy in patients with suspected small-bowel vascular malformations. Endoscopy 2011; 43(6):477–83.

39. Messer I, May A, Manner H, et al. Prospective, randomized, single-center trial compared double-balloon enteroscopy and spiral enteroscopy in patients with suspected small-bowel disorders. Gastrointest Endosc 2012. [Epub ahead of print].

40. Lennon AM, Kapoor S, Khashab M, et al. Spiral assisted ERCP is equivalent to single balloon assisted ERCP in patients with Roux-en-Y anatomy. Dig Dis Sci 2012;57(5):1391–8.

41. Wagh MS, Draganov PV. Prospective evaluation of spiral overtube-assisted ERCP in patients with surgically altered anatomy. Gastrointest Endosc 2012;76(2): 439–43.

42. Moreels TG, Pelckmans PA. Comparison between double-balloon and single-balloon enteroscopy in therapeutic ERC after Roux-en-Y entero-enteric anastomosis. World J Gastrointest Endosc 2010;2(9):314–7.

43. Gerson LB, Tokar J, Chiorean M, et al. Complications associated with double balloon enteroscopy at nine US centers. Clin Gastroenterol Hepatol 2009;7(11): 1177–82.

44. Nguyen DM, El-Sarag HB. The big burden of obesity. Gastrointest Endosc 2009; 70(4):752–7.

45. Birkmeyer NJ, Dimick JB, Share D, et al. Hospital complication rates with bariatric surgery in Michigan. JAMA 2010;304:435–42.

46. Shiffman ML, Sugerman HJ, Kellum JM, et al. Gallstone formation after rapid weight loss: a prospective study in patients undergoing gastric bypass surgery for treatment of morbid obesity. Am J Gastroenterol 1991;86(8):1000–5.

47. Baron TH, Vickers SM. Surgical gastrostomy placement as access for diagnostic and therapeutic ERCP. Gastrointest Endosc 1998;48:640–1.

48. Gutierrez JM, Lederer H, Krook JC, et al. Surgical gastrostomy for pancreatobiliary and duodenal access following Roux-en-Y gastric bypass. J Gastrointest Surg 2009;13(12):2170–5.

49. Tekola B, Wang AY, Ramanath M, et al. Percutaneous gastrostomy tube placement to perform transgastrostomy endoscopic retrograde cholangiopancreatography in patients with Roux-en-Y anatomy. Dig Dis Sci 2011;56(11):3364–9.

50. Saleem A, Levy MK, Petersen BT, et al. Laparoscopic assisted ERCP in Roux-en-Y gastric bypass (RYGB) surgery patients. J Gastrointest Surg 2012;16(1):203–8.
51. Falcao M, Campos JM, Galvao Neto M, et al. Transgastric endoscopic retrograde cholangiopancreatography for the management of biliary tract disease after Roux-en-Y gastric bypass treatment for obesity. Obes Surg 2012;22(6):872–6.
52. Schreiner MA, Chang L, Gluck M, et al. Laparoscopy-assisted versus balloon enteroscopy-assisted ERCP in bariatric post-Roux-en-Y gastric bypass patients. Gastrointest Endosc 2012;75(4):748–56.
53. Adler DG, Conway JD, Farraye FA, et al. Biliary and pancreatic stone extraction devices. Gastrointest Endosc 2009;70(4):603–9.
54. DiSario J, Chuttani R, Croffie J, et al. Biliary and pancreatic lithotripsy devices. Gastrointest Endosc 2007;65(6):750–6.
55. Somoqyi L, Chuttani R, Croffie J, et al. Guidewires for use in GI endoscopy. Gastrointest Endosc 2007;65(4):571–6.
56. Somoqyi L, Chuttani R, Croffie J, et al. Biliary and pancreatic stents. Gastrointest Endosc 2006;63(7):910–9.
57. Kethu SR, Adler DG, Conway JD, et al. ERCP cannulation and sphincterotomy devices. Gastrointest Endosc 2010;71(3):435–45.
58. Hintze RE, Veltzke W, Adler A, et al. Endoscopic sphincterotomy using an S-shaped sphincterotome in patients with a Billroth II or Roux-en-Y gastrojejunostomy. Endoscopy 1997;29(2):74–8.
59. Costamagna G, Multignani M, Perri V, et al. Diagnostic and therapeutic ERCP in patients with Billroth II gastrectomy. Acta Gastroenterol Belg 1994;57(2):155–62.
60. Kim GH, Kang DH, Song GA, et al. Endoscopic removal of bile-duct stones by using a rotatable papillotome and a large-balloon dilator in patients with a Billroth II gastrectomy (with video). Gastrointest Endosc 2008;67(7):1134–8.
61. Van Buuren HR, Boender J, Nix GA, et al. Needle-knife sphincterotomy guided by a biliary endoprosthesis in Billroth II gastrectomy patients. Endoscopy 1995; 27(3):229–32.
62. Feng Y, Zhu H, Chen X, et al. Comparison of endoscopic papillary large balloon dilation and endoscopic sphincterotomy for retrieval of choledocholithiasis: a meta-analysis of randomized controlled trials. J Gastroenterol 2012;47(6):655–63.
63. Liu Y, Su P, Lin S, et al. Endoscopic papillary balloon dilatation versus endoscopic sphincterotomy in the treatment for choledocholithiasis: a meta-analysis. J Gastroenterol Hepatol 2012;27(3):464–71.
64. Lee TH, Hwang JC, Choi HJ, et al. One-step transpapillary balloon dilation under cap-fitted endoscopy without a preceding sphincterotomy for the removal of bile duct stones in Billroth II gastrectomy. Gut Liver 2012;6(1):113–7.
65. Choi CW, Choi JS, Kang DH, et al. Endoscopic papillary large balloon dilation in Billroth II gastrectomy patients with bile duct stones. J Gastroenterol Hepatol 2012;27(2):256–60.
66. Itoi T, Ishii K, Itokawa F, et al. Large balloon papillary dilation for removal of bile duct stones in patients who have undergone a Billroth II gastrectomy. Dig Endosc 2010;22(Suppl 1):S98–102.
67. Bergman JJ, Van Berkel AM, Bruno MJ, et al. A randomized trial of endoscopic balloon dilation and endoscopic sphincterotomy for removal of bile duct stones in patients with a prior Billroth II gastrectomy. Gastrointest Endosc 2001;53(1): 19–26.
68. Koo HC, Moon JH, Choi HJ, et al. The utility of a multibending endoscope for selective cannulation during ERCP in patients with a Billroth II gastrectomy (with video). Gastrointest Endosc 2009;69(4):931–4.

69. Weilert F, Binmoeller KF, Marson F, et al. Endoscopic ultrasound-guided antero-grade treatment of biliary stones following gastric bypass. Endoscopy 2011;43:1105–8.
70. Koshitani T, Matsuda S, Takai K, et al. Direct cholangioscopy combined with double-balloon enteroscope-assisted endoscopic retrograde cholangiopancrea-tography. World J Gastroenterol 2012;18(28):3765–9.
71. Akerman PA, Demarco DC, Pangtay J, et al. A novel motorized spiral entero-scope can advance rapidly, safely and deeply into the small bowel. Gastrointest Endosc 2011;73(Suppl 4):AB446.
72. Akerman PA, Demarco DC, Bhattacharya K, et al. Endoscopic visualization of the entire small intestine in 27 consecutive patients using novel motorized spiral endoscope. Gastrointest Endosc 2012;75(Suppl 4):AB134.
73. Baron TH, Song LM, Ferreira LE, et al. Novel approach to therapeutic ERCP after long-limb Roux-en-Y gastric bypass surgery using transgastric self-expandable metal stents: experimental outcomes and first human case study (with videos). Gastrointest Endosc 2012;75(6):1258–63.

Endoscopic Approach to the Patient with Congenital Anomalies of the Biliary Tract

Quin Y. Liu, MD[a,b,]*, Vivien Nguyen, MD[b]

KEYWORDS

- Neonatal cholestasis • Biliary atresia • Alagille syndrome • Choledochal cysts
- Congenital biliary tract diseases • Infant ERCP

KEY POINTS

- Prompt and accurate diagnosis of neonatal cholestatic diseases is required to avoid potentially high morbidity and mortality.
- Endoscopic retrograde cholangiopancreatography (ERCP) and endoscopic ultrasonography (EUS) can help in the diagnosis, classification, and surgical treatment of choledochal cysts.
- ERCP can aid in the diagnosis and exclusion of biliary atresia and other congenital biliary tract diseases, although its role is not standardized and remains controversial in the evaluation of neonatal cholestasis.

INTRODUCTION

Congenital biliary tract diseases are rare in children compared to adults. Presenting signs and symptoms in toddlers and older children are often nonspecific, and diagnostic findings may be incidental. Congenital biliary tract diseases typically manifest themselves with cholestasis in the neonatal period, and prompt diagnosis and management are essential in ensuring optimal outcomes. Given the rarity of these disorders and the subtle nuances differentiating them, infants with cholestatic liver disease benefit from evaluation at a multispecialty pediatric center.

Funding sources: None.
Conflict of interest: None.
[a] Keck School of Medicine, University of Southern California, Children's Hospital Los Angeles, 4650 Sunset Boulevard, Los Angeles, CA 90027, USA; [b] Division of Gastroenterology and Nutrition, Children's Hospital Los Angeles, 4650 Sunset Boulevard, Mailstop #78, Los Angeles, CA 90027, USA
* Corresponding author. Division of Gastroenterology and Nutrition, Children's Hospital Los Angeles, 4650 Sunset Boulevard, Mailstop #78, Los Angeles, CA 90027.
E-mail address: qliu@chla.usc.edu

The differential diagnosis for neonatal cholestasis is broad and includes congenital anatomic abnormalities, infection, endocrine disorders, neonatal hepatitis, and metabolic and genetic diseases (**Box 1**). Despite a usually extensive evaluation for neonatal cholestasis, the cause may remain unclear. Because of the importance of a prompt and accurate diagnosis, endoscopy can aid in the diagnosis of congenital biliary tract diseases, and at times, definitively treat the anomaly. As in adults, the endoscopic

Box 1 **Cause of neonatal cholestasis**
Obstructive
Biliary atresia
Choledochal cyst
Inspissated bile
Genetic/metabolic
Hypothyroidism
Alpha1-antitrypsin deficiency
Neonatal hemochromatosis
Bilirubin metabolism disorders
Galactosemia
Tyrosinemia
Lysosomal storage diseases
Fatty acid oxidation disorders
Peroxisomal disorders
Urea cycle defects
Progressive familial intrahepatic cholestasis (PFIC)
Alagille syndrome
Cystic fibrosis
Infectious
TORCH infections
Mycobacterium tuberculosis
Urinary tract infection
Epstein-Barr virus
Cytomegalovirus
Autoimmune
Neonatal sclerosing cholangitis
Infiltrative/tumor
Sarcoma botryoides
Leukemia
Toxicity
Drug-induced toxicity
Total parenteral nutrition cholestasis

approach to children with congenital biliary tract diseases may involve ERCP. When performed by an experienced endoscopist, pediatric ERCP is technically successful, safe, and therapeutically effective for a broad range of pancreaticobiliary diseases.[1–5] ERCP with a therapeutic duodenal scope is usually feasible in children weighing more than 10 kg. With the availability of smaller pediatric duodenoscopes ranging from 7.5 to 8 mm in diameter, infant ERCP has also been shown to be technically feasible and safe, with a success rate ranging from 87% to 93%.[6–11] But with a 2-mm working channel, therapeutic accessories for the pediatric duodenoscopes are limited. More recently, EUS with fine-needle aspiration has also been shown to be technically feasible and safe while providing diagnostic information in children with pancreaticobiliary diseases.[4,12–15] Unfortunately, because of the small size of infants and the relatively large size of the current EUS echoendoscopes (insertion tube diameters ranging from 11.8 to 12.8 mm), EUS has limited diagnostic value in infants with congenital biliary tract diseases. This article discusses the role of endoscopy in the diagnosis and management of various congenital biliary tract anomalies.

BILIARY ATRESIA

Biliary atresia is a neonatal cholestatic disease in which a fibroinflammatory process leads to complete obliteration of all or part of the extrahepatic biliary system. Incidence is higher in Asians and ranges from 1 in 5000 to 1 in 18,000.[16] Presentation occurs within the first 2 to 3 weeks of life with prolonged neonatal jaundice, conjugated hyperbilirubinemia, acholic stools, and hepatomegaly. Affected infants are usually otherwise well for the first few months of life. Biliary atresia can also present in a syndromic form with splenic malformation, intestinal malrotation, preduodenal portal vein, and congenital cardiac defects. Untreated biliary atresia leads to liver failure and progressive biliary cirrhosis with a 100% mortality rate. Surgical treatment with a portoenterostomy biliary diversion, first described by Kasai and Suzuki in 1950, reestablishes bile flow by resecting the fibrosed bile duct and anastomosing a Roux limb to patent intrahepatic bile ducts within the porta hepatis.[17] Although the procedure has since been refined, diagnosis remains time sensitive because delayed surgical treatment is associated with poor outcome.[18,19] Despite timely surgical intervention, the chronic inflammatory process continues to progress and biliary atresia remains the leading cause for pediatric liver transplantation.[20]

The diagnosis of biliary atresia is considered when evaluating infants with cholestasis, and several studies are typically carried out, including laboratory tests, abdominal ultrasonography, hepatobiliary iminodiacetic acid (HIDA) scan, and percutaneous liver biopsy. Despite this extensive evaluation, the diagnosis of biliary atresia occurs before cholangiography in approximately 86% of cases.[21] Definitive diagnosis requires an intraoperative cholangiogram to distinguish this obliterative cholangiopathy from other neonatal cholestatic diseases. Because the gold standard for diagnosis involves surgery, studies have assessed the role of ERCP as a minimally invasive means of evaluating cholestatic infants suspected to have biliary atresia.

There are 3 main variants of biliary atresia: type 1, atresia of the common bile duct; type 2, atresia of the common hepatic duct; and type 3, atresia of the hepatic ducts within the porta hepatitis.[22] Guelrud and colleagues[23] reported 3 ERCP findings suggesting the different variants of biliary atresia (**Fig. 1**): type 1, opacification of the pancreatic duct only with no visualization of the bile duct; type 2, opacification of the common bile duct and gallbladder with no visualization of the common hepatic and intrahepatic ducts; and type 3, opacification of the common bile duct, gallbladder, and hepatic duct with bile lakes at the porta hepatitis (**Fig. 2**). In this prospective study,

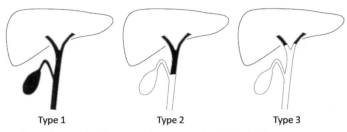

Type 1   Type 2   Type 3

Fig. 1. Anatomic variants of biliary atresia seen with ERCP. Black area represents the atretic biliary segment not visualized on cholangiogram by ERCP.

the investigators were able to demonstrate a normal biliary tract in 10 patients who had findings of liver biopsy suggesting extrahepatic biliary atresia, therefore avoiding surgery for those patients.

Further studies have shown the utility of ERCP for diagnosing and excluding biliary atresia (**Table 1**). ERCP demonstrating a normal and patent biliary system can exclude biliary atresia and prevent unnecessary surgery in 12% to 43% of infants with an indeterminate precholangiogram evaluation.[8,9,24–26] For diagnosis of biliary atresia, ERCP has been reported to have a sensitivity of 86% to 100%, specificity of 73% to 94%, positive predictive value of 86% to 88%, and negative predictive value of 100%.[8,9,26] Although Petersen and colleagues[8] include ERCP in their algorithm for all infants suspected with biliary atresia, its use remains uncommon when evaluating for biliary atresia. Centers that have studied the use of ERCP in biliary atresia recommend its selective use in infants in whom the precholangiogram evaluation is indeterminate and the diagnosis of biliary atresia is not certain. Yet, most pediatric gastroenterologists continue to rely on the clinical presentation, laboratory values, ultrasonography, HIDA scan, and liver biopsy to determine if a cholestatic infant requires a surgical intraoperative cholangiogram.

ALAGILLE SYNDROME

Paucity of bile ducts can be divided into nonsyndromic and syndromic (Alagille syndrome). Diagnosis of paucity of bile ducts is made on liver biopsy when the bile-duct-to-portal-tract ratio is less than 0.9. There should be at least 6 to 10

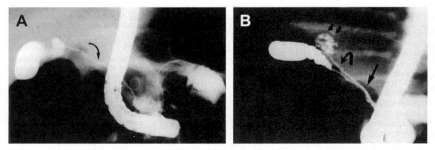

Fig. 2. Cholangiogram of infants with biliary atresia. (*A*) Type 2 ERCP finding with the gallbladder and common bile duct opacified (*curved arrow*). (*B*) Type 3 ERCP finding with gallbladder, common bile duct (*straight arrow*), common hepatic duct (*curved arrow*), and bile lakes (*double arrows*). (*From* Guelrud M, Jaen D, Mendoza S, et al. ERCP in the diagnosis of extrahepatic biliary atresia. Gastrointest Endosc 1991;37(5):525; from Elsevier with permission.)

Table 1
ERCP in the evaluation of infants with neonatal cholestasis suspicious for BA

Author	No. of ERCPs	Successful Cannulation	Complete Biliary Tree Visualized	Incomplete or No Biliary Tree Visualized (Suggestive of BA)	BA Confirmed with IOC/BA Suggested by ERCP
Guelrud et al,[23] 1991	32	30 (94%)	10 (31%)	20 (63%)	20/20 (100%)
Ohnuma et al,[7] 1997	75	66 (75%)	19 (25%)	46 (61%)[a]	46/46 (100%)
Aabakken et al,[6] 2009	23	20 (87%)	14 (61%)	6 (26%)	6/6 (100%)
Vegting et al,[25] 2009	26	26 (100%)	3 (12%)	23 (88%)	21/23 (91%)
Petersen et al,[8] 2009	140	122 (87%)	34 (28%)	88 (72%)	72/88 (82%)
Shanmugam et al,[9] 2009	48	45 (94%)	20 (42%)	25 (52%)	22/25 (88%)
Keil et al,[26] 2010	104	95 (91%)	44 (42%)	51 (49%)	49/51 (96%)
Shteyer et al,[24] 2012	21	18 (86%)	4 (19%)	14 (67%)	13/14 (93%)

Abbreviations: BA, biliary atresia; IOC, intraoperative cholangiogram.
[a] One cholangiogram excluded because of poor-quality radiograph.

microscopic portal tracts present in the core needle biopsy specimen for an accurate analysis.[27,28] Although nonsyndromic bile duct paucity can be seen in other infectious, metabolic, or inflammatory diseases, Alagille syndrome is an autosomal dominant disorder that also includes congenital cardiac, renal, vertebral, and ocular diseases. Patients may also have characteristic facial features including prominent forehead, deep-set eyes, and pointed chin.[29,30] Mutations in *JAG1* and *Notch2* have been shown to cause Alagille syndrome, and detection of the mutations can aid in diagnosis.[31–33]

The features of Alagille syndrome frequently become apparent in the neonatal period or during early infancy and are nearly indistinguishable from those of biliary atresia. During childhood, jaundice may wax and wane and children may show signs of malnutrition and growth failure.[34] Pruritus is the most unbearable symptom, leading to excoriation of the skin, difficulty with sleep, and poor concentration. Severe pruritus can be treated at experienced pediatric liver centers with an externalized surgical biliary diversion, which is thought to ameliorate the condition by decreasing enterohepatic recirculation of bile salts.[35]

Paucity of bile ducts on liver biopsy, along with the extrahepatic features noted above, can differentiate Alagille syndrome from other neonatal cholestatic diseases. As mentioned, it is not uncommon for the presentation of Alagille syndrome to resemble that of biliary atresia in young infants. Infants with Alagille syndrome may have indeterminate results of liver biopsies and also abnormal HIDA scan results. It is important to make a timely and proper diagnosis to ensure that patients are not incorrectly diagnosed with biliary atresia because the Kasai portoenterostomy is not beneficial for patients with Alagille syndrome and it may actually worsen their outcomes.[36] As with patients with biliary atresia, in patients with an indeterminate diagnosis, ERCP may be helpful in diagnosing Alagille syndrome while at the same time excluding biliary atresia. In patients with Alagille syndrome, ERCP can show a normal or diffuse narrowing of the extrahepatic biliary ducts and narrowing of the intrahepatic ducts with reduced arborization.[37]

CHOLEDOCHAL CYST

Choledochal cysts are structural anomalies consisting of cystic dilations of the biliary tree. Although classified as congenital, there is speculation that the cysts may result from the reflux of pancreatic enzymes into the bile duct secondary to an anomalous pancreaticobiliary duct junction proximal to the sphincter of Oddi.[38]

Choledochal cysts occur more frequently in females than in males and are more common in Asians than in other populations, with an incidence as high as 1:1000.[39] Most cysts present during childhood, and symptoms may vary with age. Infants may present with the classical triad of jaundice, abdominal pain, and a palpable abdominal mass, although the concomitant presence of all the 3 symptoms is rare.[40] Older children may present with abdominal pain, jaundice, cholangitis, and pancreatitis. Patients sometimes do not present until early adulthood, with symptoms similar to older children. Choledochal cysts have also been known to be diagnosed incidentally in both children and adults during evaluation for unrelated symptoms—from our experience, it is not uncommon to encounter a choledochal cyst on abdominal ultrasonography obtained during evaluation of renal disease.

There are several types of congenital choledochal cysts (**Fig. 3**).[41] Type I cysts are the most common, representing approximately 77% of all biliary cysts. Type I cysts are subdivided into the following subtypes: A, cystic dilation of the common bile duct; B, smaller segmental cystic dilation; and C, cylindrical fusiform dilation. Type II cysts are diverticuli of the bile duct. Type III cysts are intraduodenal choledochoceles, of which there are 2 variants (**Fig. 4**).[42] Type IV cysts are multiple intrahepatic and extrahepatic cyst. Type V cysts, also referred to as Caroli disease, are intrahepatic

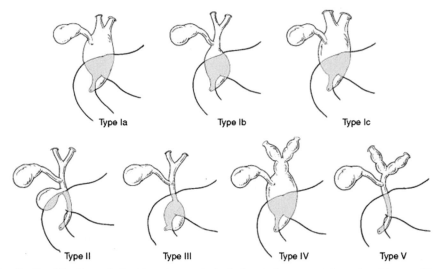

Type Ia   Type Ib   Type Ic

Type II   Type III   Type IV   Type V

Fig. 3. Classification of the 5 major choledochal cyst forms and type 1 subtypes. (*From* Gonzales KD, Lee H. Choledocal cyst. In: Coran AG, Editor. Pediatric Surgery. Philadelphia: Elsevier Saunders; 2012, with permission.)

A

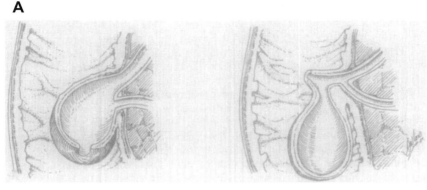

Type 1   Type 2

B   C

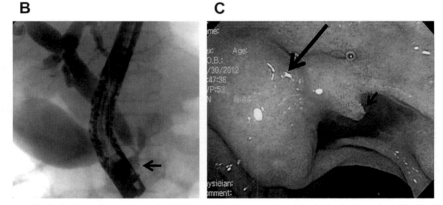

Fig. 4. Choledochocele variants. (A) Schematic of types 1 and 2 choledochoceles. (B) Cholan-giogram of type 1 choledochocele (arrow). (C) Endoscopic view of type 2 choledochocele (long arrow) and papilla with bile drainage (short arrow). ([A] From O'Neill JA Jr. Choledo-chal cyst. Curr Probl Surg 1992;29(6):374; by Mosby, an imprint of Elsevier Inc. with permission.)

biliary cysts. Caroli disease is frequently associated with congenital hepatic fibrosis and polycystic kidney disease. The management of Caroli disease usually requires a multidisciplinary approach, including pediatric hepatologists and nephrologists.

As stated earlier, an anomalous pancreaticobiliary duct junction may play a role in the pathogenesis of congenital choledochal cysts, specifically types I to IV. Normally, the common bile duct and pancreatic duct enter the duodenum separately or as a common channel. But the common bile duct joining into the pancreatic duct, or the pancreatic duct joining into the common bile duct, is classified as an anomalous pancreaticobiliary duct junction.[43] An abnormally long common channel, especially one with the pancreaticobiliary duct junction proximal to the sphincter of Oddi, is also thought to be anomalous. Normal common channel length can range from 1 to 3 mm in infants younger than 1 year.[38,44] In adults, a common channel is normally 4 to 6 mm in length and can range from 2 to 10 mm.[45] Many consider a common channel greater than 15 mm to be abnormal, although a length of 8 mm or greater has been considered abnormal.[46] There are also reports of children with anomalous pancreati-cobiliary duct junction without cystic dilation of the bile duct. These children may present with similar symptoms of abdominal pain, emesis, and jaundice, which are thought to be due to obstruction of the common channel by proteinaceous plugs.[47,48]

Initial evaluation usually consists of ultrasonography and magnetic resonance cholangiopancreatography (MRCP). Although both modalities can be highly suggestive in diagnosing a choledochal cyst, ERCP is, at times, required to confirm the diagnosis. ERCP has been shown to be more sensitive than MRCP in identifying and classifying anomalous pancreaticobiliary duct junctions and aids in optimal surgical planning for cyst resection.[43,49,50] EUS can also aid in surgical planning by better defining the involvement of the cystic lesion in relationship to the pancreatic head (**Fig. 5**). In patients with congenital choledochal cyst, who present with obstructive jaundice, cholangitis, or exacerbating symptoms refractory to noninvasive management, ERCP can also serve as a bridge to first stabilize the patient and decompress the biliary system before definitive surgery. ERCP with sphincterotomy and stone debris removal, with or without stent placement, has been shown to be safe and effective in relieving symptoms and extracting obstructing stone debris while aiding in surgical planning of cyst resection.[47,48,51,52] Stone debris in the biliary tract or common channel in patients with congenital choledochal cyst have been found to be not only biliary stones but also pancreatic proteinaceous plugs, similar to those seen in patients with anomalous pancreaticobiliary duct junction without biliary cysts.[52,53] The definitive treatment of choice for people with types I, II, and IV cysts is complete surgical excision with a hepaticojejunostomy because of the increased risk of biliary neoplasia. The incidence of malignant change in patients diagnosed within the first decade of life is less than 1%; however, the risk increases to 14% in those diagnosed after the age of 20 years.[54] An increased risk of biliary malignancy persists even after cyst resection, with the risk of biliary carcinoma reported as high as 121 times greater than the general population.[55]

ERCP has also been used to treat and initially diagnose a patient with Caroli disease who presented with jaundice and cholangitis.[56] Caroli disease is also associated with an increased risk of malignancy and cirrhosis; therefore, lobectomy has been performed in intrahepatic cystic lesions isolated from a single hepatic lobe and liver transplant has been successful for patients with diffuse Caroli disease.[57,58] This is different from type III choledochal cysts because their risk of malignancy is considered much lower. Therefore, it is important to accurately diagnose type III choledochal cysts because they can be managed with endoscopic sphincterotomy or unroofing of the cyst to achieve drainage.[59,60]

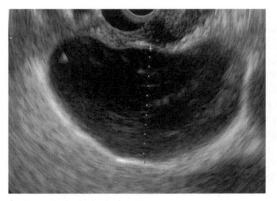

Fig. 5. EUS image of a type 1 choledochal cyst.

INSPISSATED BILE SYNDROME

Inspissation of bile and mucus may cause obstruction of the biliary system in infants. Inspissated bile can be considered along the spectrum of neonatal cholelithiasis. When found incidentally in asymptomatic infants, neonatal cholelithiasis should be followed up clinically because spontaneous resolution of lithiasis can occur.[61–63] Although inspissated bile syndrome may be considered an acquired biliary disease, it has been found to occur in infants secondary to congenital or genetic diseases, particularly cystic fibrosis. The condition has also been described in otherwise healthy neonates; however, prematurity, use of diuretics, and prolonged dependence on parenteral nutrition seem to be predisposing factors. Bile stasis, infection, and increased bilirubin load are thought to be involved in the pathogenesis of the syndrome.[64] With the development of measures to prevent Rh and ABO incompatibilities, the contribution of the latter has declined.

The clinical presentation of inspissated bile syndrome is similar to that of biliary atresia, with jaundice, conjugated hyperbilirubinemia, dark urine, and acholic stools. Hepatobiliary scintigraphy may show absence of radionuclide excretion into the intestinal lumen, but ultrasonography may demonstrate dilatation of the intrahepatic biliary ducts with biliary sludge, which can distinguish it from biliary atresia.[65] Most cases of inspissated bile syndrome are managed conservatively, surgically, or percutaneously with flushing of the biliary tree with saline or mucolytic agent.[65–67] However, ERCP presents a potential alternative to these invasive procedures and shows areas of biliary system dilation (**Fig. 6**). As noted by Guelrud and colleagues,[68] improvement in the clinical status of patients with inspissated bile syndrome after ERCP raises the question of whether irrigation of the biliary tree may be therapeutic as well.[68]

NEONATAL SCLEROSING CHOLANGITIS

The clinical features of neonatal sclerosing cholangitis (NSC) are nearly indistinguishable from those of biliary atresia. Infants present with jaundice, cholestasis, hepatosplenomegaly, and variable stool pigmentation. HIDA scan may assist in diagnosis if radionuclide excretion is noted, but histological studies demonstrate nonspecific evidence of large-duct obstruction.[69] The advent of direct cholangiography has

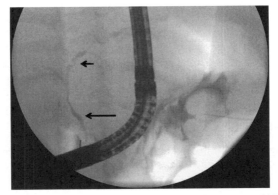

Fig. 6. ERCP in an 8-month-old child with cystic fibrosis and inspissated bile syndrome. Cholangiogram shows dilation of the common bile duct (*long arrow*) and intrahepatic bile duct (*short arrow*). (*Courtesy of* Douglas Fishman, MD, Texas Children's Hospital, Baylor College of Medicine, Houston, TX.)

allowed for refinement in identification of the disorder. ERCP findings include rarefaction of segmental intrahepatic and extrahepatic bile ducts, stenosis, and focal dilatation.[9,70]

Although most affected infants are nonsyndromic, without other extrahepatic anomalies, NSC may occur in the setting of diseases such as human immunodeficiency virus infection, autoimmune hepatitis, cystic fibrosis, and sickle cell disease. A familial form of NSC associated with abnormalities of the epidermis has also been described. Neonatal ichthyosis and sclerosing cholangitis syndrome (NISCH) is a rare autosomal recessive disease characterized by neonatal-onset sclerosing cholangitis, ichthyosis, hypotrichosis, and dental anomalies. NISCH is caused by mutations in *CLDN1* encoding claudin-1, an integral tight-junction protein.[71] Absence of claudin-1 in the biliary epithelium is thought to lead to increased paracellular permeability and hepatocyte injury secondary to paracellular leakage of bile constituents.[72] Cholestasis and fibrosis without fatty infiltration or ductular proliferation are found on liver biopsy, whereas transmission electron microscopy of the skin shows disruption in the anchoring plaques of desmosomes.

Medical management of this condition focuses on enhancing bile flow with ursodeoxycholic acid and ameliorating the nutritional sequelae of cholestasis with fat-soluble vitamin and medium-chain triglyceride supplementation. Response to conservative measures remains variable, and a significant proportion of affected children require liver transplant because of progressive biliary cirrhosis.

SUMMARY

The cause of neonatal cholestasis is vast with an evaluation that can be broad and extensive for congenital biliary tract anomalies. Evaluation of a cholestatic infant must be prompt and accurate to avoid high morbidity and mortality related to late or incorrect diagnosis. Although endoscopy is not required for most patients with neonatal cholestasis, ERCP and EUS are integral in the diagnosis of choledochal cysts, because both modalities are able to clearly delineate anomalies of the biliary tree, thereby guiding definitive surgical treatment. Therapeutic ERCP can also relieve symptoms in patients with choledochal cysts and biliary obstruction. The role of ERCP in the evaluation and management biliary atresia and other congenital biliary tract anomalies presenting during infancy is less clear. Although studies show that ERCP aids in the diagnosis and exclusion of biliary atresia and other infant biliary diseases, its integration into the diagnostic algorithm for neonatal cholestasis is not well established and its routine use has been limited to a few pediatric liver centers. Therefore, it is important that infants with prolonged neonatal cholestasis be evaluated at an experienced pediatric liver center, where endoscopy and other modalities are used appropriately. As ERCP is further studied in the evaluation of biliary atresia and neonatal cholestasis, its role will be better defined.

ACKNOWLEDGMENTS

The authors covey special thanks to Dr Dan Thomas, MD, for his contributions to this article.

REFERENCES

1. Fox VL, Werlin SL, Heyman MB. Endoscopic retrograde cholangiopancreatography in children. Subcommittee on Endoscopy and Procedures of the Patient Care

Committee of the North American Society for Pediatric Gastroenterology and Nutrition. J Pediatr Gastroenterol Nutr 2000;30(3):335–42.

2. Jang JY, Yoon CH, Kim KM. Endoscopic retrograde cholangiopancreatography in pancreatic and biliary tract disease in Korean children. World J Gastroenterol 2010;16(4):490–5.

3. Otto A, Neal M, Slivka A, et al. An appraisal of endoscopic retrograde cholangio-pancreatography (ERCP) for pancreaticobiliary disease in children: our institutional experience in 231 cases. Surg Endosc 2011;25(8):2536–40.

4. Varadarajulu S, Wilcox CM, Hawes RH, et al. Technical outcomes and complications of ERCP in children. Gastrointest Endosc 2004;60(3):367–71.

5. Rocca R, Castellino F, Daperno M, et al. Therapeutic ERCP in paediatric patients. Dig Liver Dis 2005;37(5):357–62.

6. Aabakken L, Aagenaes I, Sanengen T, et al. Utility of ERCP in neonatal and infant cholestasis. J Laparoendosc Adv Surg Tech A 2009;19(3):431–6.

7. Ohnuma N, Takahashi T, Tanabe M, et al. The role of ERCP in biliary atresia. Gastrointest Endosc 1997;45(5):365–70.

8. Petersen C, Meier PN, Schneider A, et al. Endoscopic retrograde cholangiopan-creaticography prior to explorative laparotomy avoids unnecessary surgery in patients suspected for biliary atresia. J Hepatol 2009;51(6):1055–60.

9. Shanmugam NP, Harrison PM, Devlin J, et al. Selective use of endoscopic retrograde cholangiopancreatography in the diagnosis of biliary atresia in infants younger than 100 days. J Pediatr Gastroenterol Nutr 2009;49(4): 435–41.

10. Guelrud M, Jaen D, Torres P, et al. Endoscopic cholangiopancreatography in the infant: evaluation of a new prototype pediatric duodenoscope. Gastrointest Endosc 1987;33(1):4–8.

11. Kato S, Kamagata S, Asakura T, et al. A newly developed small-caliber videoduo-denoscope for endoscopic retrograde cholangiopancreatography in children. J Clin Gastroenterol 2003;37(2):173–6.

12. Al-Rashdan A, LeBlanc J, Sherman S, et al. Role of endoscopic ultrasound for evaluating gastrointestinal tract disorders in pediatrics: a tertiary care center experience. J Pediatr Gastroenterol Nutr 2010;51(6):718–22.

13. Attila T, Adler DG, Hilden K, et al. EUS in pediatric patients. Gastrointest Endosc 2009;70(5):892–8.

14. Cohen S, Kalinin M, Yaron A, et al. Endoscopic ultrasonography in pediatric patients with gastrointestinal disorders. J Pediatr Gastroenterol Nutr 2008;46(5): 551–4.

15. Roseau G, Palazzo L, Dumontier I, et al. Endoscopic ultrasonography in the evaluation of pediatric digestive diseases: preliminary results. Endoscopy 1998; 30(5):477–81.

16. Sokol RJ, Shepherd RW, Superina R, et al. Screening and outcomes in biliary atresia: summary of a National Institutes of Health workshop. Hepatology 2007; 46(2):566–81.

17. Kasai M, Suzuki S. A new operation for "non-correctable" biliary atresia, hepatic portoenterostomy. Shujitsu 1959;13:733–9.

18. Davenport M, Kerkar N, Mieli-Vergani G, et al. Biliary atresia: the King's College Hospital experience (1974-1995). J Pediatr Surg 1997;32(3):479–85.

19. Mieli-Vergani G, Howard ER, Portman B, et al. Late referral for biliary atresia-missed opportunities for effective surgery. Lancet 1989;1(8635):421–3.

20. McEvoy CF, Suchy FJ. Biliary tract disease in children. Pediatr Clin North Am 1996;43(1):75–98.

21. Manolaki AG, Larcher VF, Mowat AP, et al. The prelaparotomy diagnosis of extra-hepatic biliary atresia. Arch Dis Child 1983;58(8):591–4.
22. Ohi R, Ibrahim M. Biliary atresia. Semin Pediatr Surg 1992;1(2):115–24.
23. Guelrud M, Jaen D, Mendoza S, et al. ERCP in the diagnosis of extrahepatic biliary atresia. Gastrointest Endosc 1991;37(5):522–6.
24. Shteyer E, Wengrower D, Benuri-Silbiger I, et al. Endoscopic retrograde cholangiopancreatography in neonatal cholestasis. J Pediatr Gastroenterol Nutr 2012; 55(2):142–5.
25. Vegting IL, Tabbers MM, Taminiau JA, et al. Is endoscopic retrograde cholangio-pancreatography valuable and safe in children of all ages? J Pediatr Gastroen-terol Nutr 2009;48(1):66–71.
26. Keil R, Snajdauf J, Rygl M, et al. Diagnostic efficacy of ERCP in cholestatic infants and neonates–a retrospective study on a large series. Endoscopy 2010;42(2): 121–6.
27. Kahn E. Paucity of interlobular bile ducts. Arteriohepatic dysplasia and nonsyn-dromic duct paucity. Perspect Pediatr Pathol 1991;14:168–215.
28. Hadchouel M. Paucity of interlobular bile ducts. Semin Diagn Pathol 1992;9(1): 24–30.
29. Alagille D, Borde J, Habib EC, et al. Surgical attempts in atresia of the intrahe-patic bile ducts with permeable extrahepatic bile duct. Study of 14 cases in chil-dren. Arch Fr Pediatr 1969;26(1):51–71 [in French].
30. Alagille D, Odievre M, Gautier M, et al. Hepatic ductular hypoplasia associated with characteristic facies, vertebral malformations, retarded physical, mental, and sexual development, and cardiac murmur. J Pediatr 1975;86(1):63–71.
31. Krantz ID, Colliton RP, Genin A, et al. Spectrum and frequency of jagged1 (JAG1) mutations in Alagille syndrome patients and their families. Am J Hum Genet 1998; 62(6):1361–9.
32. Li L, Krantz ID, Deng Y, et al. Alagille syndrome is caused by mutations in human Jagged1, which encodes a ligand for Notch1. Nat Genet 1997;16(3):243–51.
33. Oda T, Elkahloun AG, Pike BL, et al. Mutations in the human Jagged1 gene are responsible for Alagille syndrome. Nat Genet 1997;16(3):235–42.
34. Sokol RJ, Stall C. Anthropometric evaluation of children with chronic liver disease. Am J Clin Nutr 1990;52(2):203–8.
35. Emerick KM, Whitington PF. Partial external biliary diversion for intractable pruritus and xanthomas in Alagille syndrome. Hepatology 2002;35(6):1501–6.
36. Kaye AJ, Rand EB, Munoz PS, et al. Effect of Kasai procedure on hepatic outcome in Alagille syndrome. J Pediatr Gastroenterol Nutr 2010;51(3):319–21.
37. Morelli A, Pelli MA, Vedovelli A, et al. Endoscopic retrograde cholangiopancrea-tography study in Alagille's syndrome: first report. Am J Gastroenterol 1983;78(4): 241–4.
38. Miyano T, Suruga K, Suda K. Abnormal choledocho-pancreatico ductal junction related to the etiology of infantile obstructive jaundice diseases. J Pediatr Surg 1979;14(1):16–26.
39. Yamaguchi M. Congenital choledochal cyst. Analysis of 1,433 patients in the Japanese literature. Am J Surg 1980;140(5):653–7.
40. Stringer MD, Dhawan A, Davenport M, et al. Choledochal cysts: lessons from a 20 year experience. Arch Dis Child 1995;73(6):528–31.
41. Todani T, Watanabe Y, Narusue M, et al. Congenital bile duct cysts: classification, operative procedures, and review of thirty-seven cases including cancer arising from choledochal cyst. Am J Surg 1977;134(2):263–9.
42. O'Neill JA Jr. Choledochal cyst. Curr Probl Surg 1992;29(6):371–410.

43. Komi N, Takehara H, Kunitomo K, et al. Does the type of anomalous arrangement of pancreaticobiliary ducts influence the surgery and prognosis of choledochal cyst? J Pediatr Surg 1992;27(6):728–31.

44. Guelrud M, Morera C, Rodriguez M, et al. Normal and anomalous pancreaticobiliary union in children and adolescents. Gastrointest Endosc 1999;50(2):189–93.

45. Kimura K, Ohto M, Saisho H, et al. Association of gallbladder carcinoma and anomalous pancreaticobiliary ductal union. Gastroenterology 1985;89(6): 1258–65.

46. Misra SP, Dwivedi M. Pancreaticobiliary ductal union. Gut 1990;31(10):1144–9.

47. Ando H, Ito T, Nagaya M, et al. Pancreaticobiliary maljunction without choledochal cysts in infants and children: clinical features and surgical therapy. J Pediatr Surg 1995;30(12):1658–62.

48. Miyano T, Ando K, Yamataka A, et al. Pancreaticobiliary maljunction associated with nondilatation or minimal dilatation of the common bile duct in children: diagnosis and treatment. Eur J Pediatr Surg 1996;6(6):334–7.

49. De Angelis P, Foschia F, Romeo E, et al. Role of endoscopic retrograde cholangiopancreatography in diagnosis and management of congenital choledochal cysts: 28 pediatric cases. J Pediatr Surg 2012;47(5):885–8.

50. Sharma AK, Wakhlu A, Sharma SS. The role of endoscopic retrograde cholangiopancreatography in the management of choledochal cysts in children. J Pediatr Surg 1995;30(1):65–7.

51. Houben CH, Chiu PW, Lau J, et al. Preoperative endoscopic retrograde cholangiopancreatographic treatment of complicated choledochal cysts in children: a retrospective case series. Endoscopy 2007;39(9):836–9.

52. Tsuchiya H, Kaneko K, Itoh A, et al. Endoscopic biliary drainage for children with persistent or exacerbated symptoms of choledochal cysts. J Hepatobiliary Pancreat Sci 2012. [Epub ahead of print].

53. Kaneko K, Ando H, Ito T, et al. Protein plugs cause symptoms in patients with choledochal cysts. Am J Gastroenterol 1997;92(6):1018–21.

54. Benjamin IS. Biliary cystic disease: the risk of cancer. J Hepatobiliary Pancreat Surg 2003;10(5):335–9.

55. Kobayashi S, Asano T, Yamasaki M, et al. Risk of bile duct carcinogenesis after excision of extrahepatic bile ducts in pancreaticobiliary maljunction. Surgery 1999;126(5):939–44.

56. Pezzilli R, Carini G, Cennamo V. Education and imaging. Hepatobiliary and pancreatic: Caroli's disease. J Gastroenterol Hepatol 2008;23(10):1621.

57. Lendoire JC, Raffin G, Grondona J, et al. Caroli's disease: report of surgical options and long-term outcome of patients treated in Argentina. Multicenter study. J Gastrointest Surg 2011;15(10):1814–9.

58. Ulrich F, Pratschke J, Pascher A, et al. Long-term outcome of liver resection and transplantation for Caroli disease and syndrome. Ann Surg 2008;247(2): 357–64.

59. Lopez RR, Pinson CW, Campbell JR, et al. Variation in management based on type of choledochal cyst. Am J Surg 1991;161(5):612–5.

60. Ulas M, Polat E, Karaman K, et al. Management of choledochal cysts in adults: a retrospective analysis of 23 patients. Hepatogastroenterology 2012;59(116): 1155–9.

61. Debray D, Pariente D, Gauthier F, et al. Cholelithiasis in infancy: a study of 40 cases. J Pediatr 1993;122(3):385–91.

62. St-Vil D, Yazbeck S, Luks FI, et al. Cholelithiasis in newborns and infants. J Pediatr Surg 1992;27(10):1305–7.

63. Wendtland-Born A, Wiewrodt B, Bender SW, et al. Prevalence of gallstones in the neonatal period. Ultraschall Med 1997;18(2):80–3 [in German].
64. Suchy F. Pediatric disorders of the bile ducts. In: Feldman M, Friedman LS, Brand LJ, editors. Sleisenger and Fordtran's gastrointestinal and liver disease. Philadelphia: Saunders; 2010. p. 1045–66.
65. Mahr MA, Hugosson C, Nazer HM, et al. Bile-plug syndrome. Pediatr Radiol 1988;19(1):61–4.
66. Brown DM. Bile plug syndrome: successful management with a mucolytic agent. J Pediatr Surg 1990;25(3):351–2.
67. Duman L, Buyukyavuz BI, Akcam M, et al. Percutaneous management of bile-plug syndrome: a case report. J Pediatr Surg 2011;46(12):e37–41.
68. Guelrud M, Carr-Locke D, Fox VL. Acquired diseases. ERCP in pediatric practice. Diagnosis and treatment. Oxford (United Kingdom): Isis Medical Media Ltd; 1997.
69. Mieli-Vergani G, Hadzic N. Biliary atresia and neonatal disorders of the bile ducts. In: Wyllie R, Hyams JS, editors. Pediatric gastrointestinal and liver diseases. Philadelphia: Elsevier Saunders; 2011. p. 741–51.
70. Charlesworth P, Thompson R. Neonatal sclerosing cholangitis: Kings College Hospital experience. J Pediatr Gastroenterol Nutr 2006;42(5):E77.
71. Shah I, Bhatnagar S. NISCH syndrome with hypothyroxinemia. Ann Hepatol 2010; 9(3):299–301.
72. Grosse B, Cassio D, Yousef N, et al. Claudin-1 involved in neonatal ichthyosis sclerosing cholangitis syndrome regulates hepatic paracellular permeability. Hepatology 2012;55(4):1249–59.

Index

Note: Page numbers of article titles are in **boldface** type.

A

Gastrointest Endoscopy Clin N Am 23 (2013) 519–534
http://dx.doi.org/10.1016/S1052-5157(13)00050-0
1052-5157/13/$ – see front matter © 2013 Elsevier Inc. All rights reserved.

Moving?

Make sure your subscription moves with you!

To notify us of your new address, find your **Clinics Account Number** (located on your mailing label above your name), and contact customer service at:

Email: journalscustomerservice-usa@elsevier.com

800-654-2452 (subscribers in the U.S. & Canada)
314-447-8871 (subscribers outside of the U.S. & Canada)

Fax number: 314-447-8029

Elsevier Health Sciences Division
Subscription Customer Service
3251 Riverport Lane
Maryland Heights, MO 63043

*To ensure uninterrupted delivery of your subscription, please notify us at least 4 weeks in advance of move.